Statistics in Human Genetics

$$P^2 \uparrow$$

$$\frac{1}{\uparrow}$$

$$\leftarrow P \ (AA) \cdot P(\text{siak.}|AA) \cdot P\ell \quad \overline{0.5}$$

$$\nearrow {}^{1\text{-}P} \cdot {}^{P^2} \uparrow$$

$$P(M, F, k) = P(M) \cdot P(F|M)(P \, \omega|MF)$$

D1405130

Arnold Applications of Statistics Series

Series Editor: **BRIAN EVERITT**
Department of Biostatistics and Computing, Institute of Psychiatry, London, UK

This series offers titles which cover the statistical methodology most relevant to particular subject matters. Readers will be assumed to have a basic grasp of the topics covered in most general introductory statistics courses and texts, thus enabling the authors of the books in the series to concentrate on those techniques of most importance in the discipline under discussion. Although not introductory, most publications in the series are applied rather than highly technical, and all contain many detailed examples.

Statistics in Human Genetics

Pak Sham
Institute of Psychiatry, London, UK

A member of the Hodder Headline Group
LONDON • NEW YORK • SYDNEY • AUCKLAND

Copublished in North, Central and South America
by John Wiley & Sons Inc.
New York • Toronto

First published in Great Britain in 1998 by Arnold,
a member of the Hodder Headline Group,
338 Euston Road, London, NW1 3BH
http://www.arnoldpublishers.com

Copublished in North, Central and South America by
John Wiley & Sons, Inc., 605 Third Avenue,
New York, NY 10158–0012

© 1998 Pak Sham

All rights reserved. No part of this publication may be reproduced or transmitted
in any form or by any means, electronically or mechanically, including
photocopying, recording or any information storage or retrieval system,
without either prior permission in writing from the publishers or a licence permitting
restricted copying. In the United Kingdom such licences are issed by the Copyright
Licensing Agency: 90 Tottenham Court Road, London W1P 9HE

British Library Cataloging in Publication Data
A catalogue record for this book is available from the British Library

Library of Congress Cataloguing-in-Publication Data
A catalog record for this book is available from the Library of Congress

ISBN: 0 340 66241 7
ISBN: 0 471 19488 3 (Wiley)

Publisher: Nicki Dennis
Production Editor: Wendy Rooke
Production Controller: Sarah Kett
Cover design: M2

Typeset in 10/11 Times by MCS Limited, Salisbury, Wiltshire
Printed and bound in Great Britain by J W Arrowsmith Ltd., Bristol

Contents

Preface

Research in human genetics poses many interesting statistical problems for which specialized analytic methods have been, and are being, developed. The purpose of this book is to provide an introduction to some of these methods. It is intended primarily for research workers and postgraduate students, although some of the material may also be suitable for specialist options in undergraduate courses. No background knowledge of genetics is assumed, but the reader is expected to have an understanding of basic statistical concepts.

A great variety of statistical methods are used in human genetic research. This book focuses on methods whose aim is to unravel the genetic basis of diseases and other traits. The main topics are segregation ratios, population frequencies, genetic linkage, allelic associations, and continuous and quasi-continuous traits. There is a vast literature on these topics, scattered in numerous books and periodicals devoted to the various overlapping branches of genetics such as medical genetics, population genetics, quantitative genetics, behavioural genetics, molecular genetics, and genetic epidemiology. By providing an introduction to these topics, it is hoped that the present volume will serve as a useful addition to this literature.

The emphasis of this book is on principles of study design and data analysis, rather than mathematical or computational details. The aim is to convey to the reader a sense of the nature of the scientific questions and the associated statistical problems; and the rationales, stengths and limitations of the methods used to tackle these problems. The text, concerned mainly with general principles, is interspersed with examples to illustrate the application of these principles in specific situations.

I wish to express my gratitude to the many people who have made this book possible. I am indebted to my head of department, Professor Robin Murray, for his continuous support and encouragement of my research over the past nine years. I am also grateful to Professor Brian Everitt for his advice and patience during the writing of this book. I have also had the good fortune to have worked with, and learned from, many geneticists and statisticians, including Professor Newton Morton at the University of Southampton; Professors

Kenneth Kendler, Lindon Eaves, Charles MacLean and Michael Neale at the Medical College of Virginia; Professors Robert Plomin and David Fulker and Dr Andrew Pickles at the Institute of Psychiatry; Professor Graham Dunn at the University of Manchester; Professor Peter McGuffin at the University of Wales and Dr David Curtis at the Royal London Hospital. Dr Curtis, in particular, made many valuable comments and suggestions during the writing of this book. Thanks are due also to Drs Alison Macdonald, Ming Wei Lin, Tao Li, Sanobar Shaikh and Homero Vallada for making their data available for use as examples, to Dr Jing Hua Zhao for providing technical and computing assistance, to Stephanie Hamer and Muriel Walshe for secretarial assistance, and to Iman Abusaad for providing Figure 1.4. Finally, I would like to thank The Wellcome Trust for funding me over the past eight years through a Training Fellowship and then a University Award.

Pak Sham
London
May 1997

1
Introduction

The importance of statistics in human genetic research is clear. Many articles in prominent human genetics journals are devoted to the development of new statistical methods, and the majority of the others involve some form of data analysis. In fact, there is a long historical link between genetics and statistics. Karl Pearson and Ronald Fisher, two of the most important pioneers of modern statistics, were both involved in genetics at some point in their careers. In the first issue of *Biometrika* (1901), founded by Karl Pearson together with Francis Galton and William Weldon, the editorial stated that:

> The biologist, the mathematician, and the statistician have hitherto had widely differentiated fields of work .... Patient endeavour to understand each other's methods, and to bring them into harmony for united ends and common profits – this is the only method by which we can earn for biometry a recognised place in the world of Science ....

Despite this strong historical link, genetic statistics is often regarded as a difficult area by both geneticists and statisticians. Geneticists are often bewildered by novel statistical methods, and some statisticians are put off by the technical jargon of genetics. This is clearly an unsatisfactory state of affairs.

In subsequent chapters, we attempt to explain the statistical ideas and methods that are fundamental to some of the most important research tools in human genetics. Before proceeding further, however, we provide a brief outline of the physical structure of the genetic material and the mechanisms of genetic transmission. We also introduce some basic but potentially confusing terminology.

1.1 The physical structure of the gene

The science of genetics has made enormous advances in recent decades. There is now a huge amount of information regarding the precise molecular mechanisms of genetic transmission from parent to offspring. Here, we are content to present a brief outline, at a level appropriate for the research methods to be described in this book.

The concept that human characteristics are inherited from parents to offspring in discrete units called *genes* is now so well established that it may appear self-evident to many people. In fact, up until the early part of this century, the gene concept was virtually unknown, and most experts believed in a theory of inheritance called pangenesis. This theory supposes that each gamete (i.e. a sperm or an ovum) contains minute quantities of every organ of the parent, and that these constitute the raw materials from which the organs of the offspring are developed. This theory can be traced back as far as Hippocrates (about 400 BC):

> the seeds come from all parts of the body, healthy seed from healthy parts, diseased seed from diseased parts.   Hippocrates (1849)

Charles Darwin reviewed the state of knowledge on heredity in 1868 in his book *The Variation of Animals and Plants under Domestication*. He distinguished between continuous and discontinuous variations, but unfortunately placed more emphasis on the former, for it was the study of discontinuous characters in the garden pea by Gregor Mendel that provided the first convincing demonstration of the existence of genes. The importance of Mendel's discovery later earned him the title of 'father of genetics'. The gene concept was popularized by Bateson (1901) for being as fundamental to genetics as the concept of the atom is to chemistry.

> We thus reach the conception of unit characters, which may be rearranged in the formation of reproductive cells. It is hardly too much to say that the experiments which led to this advance in knowledge are worthy to rank with those that laid the foundations of the atomic laws of chemistry.   Bateson (1901)

The gene did not remain a theoretical construct for long. The physical location of the genes was soon established to be the *chromosomes* in the cell nucleus. Subsequently, the chemical structure of the gene was discovered to be *deoxyribonucleic acid* (DNA). Leaving aside the interesting historical details of these discoveries, we now describe briefly the present state of knowledge about the structure and function of chromosomes and DNA.

The genetic blueprint of an individual is contained in 23 pairs of chromosomes. There is a set of these 23 pairs of chromosomes in the nucleus of every cell. During normal cell division, called *mitosis*, each chromosome is duplicated so that a full set of the 23 pairs of chromosomes is distributed to each of the two daughter cells. The duplication of each chromosome into two identical chromosomes is made possible by the peculiar structure of DNA (Figure 1.1). Each chromosome contains two very long strands of DNA which are normally bound to each other lengthwise by hydrogen bonds and are twisted around each other as a double helix. Each strand of DNA is a long molecule made up of a linear sequence of subunits. The subunits are called *nucleotides*, which are made up of three parts: a sugar (deoxyribose), a

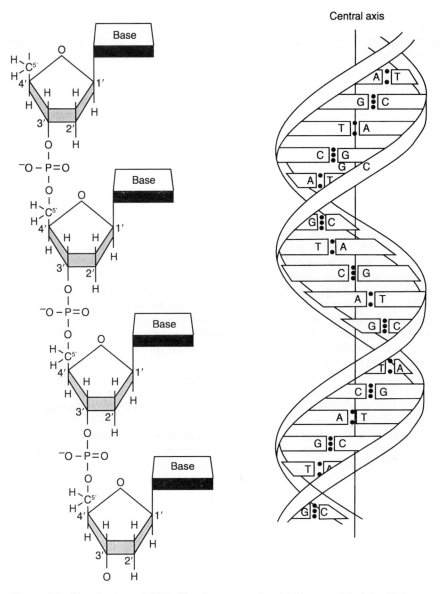

Figure 1.1 The structure of DNA. The diagram on the right is a model of the Watson–Crick DNA double helix. The two bands represent the sugar phosphate backbones of the two strands, which run in opposite directions. The vertical line represents the central axis around which the strands wind. The positions of the four nucleotide bases, C, A, T and G are shown, together with the hydrogen bonds (●) which link them together. The diagram on the left represents the structure of part of a DNA chain. It shows the chain-linked deoxyribose and phosphate residues that form the sugar-phosphate backbone.

nitrogenous base, and phosphates. There are four different *nitrogenous bases*, called adenine (A), guanine (G), cytosine (C) and thymine (T). The nucleotides containing these bases are called dATP, dGTP, dCTP and dTTP, respectively. A single strand of DNA consists of a linear array of these nucleotides, where the carbon atom at the 3′ position of the deoxyribose of one nucleotide is joined to 5′ carbon of the deoxyribose of the next by a phosphodiester bond.

The variability introduced by having four different nitrogenous bases is crucial for the ability of DNA to store information. In simple terms, a DNA molecule is like a very long word in a language that has an alphabet of only four different letters. This language is translated into *protein* molecules, through which DNA exerts its control over cellular functions. Each protein molecule is a linear chain of subunits called *amino acids*, of which there are 20 different forms. The physical and chemical properties of a protein molecule are largely determined by its sequence of amino acids. Having 20 different amino acids as building blocks means that an enormous number of different protein molecules with diverse physical and chemical properties can be constructed. This diversity enables protein molecules to perform all kinds of different structural and biochemical functions. Proteins are therefore the ideal agents for executing the genetic programs stored in DNA.

Roughly speaking, a gene is a segment of DNA within a chromosome that specifies the amino acid sequence, and therefore the structure and function, of a single subunit of a protein. Since the chromosomes are in the cell nucleus and the sites of protein synthesis, the ribosomes, are in the cytoplasm, the decoding of the information in the DNA into proteins involves two stages called *transcription* and *translation* (Figure 1.2).

Transcription is the process in which a segment of one of the two strands of a DNA double helix is used as a template to synthesize a single-stranded *ribonucleic acid* (RNA) molecule. RNA differs from DNA in having ribose instead of deoxyribose, and uracil (U) instead of thymine (T). The molecular mechanism of transcription is crucially dependent on a special property of DNA (and RNA) called complementarity, discovered by Watson and Crick in 1953. The bases A and T (or A and U) can be joined up by two hydrogen bonds. Similarly, the bases G and C can be joined up by three hydrogen bonds. Because of this, the two strands of DNA that constitute a double helix are complementary in sequence, where A is always paired with T, and G with C. For example, if one strand has the sequence TAGACC, then the other strand must have the complementary sequence ATCTGG. During transcription, the double helix splits open, and fresh ribonucleotides are bonded to one of the two exposed DNA strands (called the template strand) in a complementary fashion to synthesize a single-stranded RNA molecule. Thus, if the template DNA strand is TAGACC, then the RNA transcript is AUCUGG.

This crucial property of DNA also provides an obvious way in which DNA can be replicated. The two DNA strands of a double helix are separated, and fresh deoxyribonucleotides are bound to the exposed nucleotides of these two single strands in a complementary fashion to form two new DNA strands. This results in two double-strands, each consisting of an original strand and a newly synthesized strand. During mitosis, all 46 chromosomes in the parent cell undergo this process of replication, producing two identical sets of 46

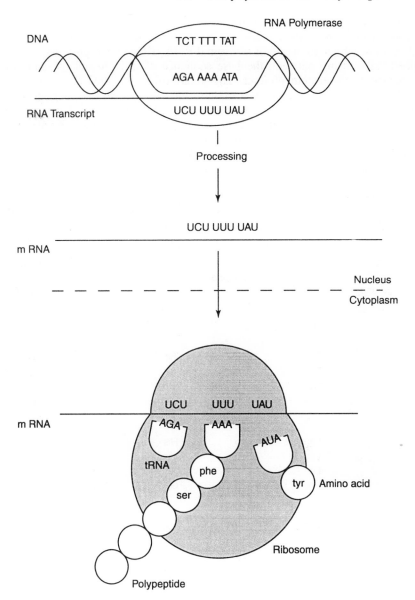

Figure 1.2   DNA function. Transcription and translation (protein synthesis).

chromosomes. These two sets of chromosomes are separated and distributed into two daughter cells. Each daughter cell therefore contains an entire copy of the genetic blueprint of the organism.

Returning to protein synthesis, the stage after transcription is called translation. However, before translation can take place, RNA transcripts are processed by the addition of chemicals at either ends ('caps' and 'tails') and the deletion of certain non-coding sequences ('splicing'). The processed RNA chains, called messenger RNA (abbreviated as mRNA), are transported to ribosomes, which are made of ribosomal RNA (rRNA) and proteins. There is a direct relationship between the base sequence of mRNA and the amino acid sequence of its protein product. This relationship is called the genetic code. Each 'codeword' (or codon) is a triplet of nucleotides, so that there are 4^3 (i.e. 64) possible codewords. Since there are only 20 amino acids, the genetic code is degenerate, with each amino acid being specified on average by about three different codons. Translation proceeds from the 5′ end to the 3′ end of the mRNA, starting at the initiation codon AUG (which also codes for methionine). It proceeds one codon at a time, with no overlap or gap between consecutive codons, until a termination codon (UGA, UAA or UAG) is reached (Figure 1.3).

The molecular mechanism of translation involves another class of RNA molecules called transfer RNA (abbreviated as tRNA). There are 30 different

First position (5′ end)	Second position				Third position (3′ end)
	U	C	A	G	
U	Phe	Ser	Tyr	Cys	U
	Phe	Ser	Tyr	Cys	C
	Leu	Ser	Stop	Stop	A
	Leu	Ser	Stop	Trp	G
C	Leu	Pro	His	Arg	U
	Leu	Pro	His	Arg	C
	Leu	Pro	Gln	Arg	A
	Leu	Pro	Gln	Arg	G
A	Ile	Thr	Asn	Ser	U
	Ile	Thr	Asn	Ser	C
	Ile	Thr	Lys	Arg	A
	Met	Thr	Lys	Arg	G
G	Val	Ala	Asp	Gly	U
	Val	Ala	Asp	Gly	C
	Val	Ala	Glu	Gly	A
	Val	Ala	Glu	Gly	G

Figure 1.3 The genetic code. The codons are given as they appear in mRNA. The abbreviations for the different amino acids are the first three letters of each amino acid except in the case of Asn, asparagine; Gln, glutamine; Ile, isoleucine; and Trp, tryptophane.

types of tRNA molecules, each of which is characterized by a specific triplet of nucleotides (the 'anticodon') at one end, and the ability to 'carry' a specific amino acid at the other. The pairing of codons with anticodons follows the normal A-U and G-C rules for the first two base positions, but is more flexible at the third position where G-U base pairs are also admitted. A series of codons on a mRNA molecule attracts a series of tRNA molecules with complementary anticodons, and therefore leads to the formation of a corresponding series of amino acids. These amino acids are polymerized to form a specific polypeptide molecule.

1.2 The inheritance of chromosomes

All the cells of an adult human are ultimately derived from a single cell called the *zygote* which is formed by the union of two *gametes*, the ovum and the sperm. Each gamete contributes a half (or *haploid*) set of 23 chromosomes, so that the zygote receives a full (or *diploid*) set of 23 pairs of chromosomes. Normal gametes contain 22 *autosomes* and a *sex chromosome*. The 22 autosomes are numbered in order of decreasing length from 1 to 22 (except that chromosome 21 is slightly shorter than chromosome 22). There are two types of sex chromosome, a long type called X and a much shorter type called Y. The sex chromosome in a normal ovum is always X, but that in a normal sperm is equally likely to be X or Y. If a zygote contains a Y chromosome, then it will normally develop into a male, otherwise it will normally develop into a female.

Two chromosomes are said to be *homologous* if they belong to the same family of chromosomes (e.g. both chromosome 21). Two homologous chromosomes are not only similar in length, but are also similar in sequence. This similarity between homologous chromosomes means that diploid organisms such as humans have two copies of every gene, except for those on the X or Y chromosomes.

The chromosomes are visible using an optical microscope only when the nucleus is undergoing division. The chromosomes can then be seen to occur in pairs attached to each other at a region called the *centromere*, which divides the chromosome into two arms, the shorter of which is labelled p and the longer labelled q. The tips of these arms are called the telomeres. When treated with special stains, each arm appears to be divided into a number of bands, which are numbered from the centromere. The approximate location of a gene is therefore specified by the chromosome number (i.e. $1, 2, ..., 22, X, Y$), the arm (p, q) and the band $(1, 2, 3, ...)$ (Figure 1.4).

The 23 pairs of chromosomes in the zygote are duplicated every time a cell division occurs. A copy of the entire set of these 23 pairs of chromosomes is therefore contained in every cell nucleus of the body. The only exceptions to this rule are the gametes, which are produced by the sex organs (testes and ovaries). Gametes are produced by a special form of cell division called meiosis. Unlike mitosis, meiosis gives rise to daughter cells which contain only a haploid set of 22 autosomes and a sex chromosome. This ensures that the union of two gametes will produce the correct number of 23 chromosome pairs. In addition, meiosis involves the reshuffling of genetic material. This

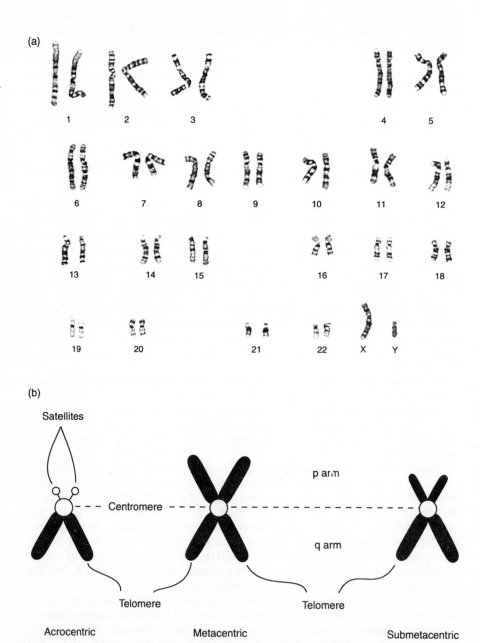

Figure 1.4 Human chromosomes. (a) The normal human male karyotype. The chromosomes are identified by their size, banding patterns and position of centromere. Trypsin-Giemsa banding. (b) The anatomy of human chromosomes. Reproduced with permission from *The New Genetics and Clinical Practice*, third edition. D. J. Weatherall (1991).

reshuffling is achieved by the exchange of genetic material between a chromosome of paternal origin and the corresponding chromosome of maternal origin (i.e. between homologous chromosomes). This exchange produces chromosomes which consist of alternating segments of paternally and maternally derived DNA. The 23 pairs of newly reconstituted chromosomes segregate independently into two daughter cells. These daughter cells develop into gametes that ensure the continued survival of the genetic material into the next generation.

1.3 The human genome

The totality of DNA characteristic of a species is called its *genome*. The human genome has about 3 000 000 000 base pairs per haploid nucleus. However, about 97% of the human genome is non-coding, so that the remaining 3% is responsible for specifying the sequences of approximately 80 000 proteins. Of these 80 000 genes, over 5 000 have been identified and catalogued (McKusick, 1994). These genes vary enormously in length, ranging from less than a thousand to over a million base pairs. However, the position of a particular gene within the genome is constant. For instance, the genes coding for the α and β subunits of haemoglobin are located on the short arm of chromosome 16 and the short arm of chromosome 11, respectively. This is an example of two functionally similar genes that are located on different chromosomes. A representation of gene locations on the chromosomes is called a *genetic map*.

Some genes do not form a continuous sequence, but consist of several segments separated by non-coding sequences. The coding segments of a gene are called *exons*, and the non-coding segments between exons are called *introns*. Introns and other non-coding regions contain what is sometimes called 'junk' DNA, although some of these sequences may not be without function. Some non-coding sequences are, for example, known to be involved in the regulation of nearby coding sequences. Non-coding DNA contains both irregular sequences and repetitions of simple short sequences.

1.4 Genetic variation

The remarkable structure of DNA allows accurate copies of it to be made. This accuracy is crucial because changes in the DNA may disrupt a coding sequence and lead to the production of a protein that is not able to perform its normal function, or a protein that has a harmful effect on the cell. Nevertheless, changes in the DNA do occur from time to time, and such *mutations* introduce diversity into the population. Despite the rarity of such events, the size of the genome ensures that most individuals will carry some uncommon genetic features. During meiosis, the genetic material is reshuffled, giving rise to offspring that have different combinations of these features. The processes of mutation and *recombination* are responsible for the generation of genetic diversity between individuals.

There are several different types of mutation. The simplest example is the replacement of one base pair by another, called nucleotide *substitution*. Other types of mutations include the *deletion* of one or more base pairs, the *insertion* of an extra segment of DNA, and the *translocation* of a DNA segment from one chromosomal region to another. Such mutations may involve very small stretches of DNA, down to a single base pair, or much larger segments, up to an entire chromosome. At certain points during evolution whole chromosomes must have been gained or lost, since different species have different numbers of chromosomes. Abnormalities in the number of chromosomes is known as *aneuploidy*, and are responsible for some cases of Down's syndrome (triple 21), Turner's syndrome (X0) and Klinefelter's syndrome (XXY). At other times in evolution whole genes have been duplicated and then the different copies have evolved separately, accounting for the occurrence of *gene families* – genes coding for distinct proteins but having a certain degree of similarity to each other. An example of a gene family is the HLA (Human Leucocyte Antigens) system involved in immune responses.

Variations in non-coding DNA usually have no discernible effect on the individual. Some point mutations in coding regions also have no effect if the new triplet codes for the same amino acid as the original. Mutations that cause a change in the amino acid sequence of a protein product are called *missense mutations*. The effect of such a mutation depends on the physico-chemical properties of the resulting protein. Sometimes the mutation has little effect because the resulting protein has similar properties to the original. Sometimes the mutation causes a dominant disorder because of the effects of the accumulation of a harmful protein. At other times there is merely a reduction in biochemical activity, in which case the individual may not be severely affected unless the genes inherited from the father and mother are both of the mutant form.

Although most fresh mutations are neutral or deleterious, there may be advantages to the species in maintaining a level of genetic diversity. A clear example of this is the genetic control of an organism's immunological profile. This consists of a specific pattern of proteins unique to the organism which allows the immune system to distinguish host tissue from foreign material. This enables an immune response to be mounted against parasitic infections without harming host tissues. If all members of a species shared the same immunological profile then it would be a relatively simple task for a parasite to mimic this profile and render itself immune from attack. The genetic diversity at the loci controlling immune profile is therefore an important safeguard against infection. Another example is the sickle cell mutation, which in heterozygote individuals is protective against malaria. The increased survival of heterozygotes leads to the preservation of both the normal and the sickle variants in the population.

1.5　Genetic terminology

There is often a mismatch between the above simplified account of our current understanding of the mechanisms of heredity, and some of the technical terms commonly used in genetics. One of the reasons for this discrepancy is that many genetic terms were introduced prior to the discovery of DNA. Another source of confusion is that it is not unusual for a term to be used in several different ways rather than in strict accordance to its formal definition.

The term 'gene' was itself introduced long before the discovery of DNA and the understanding of its structure and function. Initially, a gene was conceptualized as a discrete unit which is inherited from parent to offspring and which exerts control on a single character. Subsequently, with the discovery that genetic material is exchanged between chromosomes during meiosis, genes could no longer be viewed as distinct entities, and it was necessary to re-conceptualize them as the basic units for genetic recombination. Thus, a chromosome was thought to be rather like a collection of beads strung together by a piece of string. In this model, genetic recombination involves simply the exchange of beads between two strings. This model, however, is now known to be inaccurate, because the breakpoints for recombination can occur between any two base pairs on a chromosome and hence may fall within a gene. Later still, with the discovery of DNA and the mechanism of protein synthesis, the gene was re-defined as a segment of DNA that codes for a protein subunit. Even this definition is not entirely satisfactory, because some non-coding sequences may serve some regulatory roles (e.g. in controlling the switching and the switching off of transcription) that have an important impact on the organism. Moreover, whether a DNA segment is functional or not is irrelevant to its behaviour in mitosis or meiosis, so that for some purposes the distinction between genes and non-functional DNA segments is superfluous. Thus, it is not unusual to refer to the frequency of a particular non-functional DNA segment in the population as a gene frequency.

Another difficulty is that the word gene may be used to refer to the general concept of a functional DNA segment, or to a particular class of DNA segments that have the same position, structure and function (e.g. the gene that codes for the α chain of haemoglobin), or to a specific functional DNA segment that is present in an individual. Matters are complicated further by the fact that a gene in an offspring may be a replicate of a gene in a parent, so that sometimes they are spoken of as two genes while at other times they are spoken of as one gene.

The word gene is sometimes also confused with the frequently used terms locus and allele. A *locus* is defined as a specific position in the genome. The presence of different DNA sequences at the same locus in a population is known as a genetic *polymorphism* (while the absence of such variation is sometimes called a genetic monomorphism). The alternative DNA sequences at a locus are known as *alleles*. Despite these definitions, the distinctions between the words gene, locus and allele are not always clear. A particular gene (for example, the DNA segment that codes for the enzyme amylase) usually occurs at the same position in the genome, so that the gene and its locus are sometimes used in an almost synonymous fashion (for example, the amylase gene and the amylase locus have much the same meaning). Similarly, when a locus contains a functional DNA segment, then the different sequence variants that are present at the locus are often referred to as genes, although they are strictly speaking alleles. Thus, the terms gene frequency and allele frequency are basically synonymous.

Although the word allele is defined as one form of the alternative sequences at a locus, it is sometimes used to describe a particular DNA segment. Thus, it is quite common to speak of an allele being transmitted from a parent to an offspring, or to ask whether two alleles are replicates of the same ancestral allele. The word gene is sometimes used in the same way, although some geneticists will say that this usage is incorrect if the DNA segment is non-functional. There are many similar examples in genetics where a simple and precise term for a concept or an object is lacking. These situations are often dealt with by the flexible use of the terms that are available, rather than by an attempt to develop an entirely consistent system of terminology.

1.6 Conclusions

The main purpose of this chapter is to provide an overview of the structure and function of the genetic material, DNA. This description is, needless to say, a gross simplification. The interested reader is referred to standard texts on molecular genetics for further details (Watson *et al.*, 1987; Strachan and Read, 1996). On the other hand, even this level of detail is often unnecessary for some of the research methods to be described in later chapters, many of which were developed prior to the molecular revolution in genetics. This is not to say that statistical genetics is independent of molecular biology. Indeed, there is a constant interaction between statistics and molecular biology such that new statistical methods are stimulated by laboratory developments, and the design of molecular studies is guided by statistical principles.

In the next chapter, we turn our attention to the statistical analysis of the genetic transmission at a single locus, and of the frequency distribution of genes in the population.

2

The Analysis of Segregation and Population Frequencies

The demonstration by Gregor Mendel of the existence of genes was based on the regular occurrence of certain characteristic ratios of dichotomous characters among the offspring of crosses between parents of various characteristics and lineages. These ratios were known as *segregation ratios*, and they led to the theory known as the *law of segregation*. Although this monumental work was published in 1866, it received little attention until 1900, when it was independently 'rediscovered' by three botanists: De Vries, Correns and Tshermak. Mendel's original article and the subsequent papers by De Vries, Correns and Tshermak can be found in a special supplement of *Genetics* (Mendel *et al.*, 1950).

The analysis of segregation ratios remains an important research tool in human genetics. The demonstration of such ratios for a discrete trait among the offspring in certain types of families constitutes strong evidence that the trait has a simple genetic basis. Furthermore, since these ratios have predictable consequences for the frequency distribution of the trait in the population, the examination of population frequencies may also provide evidence for single locus inheritance of the trait. In this chapter, we describe the principles and methods for the statistical analysis of segregation ratios and population frequencies. We start, however, by stating the law of segregation and defining some associated terminology.

2.1 The law of segregation

The genetic model proposed by Mendel is as follows. Certain discrete observable traits (called *phenotypes*) are determined by discrete entities (called *genes*) inherited from parents. Each gene can take a number of different forms (called *alleles*), denoted by letters such as $A_1, A_2, \ldots$. An individual has two genes for each trait, and these genes are defined as his or her *genotype* for the trait. When the two genes are identical (e.g. A_1A_1, A_2A_2), then the genotype is said to be *homozygous*, otherwise it is said to be *heterozygous* (e.g. A_1A_2). If individuals with genotype A_1A_2 are phenotypically the same as individuals with genotype A_1A_1, but different from individuals with genotype A_2A_2, then allele A_1 is said to be dominant to allele A_2, or equivalently, allele A_2 is said to be recessive to allele A_1. In addition, the phenotype associated with A_1A_1 is said to be dominant, and the phenotype associated with A_2A_2 is said to be recessive. If A_1A_2 yields a phenotype that is different from the phenotypes of both A_1A_1 and A_2A_2, then alleles A_1 and A_2 are said to be *codominant*.

During reproduction, an individual receives with equal probability one of the two genes from the genotype of the mother, and likewise one of the two genes from the genotype of the father. This is known as Mendel's first law, or the *law of segregation*. Imagine the genotype of the parent as consisting of two marbles in a box; the law of segregation is equivalent to saying that, in the formation of a gamete, one of the two marbles in the box is selected at random. Mendel also proposed that the segregation of the genes for one trait is not affected by the segregation of genes for other traits. This is known as Mendel's second law, or the *law of assortment*, although we now know that there are exceptions to this rule. In the context of our 'box model', Mendel's second law is equivalent to saying that there is a separate box for every trait, each containing two marbles, and that when a gamete is produced, the selection of a marble from one box is independent of the selection of marbles from other boxes.

The laws of segregation and assortment have obvious parallels with the behaviour of chromosomes in meiosis, as described in Chapter 1. In meiosis, following the exchange of genetic material by the 23 pairs of chromosomes, each reconstituted chromosome is randomly distributed to a daughter cell.

2.2   Segregation analysis for autosomal dominant diseases

Consider a disease that is caused by the presence of a rare mutant allele at an autosomal locus. Let the mutant, disease-causing allele be denoted as D, and the normal allele be denoted as d, then there are three possible genotypes DD, Dd and dd. If the disease is dominant, then individuals with genotypes DD and Dd will have the disease, while individuals with genotype dd will be normal. Examples of autosomal dominant diseases in humans include Huntington's chorea and neurofibromatosis. For these diseases, the correspondence between genotype and phenotype is so close that the phenotype assumes the discrete nature of the underlying genotype, allowing the operation of the law of segregation to be clearly observed.

Since a father and mother can each have genotype DD, Dd or dd, there are $3 \times 3 = 9$ possible combinations of paternal and maternal genotypes. These nine combinations can be collapsed down to six different *mating types*: DD × DD, DD × Dd, DD × dd, Dd × Dd, Dd × dd, dd × dd. Each of these mating types will produce offspring with a characteristic distribution of genotypes, and therefore phenotypes, as shown in Table 2.1.

The proportions of the different genotypes and phenotypes in the offspring of the six mating types are known as the *segregation ratios* of the mating types. The specific values of the segregation ratios can be used to test whether a disease is caused by a single autosomal dominant gene.

Table 2.1 Segregation ratios for an autosomal dominant disorder

Mating type	Genotype			Phenotype	
	DD	Dd	dd	Affected	Normal
DD × DD	1	0	0	1	0
DD × Dd	0.5	0.5	0	1	0
DD × dd	0	1	0	1	0
Dd × Dd	0.25	0.5	0.25	0.75	0.25
Dd × dd	0	0.5	0.5	0.5	0.5
dd × dd	0	0	1	0	1

Since autosomal dominant diseases are usually rare, it is reasonable to assume that the frequency of allele D is low. Most affected individuals are therefore expected to have genotype Dd rather than DD. Thus, most matings between an affected and an unaffected person will be of the type Dd × dd. Table 2.1 shows that the offspring of this mating type has probability 1/2 of being affected. This prediction can be used to test whether the disease is autosomal dominant. This constitutes a strong test, since there are few (if any) alternative explanations for a probability of disease of exactly 1/2 among the offspring of affected individuals.

Although the hypothesis that a segregation ratio is 1/2 is extremely simple, we will nevertheless introduce several alternative tests that are applicable. We do this not because all these methods are necessary in this simple case, but in order to illustrate the relationships between different types of tests and to introduce some basic principles.

2.2.1   The binomial test

Suppose that a random sample of matings between affected and unaffected individuals is obtained and that, of the total of n offspring, r are affected by the disease. We wish to test the hypothesis that the segregation ratio is 1/2.

The *binomial distribution* is readily applicable to this problem. The binomial distribution describes the probabilities of various possible numbers of 'successful' outcomes in a fixed number of 'trials', where all the trials have the same probability of success. Let the probability of success be p, then the number of successes in n trials, X, is a random variable that can take the values $0, 1, 2, ..., n$. The binomial distribution states that the probability that X is equal to a particular value x is given:

$$P(X = x) = \binom{n}{x} p^x (1 - p)^{n - x} \qquad (2.1)$$

for $x = 0, 1, 2, ..., n$.

Returning to the problem of testing whether a segregation ratio is 1/2, if we regard each offspring as a 'trial' and an affected offspring as a 'success', then testing whether a segregation ratio is 1/2 is equivalent to testing whether a binomial proportion p is 1/2. For a two-tailed test, the P-value associated with *r* affected out of *n* offspring is the sum of binomial probabilities

$$P = \sum_{x=0}^{c} \binom{n}{x}\left(\frac{1}{2}\right)^n + \sum_{x=c}^{n} \binom{n}{x}\left(\frac{1}{2}\right)^n$$

$$= \left(\frac{1}{2}\right)^{n-1} \sum_{x=0}^{c} \binom{n}{x}$$

(2.2)

where $c = r$ if $r \leqslant n/2$, and $c = n - r$ if $r > n/2$. By convention, if the *P*-value is less than 0.05, then the hypothesis of a segregation ratio of $1/2$ is rejected.

Example 2.1
A study on opalescent dentine (Neel and Schull, 1954) examined a random sample of 112 offspring of an affected parent, and found that 52 were similarly affected while the other 60 were normal. Are these observations consistent with the hypothesis that opalescent dentine is a rare autosomal dominant condition?

According to the binomial distribution, the *P*-value for the hypothesis of a segregation ratio of $1/2$ is

$$P = \left(\frac{1}{2}\right)^{111} \sum_{x=0}^{52} \binom{112}{x} = 0.5058$$

The hypothesis of a segregation ratio of $1/2$ is therefore not rejected. The data are consistent with opalescent dentine being an autosomal dominant condition.

2.2.2   The standard normal test

The hypothesis that $p = 1/2$ can also be tested with reference to a *normal distribution*. This alternative test has some practical advantages in that the binomial distribution is usually tabulated only for small values of *n*. Fortunately, as *n* increases, the binomial distribution approaches a normal distribution. The appropriate normal distribution that can be used to approximate a binomial distribution is one that has the same *mean* (μ) and the *variance* (σ^2) as the binomial distribution. The mean and variance of a random variable having a binomial distribution with *parameters n* and *p* are

$$\left.\begin{array}{r} \mu = np \\ \sigma^2 = np(1-p) \end{array}\right\}$$

(2.3)

It follows that, if *X* is a binomial variable with parameters *n* and *p*, then the variable *Z* defined by

$$Z = \frac{X - np}{(np(1-p))^{1/2}}$$

(2.4)

has a standard normal distribution. Thus, if *r* of *n* offspring are affected, then the *P*-value is twice the probability that a standard normal random variable will exceed z, where z is defined as the absolute difference between r and its mean (i.e. $n/2$), divided by its standard deviation (i.e. $(n/4)^{1/2}$)

$$z = \frac{\left| r - \dfrac{n}{2} \right|}{\left(\dfrac{n}{4} \right)^{1/2}} \tag{2.5}$$

Example 2.2
For the problem on opalescent dentine, $p = 1/2$ and $n = 112$ give $n/2 = 56$ and $(n/4)^{1/2} = 5.29$, so that the value of z is $(52 - 56)/5.29 = -0.756$. The *P*-value is the probability that a standard normal variable is less than -0.756 or greater than $+0.756$, i.e. 0.4496. This *P*-value is slightly less than that given by the binomial test (0.5085), largely because a *continuity correction* has not been used. The need for a continuity correction arises because values of X between 52 and 53 are not possible if X has a discrete, binomial distribution. It is more accurate to define the observed value of X to be the mid-point between 52 and 53, i.e. 52.5, so that $z = (52.5 - 56)/5.29 = -0.662$, which gives a *P*-value of 0.5082, in close agreement with the *P*-value from the binomial test (0.5085).

2.2.3   The Pearson chi-squared test

Yet another test for the hypothesis of $p = 1/2$ can be made by reference to a *chi-squared distribution*. The distribution of the square of a standard normal variable is defined as a chi-squared distribution with one *degree of freedom*, denoted as χ_1^2. Since the variable Z as defined above is standard normal, its square

$$Z^2 = \frac{(X - np)^2}{np(1 - p)} \tag{2.6}$$

is distributed as χ_1^2. It can be shown that this expression is equivalent to

$$Z^2 = \frac{(X - np)^2}{np} + \frac{((n - X) - n(1 - p))^2}{n(1 - p)} \tag{2.7}$$

which is the usual formula for a *Pearson chi-squared statistic*, i.e. the sum of the squares of the differences between observed and expected counts divided by expected counts.

$$Z^2 = \sum \frac{(O - E)^2}{E} \tag{2.8}$$

Thus, if r of n offspring are affected, then the *P*-value is the probability that a chi-squared random variable with one degree of freedom will exceed z^2, which is defined as

$$z^2 = \frac{\left(r - \dfrac{n}{2}\right)^2}{\dfrac{n}{4}} \qquad (2.9)$$

Example 2.3

For the opalescent dentine data, the necessary calculations for the chi-squared test can be presented in tabular format, as follows

	Affected	Not affected	Total
Observed (O)	52	60	112
Expected (E)	56	56	112
$(O - E)^2 / E$	0.2857	0.2857	0.5714

The probability that a χ_1^2 random variable will exceed 0.5714 is 0.4497. As expected, this P-value is identical to that obtained by the standard normal test without the continuity correction. A continuity correction can be applied to the test by replacing the observed counts of 52 and 60 by 52.5 and 60.5, respectively.

Since the Pearson chi-squared test produces the same result as the standard normal test, its introduction may seem somewhat redundant. However, an advantage of the Pearson chi-squared test is that it is capable of being generalized to situations involving more than two categories of individuals, by invoking chi-squared distributions with two or more degrees of freedom. In general, when there are m observed counts, the Pearson chi-squared statistic that arises from the calculation of m 'expected counts' is asymptotically chi-squared with $m - k$ degrees of freedom, where k is the number of independent numerical values obtained from the observed counts that are used in the calculation of the expected counts.

2.2.4   The likelihood-ratio chi-squared test

Finally, the hypothesis of $p = 1/2$ can be tested by considering the *likelihood* of the data as a function of the parameter p. The likelihood function, given that r affected offspring are observed out of n offspring, is defined as

$$L(p) = \binom{n}{r} p^r (1 - p)^{n - r} \qquad (2.10)$$

The relative support for two different values of p provided by the data can be assessed by the ratio of the values of the likelihood function at the two values of p. The higher the value of the likelihood function at a certain value of p, the more strongly that value of p is supported by the data. Since the binomial coefficient does not depend on the value of p, it will always cancel out when a ratio of two likelihoods is calculated. For this reason this factor is sometimes omitted from the likelihood function.

Let the maximum value of the likelihood function in the range $0 \leqslant p \leqslant 1$ be L_1, and the value of the likelihood function at the hypothetical value $p = 0.5$ be L_0, then the *likelihood ratio statistic* is defined as twice the difference between the natural logarithms of L_1 and L_0, i.e. $2(\ln L_1 - \ln L_0)$. If the hypothesis of $p = 0.5$ is true, then this likelihood ratio statistic can be shown to have symptotically a chi-squared distribution with one degree of freedom. This provides the basis of the likelihood ratio chi-squared test.

To find $\ln L_1$, the derivative of the log-likelihood function with respect to p is set to 0, and the resulting equation used to express p in terms of n and r. When this is done, it can be shown that the value of p which maximizes the log likelihood function (and therefore the likelihood function) is $\hat{p} = r/n$, i.e. the actual proportion observed in the sample. This value $\hat{p}$ is defined as the *maximum likelihood estimate* (MLE) of p. The likelihood ratio statistic $2(\ln L_1 - \ln L_0)$ is therefore

$$2(\ln L_1 - \ln L_0) = 2\left(r\ln\frac{r}{n} + (n - r)\ln\frac{n - r}{n} - n\ln\frac{1}{2}\right) \qquad (2.11)$$

The P value is then given by the probability that a chi-squared random variable with one degree of freedom will exceed $2(\ln L_1 - \ln L_0)$.

Example 2.4
For the opalescent dentine data, the log-likelihood function is

$$\ln L(p) = 52 \ln(p) + 60 \ln(1 - p)$$

The shape of this log-likelihood function is shown in Figure 2.1. The maximum likelihood estimate of p is $52/112$. The calculation of the likelihood ratio statistic can be set out in tabular form, as follows

Model	Parameter value	Likelihood	2 ln L
General	$p = 52/112$	0.07541	−5.1695
Dominant	$p = 1/2$	0.05666	−5.7414

The likelihood ratio statistic is therefore 0.5719. Referring this to a chi-squared distribution with one degree of freedom gives a P-value of 0.4495, which is extremely close to that calculated by the Pearson chi-squared method without continuity correction (i.e. 0.4497).

Again, the likelihood ratio chi-squared may seem somewhat redundant because, in this example, it gives essentially the same result as the Pearson chi-squared test. However, the likelihood ratio test requires only that a likelihood function can be defined and evaluated. Since this is possible in many complex

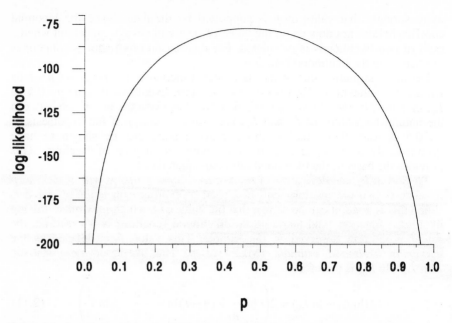

Figure 2.1   Log-likelihood function of the segregation ratio for the opalescent dentine data.

situations, the method can be generalized to cope with problems for which the simpler methods described above are not readily applicable.

2.2.5   The estimation of a segregation ratio

There are two popular methods of obtaining estimates of population parameters from sample data. These are the *method of moments* and the *method of maximum likelihood*. The method of moments expresses the theoretical values of the moments (such as the mean and variance) of certain variables in terms of the parameters to be estimated, and then equates these theoretical expressions to the values of these moments calculated from a sample of observations. These 'estimating equations' are then solved to obtain estimates of the parameters.

Given the parameter of interest p, the expected value of the number of affected offspring out of n offspring is np. If, in a sample of n offspring, r of the offspring are observed to be affected, then the method of moments estimate of p is given by the equation $np = r$, which can be rearranged to obtain the estimate $p = r/n$.

The maximum likelihood estimate of a parameter is the value of the parameter that maximizes the likelihood function. For a sample of n offspring of whom r are affected, the derivative of the log-likelihood function is

$$\frac{r}{p} - \frac{n-r}{1-p} \tag{2.12}$$

Setting this to 0 gives the maximum likelihood estimate of p as $\hat{p} = r/n$, which is identical to the methods of moments estimate. Thus, both the method of moments and the method of maximum likelihood give the sample proportion r/n as an estimate of the population proportion p.

This *point estimate* is of limited use unless it is accompanied by some measure of its accuracy. The observed value r can be regarded as a realization of the random variable X, which has a binomial distribution with parameters n and p. Since the mean and variance of X are np and $np(1-p)$, the sampling mean and variance of X/n are p and $p(1-p)/n$. The statistic X/n is therefore an unbiased estimate of p with *standard error* $[p(1-p)/n]^{1/2}$. As the true value of p is unknown, it is usual to substitute into this expression the estimate of p, giving

$$SE(p) = \left(\frac{\left(\frac{r}{n} \right)\left(1 - \frac{r}{n} \right)}{n} \right)^{1/2} \tag{2.13}$$

The standard error of p can be used to obtain a 95% *confidence interval* for p, which is the range of values of p that has 95% probability of containing the true value of p. Because of the approximate normality of r/n when n is large, a 95% confidence interval for p is the range of values within plus or minus 1.96 standard errors of r/n.

Example 2.5
Using these formulae on the opalescent dentine data, the estimate of p, and its standard error, are found to be 0.464 and 0.047, respectively. The 95% confidence interval for p is therefore (0.372, 0.557). The value of 0.5 predicted by autosomal dominant transmission is within this range, so that the data are consistent with this hypothesis.

2.3 Segregation analysis for codominant loci

A locus is said to be codominant if individuals with heterozygous genotypes at the locus are phenotypically different from individuals with homozygous genotypes. For a biallelic locus, this means that all three possible genotypes are phenotypically distinguishable from each other. Because of this, all six possible mating types can be identified, and the segregation ratios of each mating type examined to see if they are consistent with Mendelian inheritance. Since there will be three categories of offspring in some mating types, the binomial and the standard normal tests are not directly applicable. Instead, the Pearson and likelihood ratio chi-squared tests can be easily extended to deal with this situation.

Example 2.6
An example of a codominant locus in humans is MN blood types. Every person can be classified into one of three groups: MM, MN and NN. In a study of MN blood groups (Wiener, 1943), the frequencies of the blood types MM, MN and NN were found to be 71, 141 and 63, respectively, in a random sample of offspring from MN × MN matings. Do these data support Mendelian segregation for this trait?

The prediction of Mendelian segregation is that the probabilities of the types MM, MN and NN (i.e. the segregation ratios) are $1/4$, $1/2$ and $1/4$, respectively. The calculations involved in a Pearson chi-squared test can be tabulated as follows

	MM	MN	NN	Total
Observed (O)	71	141	63	275
Expected (E)	68.75	137.5	68.75	275
$(O-E)^2/E$	0.074	0.089	0.481	0.644

The chi-squared statistic is 0.644. The number of degrees of freedom is 2 because the calculation of the expected counts used one numerical value from the observed counts (namely the sum). This gives a P-value of 0.725, so that the data are consistent with the hypothesis of Mendelian segregation.

The likelihood ratio chi-squared test requires the calculation of the likelihood for values of segregation ratios that correspond to the null hypothesis of Mendelian transmission, and the maximum likelihood over all possible combinations of values of the segregation ratios. The likelihood under Mendelian segregation is proportional to $(1/4)^{71}(1/2)^{141}(1/4)^{63}$, while the maximum likelihood can be obtained by first finding (by calculus) the maximum likelihood estimates of the segregation ratios, which turn out to be simply the sample proportions, and then substituting these estimates into the likelihood equation. The maximum likelihood is therefore proportional to $(71/275)^{71}(141/275)^{141}(63/275)^{63}$. The calculations involved in the likelihood chi-squared test can be tabulated as follows.

Model	Parameter values	2 ln (likelihood)
General	71/275, 141/275, 63/275	− 566.338
Mendelian	1/4, 1/2, 1/4	− 566.994

The chi-squared statistic of 0.656 with two degrees of freedom gives a P-value of 0.720. These results are in excellent agreement with those obtained using the Pearson chi-squared test.

2.4   Segregation analysis for autosomal recessive disorders

For the segregation analysis of suspected codominant or rare dominant traits, specific mating types can be selected on the basis of the phenotypes of the parents. The situation with a rare recessive disorder is more difficult in that the mating type that one would like to examine is Dd × Dd, which is predicted to have a segregation ratio of $1/4$. However, for a recessive disorder, individuals with genotype Dd are unaffected and phenotypically indistinguishable from individuals with genotype dd, who constitute the majority of the population. It is therefore not possible to select families of the Dd × Dd mating type on the basis of the disease status of the parents. Since Dd × Dd matings can potentially produce affected offspring, it is possible to obtain such matings by selecting families with at least one affected child. This *ascertainment procedure* will, however, miss those families with the Dd × Dd mating type that by chance do not have any affected children. In the extreme case where all families are allowed only to have one child, selecting families with an affected child will mean that all the children in the selected families are affected. The need to take account of the *incomplete selection* of a mating type in segregation analysis was pointed out by Fisher in a classic paper in 1934 called 'The effect of methods of ascertainment upon the estimation of frequencies'.

> It is a statistical commonplace that the interpretation of a body of data requires a knowledge of how it was obtained .... Nevertheless, in human genetics especially, statistical methods are sometimes put forward, and their respective claims advocated with entire disregard of the conditions of ascertainment.   Fisher (1934)

2.4.1 Systematic ascertainment via probands

When families are ascertained on the basis of having at least one affected offspring, this does not necessarily mean that all such eligible families are ascertained with equal probability. For example, it is possible that the probability of ascertainment depends on the number of affected offspring in the family. Proper allowance for ascertainment is only possible if the ascertainment process is clearly defined. Human geneticists have therefore emphasized the importance of having a systematic method of ascertaining families for the segregation analysis of suspected recessive disorders. The usual procedure is to select initially a random sample of affected individuals in the population, and then to study the families of these affected individuals for additional affected members. The affected individuals initially identified, independently of other affected individuals, are called *probands*, while the additional affected individuals in the families of these probands are called *secondary cases*. It is possible for two or more probands to belong to the same family, in which case an affected individual may be a proband and at the same time also be a secondary case to another proband.

The probability that an affected individual in the population is identified as a proband is known as the ascertainment probability, and is conventionally denoted as π. It is often assumed that π is constant for all affected individuals in the population, although this is unlikely to be strictly true in reality. For example, affected individuals in families with several affected members may be more likely to be identified as probands than isolated cases. Under the assumption of a uniform π, the probability that a family with r affected offspring is not ascertained is $(1 - \pi)^r$. The probability that a family with r affected offspring is ascertained is therefore $1 - (1 - \pi)^r$.

When $\pi = 1$, $1 - (1 - \pi)^r$ is 1 regardless of the number of affected offspring. This situation is known as *complete ascertainment* because all families with affected offspring are ascertained. When π is nearly 0, the probability of ascertaining a family with r affected offspring becomes approximately $1 - (1 - r\pi) = r\pi$, so that the probability of ascertainment is approximately proportional to the number of affected offspring. Since π is very small, almost all ascertained families will have only one proband, and this situation is known as *single ascertainment*.

Example 2.7
The following dataset was presented by Fisher (1934) to illustrate the need to take account of the method of ascertainment in segregation analysis. The data consist of 340 families all with five offspring, of whom at least one is affected (because the families were ascertained through an affected offspring). For each family, the variables are the number of affected offspring, X, and the number of probands, B.

Number of probands	Number affected					
	1	2	3	4	5	Total
1	140	80	35	4	0	259
2		52	12	7	1	72
3			7	0	0	7
4				2	0	2
5					0	0
Total	140	132	54	13	1	340

From these data, it can be calculated that the total number of offspring (n_s), the total number of affected offspring (A), and the total number of probands (B), are

$$n_s = 340(5) \qquad\qquad\qquad\qquad\qquad = 1700$$

$$A = 140(1) + 132(2) + 54(3) + 13(4) + 1(5) = 623$$

$$B = 259(1) + 72(2) + 7(3) + 2(4) + 0(5) \quad = 434$$

If we were unaware of the need to take account of ascertainment, we might estimate the segregation ratio simply by the proportion of offspring who are affected, i.e. $623/1700 = 0.3665$. Moreover, we might be tempted to estimate the ascertainment probability by $434/623 = 0.6966$. However, these simple estimates are grossly inflated, and we now describe some statistical procedures that are designed to take account of ascertainment.

2.4.2   Complete ascertainment

Fisher (1934) first described a method based on the *truncated binomial distribution*, which is appropriate under complete ascertainment. The theory of the method is as follows. Consider families of mating type Dd × Dd and s offspring. The number of affected offspring in such families can vary from 0 to s. Let the number of affected offspring in such a family be a random variable denoted as X, then the distribution of X in the population is binomial with parameters s and p, where the value of p is predicted to be $1/4$ for a rare recessive disorder. In complete ascertainment, all families with one or more affected offspring, i.e. $X > 0$, are ascertained. The probability distribution of X, conditional on $X > 0$, is known as a binomial distribution truncated at 0. The conditional probability of $X = r$, where r is an integer number between 0 and s, given that $X > 0$, is defined as the joint probability that $X = r$ and $X > 0$ divided by the probability that $X > 0$. The joint probability of $X = r$ and $X > 0$ is simply the probability of $X = r$ when $1 \leq r \leq s$ (and 0 when $r = 0$), and the probability that $X > 0$ is $1 - (1 - p)^s$. Hence, for $1 \leq r \leq s$, the probability function of X is

$$P(X = r) = \frac{\binom{s}{r} p^r (1 - p)^{s - r}}{1 - (1 - p)^s} \tag{2.14}$$

The expected value of X is therefore

$$E(X) = \frac{sp(1 - p)}{1 - (1 - p)^s} \tag{2.15}$$

The only unknown in this expression is the segregation ratio p, since sibship size s is directly observable from the data. An estimate of p can be obtained by equating this theoretical mean with the observed mean in a sample of sibships of size s obtained by complete ascertainment. This turns out to be the maximum likelihood estimate of p, denoted by $\hat{p}$, as can be validated by setting the derivative of the log-likelihood function to 0. Denoting the number of families with r affected offspring by a_r, the log-likelihood function is

$$L(p) = \sum_r a_r \ln \left(\frac{\binom{s}{r} p^r (1 - p)^{s - r}}{1 - (1 - p)^s} \right) \tag{2.16}$$

where the summation is taken over $r = 1, \ldots, s$. Fisher derived the variance of the estimate of p using the '*delta method*'. Since the estimate $\hat{p}$ is a function of the mean number of affected offspring per family, $\bar{r}$, the variance of $\hat{p}$ and the variance of $\bar{r}$ are related by the formula

$$\mathrm{Var}(\hat{p}) = \left(\frac{d\hat{p}}{d\bar{r}} \right)^2 \mathrm{Var}(\bar{r}) \tag{2.17}$$

where the derivative is evaluated at the expected value of $\bar{r}$. Omitting mathematical details, the expression derived by Fisher is

$$\mathrm{Var}(\hat{p}) = \frac{p(1 - p)\,[1 - (1 - p)^s]^2}{n_s s [1 - (1 - p)^s - sp(1 - p)^{s - 1}]} \tag{2.18}$$

where n_s is the number of families with s offspring in the sample. Since p is not known it is replaced by its estimate, $\hat{p}$, in the calculation of $\mathrm{Var}(\hat{p})$.

Obtaining the value of $\hat{p}$ from the estimating equation

$$\frac{s\hat{p}(1-\hat{p})}{1-(1-\hat{p})^s} = \bar{r} \tag{2.19}$$

is not straightforward because $\hat{p}$ cannot be expressed explicitly in terms of $\bar{r}$ and s. Here, we introduce two popular numerical procedures that are often used for obtaining maximum likelihood estimates.

The EM algorithm   The *EM (expectation-maximization) algorithm* is a numerical method for finding the maximum likelihood estimates of parameters, and is applicable when the problem can be formulated as one of *incomplete data*. In other words, it is applicable to situations where the problem of estimation can be made much easier if certain additional pieces of data are available. Once the nature of the necessary missing data has been formulated, then the EM algorithm can proceed. First, the unknown parameters are assumed to take an initial set of plausible values. Then, based on these initial parameter values, the expected values of the missing data are calculated. These expected values are imputed into the missing data, so that, together with the available data, a complete data set is obtained. This is known as the *expectation step*, since expected values are imputed for missing data. From the complete data set, maximum likelihood estimates of the parameter estimates are obtained, and these constitute improved estimates of the parameters. This is known as the *maximization step*, since maximum likelihood estimates are obtained from the complete data. The improved parameter estimates are used in another expectation step to give an improved set of imputed values for the missing data. The newly imputed values are then combined with the observed data and subjected to another maximization step to give a set of even more accurate parameter estimates. This procedure of alternating expectation and maximization steps is repeated until the changes in parameter estimates are negligible for the purpose of the study.

For the problem of estimating p from families ascertained for having an affected child, the necessary missing data may be formulated as the number of Dd × Dd families in the population with s unaffected offspring. Let the number of such families be U. For a given value of the segregation ratio (p) and a given number of families with one or more affected offspring (n_s), the expected value of U is

$$E(U) = n_s \frac{(1-p)^s}{1-(1-p)^s} \tag{2.20}$$

If the total number of affected offspring in the sample is A, then for a given value of U, the maximum likelihood estimate of p is simply A divided by the sum of the number of offspring in the sample (i.e. sn_s) and the number of offspring in those U families without affected offspring (i.e. sU). If the initial estimate of U is 0, then the first two iterations of the EM algorithm consist of the steps

$$
\left.
\begin{aligned}
U_0 &= 0 \\[6pt]
p_0 &= \frac{A}{sn_s + sU_0} \\[6pt]
U_1 &= \frac{n_s(1 - p_0)^s}{1 - (1 - p_0)^s} \\[6pt]
p_1 &= \frac{A}{sn_s + sU_1} \\[6pt]
U_2 &= \frac{n_s(1 - p_1)^s}{1 - (1 - p_1)^s} \\[6pt]
p_2 &= \frac{A}{sn_s + sU_2}
\end{aligned}
\right\}
\qquad (2.21)
$$

In general, the *i*th iteration is

$$
\left.
\begin{aligned}
U_i &= \frac{n_s(1 - p_{i-1})^s}{1 - (1 - p_{i-1})^s} \\[8pt]
p_i &= \frac{A}{sn_s + sU_i}
\end{aligned}
\right\}
\qquad (2.22)
$$

These steps can be repeated until further iterations do not lead to appreciable changes in the estimate of p.

Newton–Raphson and Fisher's scoring algorithms   Two other popular numerical procedures for finding maximum likelihood estimates are the Newton–Raphson and the Fisher scoring methods. The *score function* is defined as the first derivative of the log-likelihood function with respect to the parameter

$$
S(p) = \frac{\ln(p)}{dp}
\qquad (2.23)
$$

The derivative of the score function is defined as the *Hessian function*, denoted as $H(p)$. If several parameters are involved, then the score becomes a vector of first-order derivatives, and the Hessian becomes a matrix of second-order derivatives.

For a given parameter value, say p_0, the score and the Hessian at that value provide an estimate of how far p_0 is from the maximum likelihood estimate $\hat{p}$.

For a linear score function, the Hessian is constant, and is given by

$$H = \frac{S(\hat{p}) - S(p_0)}{\hat{p} - p_0} \tag{2.24}$$

However, maximum likelihood implies a score of 0, so that $\hat{p}$ is related to p_0 by

$$\hat{p} = p_0 - \frac{S(p_0)}{H} \tag{2.25}$$

Although this simple relationship does not hold when the score function is non-linear, the quantity $p_0 - S(p_0)/H(p_0)$ remains a reasonable approximation of $\hat{p}$. If this revised estimate is denoted as p_1, then it can be subjected to the same procedure to give a second revised estimate $p_2 = p_1 - S(p_1)/H(p_1)$. The procedure is repeated until the score is deemed to be sufficiently close to 0. This algorithm is called the Newton–Raphson method.

Fisher's observed information at a certain parameter value p, denoted as $I_0(p)$ is defined as the negative of the Hessian at that value of p. The observed information is so-called because the precision of a maximum likelihood estimate is reflected by the 'sharpness' of the peak in the log-likelihood function around the maximum, which is in turn reflected by the gradient of the score function around the maximum, i.e. the Hessian. However, since the Hessian is negative near the maximum, it is convenient to define the observed information as the negative of the Hessian. In terms of Fisher's observed information, the ith revised estimate of the Newton–Raphson method is given by $p_i = p_{i-1} + S(p_{i-1})/I_0(p_{i-1})$.

Fisher's expected information, at a certain parameter value p, denoted as $I_E(p)$, is defined as the negative of the expected value of Hessian at that value of p. The calculation of the expected value of the Hessian involves summing (or integrating) over all possible values of the Hessian, weighted by the probabilities (or densities) of these values under the parameter p. Substituting expected information in place of observed information in the Newton–Raphson method, the iterative equation becomes $p_i = p_{i-1} + S(p_{i-1})/I_E(p_{i-1})$. This is known as Fisher's scoring method.

The inverse of Fisher's expected information at a given parameter value can be shown to be equal to the variance of the maximum likelihood estimate of the parameter. If several parameters are involved, then the inverse of Fisher's expected information matrix is equal to the covariance matrix of the maximum likelihood estimates. Fisher's expected information at a given parameter value can also be shown to be equal to the expectation of the square of the score function at that parameter value

$$I_E(p) = [V(p)]^{-1} = E[S(p)^2] \tag{2.26}$$

In the present problem of estimating the segregation ratio p from family data ascertained through an affected child, the score function obtained by differentiating the log-likelihood function with respect to p can be shown to be

$$S(p) = \frac{A}{p} - \frac{n_s s - A}{1 - p} - \frac{n_s s (1 - p)^s - 1}{1 - (1 - p)^s} \tag{2.27}$$

and Fisher's expected information, being the inverse of $\mathrm{Var}(\hat{p})$, is given by

$$I_E(p) = \frac{n_s s[1 - (1-p)^s - sp(1-p)^{s-1}]}{p(1-p)[1-(1-p)^s]^2} \tag{2.28}$$

Example 2.8
Although complete ascertainment clearly does not apply for the data given by Fisher, since not every affected offspring is a proband, one could nevertheless illustrate the method by ignoring the number of probands in each family. In other words, one could simply use the total number of families $(n_s = 340)$, the number of offspring per family $(s = 5)$, and the total number of affected offspring $(A = 623)$, under the assumption of complete ascertainment, to estimate the segregation ratio. The application of the EM algorithm and Fisher's scoring method to these data is illustrated as follows.

	EM algorithm		Fisher's score method			
i	p_i	U_i	p_i	$S(p_i)$	$I_E(p_i)$	d_i
0	0.3664	38.642	0.3664	−304.9	5473.8	−0.055
1	0.3290	53.496	0.3107	−12.11	5496.0	−0.002
2	0.3166	59.535	0.3085	−0.019	5500.0	−0.000
3	0.3118	62.035	0.3085	−0.000	5500.0	−0.000
4	0.3099	63.077				
5	0.3091	63.513				
6	0.3087	63.696				
7	0.3086	63.772				
8	0.3085	63.804				
9	0.3085	63.817				
10	0.3085	63.823				

Fisher's method of scoring is therefore more efficient than the EM algorithm in that convergence is reached in fewer iterations. The maximum likelihood estimate of p obtained by both methods is $\hat{p} = 0.3805$. The variance of the estimate, assuming that the true value of p is 0.25, can be obtained by substituting $p = 0.25$, $s = 5$, and $n_s = 340$ into the formula for $\mathrm{Var}(\hat{p})$. This gives

$$\mathrm{Var}(\hat{p}) = 0.0001747$$

so that the standard error of p is

$$\mathrm{SE}(\hat{p}) = \sqrt{0.0001747} = 0.0132$$

The estimate $\hat{p} = 0.3085$ is almost four standard errors from the predicted value of 0.25 under the hypothesis of recessive transmission. This would appear to be evidence against recessive transmission. However, this conclusion is justified only if the assumption of complete ascertainment is valid.

The observed counts of families with 1, 2, 3, 4 and 5 affected offspring in Fisher's data can be used to test the assumption of complete ascertainment. The expected values of these counts under complete ascertainment can be obtained by multiplying the probabilities given by the truncated binomial distribution (with an estimated parameter of 0.3085) by the total number of sibships (i.e. 340). The observed and expected numbers are as follows*

Number affected	1	2	3	4	5	Total
Observed (O)	140	132	54	13	1	340
Expected (E)	142.4	127.1	56.71	12.65	1.129	340
$(O - E)^2 / E$	0.041	0.189	0.130	0.009	0.015	0.381

The overall Pearson chi-squared statistic of 0.381 on four degrees of freedom indicates an excellent fit of the model to the data, so that there is no evidence against complete ascertainment.

2.4.3   Incomplete ascertainment

If data on the number of probands in each family were available, then the assumption of complete ascertainment could be clearly seen to be inappropriate for Fisher's data, since there are many affected offspring who are not probands. The above analysis based on the assumption of complete ascertainment is therefore inappropriate even though the numbers of affected offspring in the families do not provide evidence against this assumption. It is possible to analyse the data using the likelihood method without making the assumption of complete ascertainment, but this requires the use of a computer. Before presenting the likelihood method, we present two popular methods that are easy to use and intuitively appealing.

Fisher (1934) described a technique (originally proposed by Weinberg) which he called the '*sib method*' but now known as the '*proband method*' for the estimation of the segregation ratio, p, when both the number of affected offspring and the number of probands in each family are known. A similar method for estimating p in this situation, called the '*singles method*' was proposed by Davie (1979), generalizing the work of Li and Mantel (1968) on complete ascertainment. The basic principles of the two methods are similar; instead of simply dividing the number of affected offspring by the total number of offspring to obtain an estimate of p (as is appropriate in the case of complete selection), both the numerators and denominators are adjusted for incomplete selection. In other words, the estimate of p takes the form of a ratio R/S, where R is an adjusted number of affected offspring, and S is an adjusted total number of offspring. The two methods differ in how the adjustments are made, i.e. in how R and S are defined.

The proband method   The principle of the proband method is to treat the siblings of the probands as the 'effective observations', so that R is defined as the total number of affected siblings, and S the total number of siblings, of the probands. The probands themselves are excluded from either R or S (unless they are also siblings of other probands). The basis for this procedure is that, conditional on the parental genotype, the genotypes of the offspring are

---

*The entries in this and other tables do not always add up to the totals given owing to rounding errors.

mutually independent. In other words, if the genotypes of the parents are known, then the fact that a particular offspring is affected does not influence the probability that any other offspring is affected. This principle means that, if the hypothesis of autosomal recessive inheritance is true, then the fact that the proband is affected establishes the genotypes of the parents to be Dd × Dd, and so the probability that a sibling of the proband is affected is the segregation ratio, $1/4$. The proportion of siblings affected is therefore a reasonable estimate of the segregation ratio.

The proband method is straightforward for families containing just one proband. For such a family with r affected out of s offspring, the proband has $r - 1$ affected out of $s - 1$ siblings, and so the family contributes to $r - 1$ to R and $s - 1$ to S. For families with multiple probands the situation is less clear, because an offspring who is a proband can also be the sibling of another proband in the family. In this situation, the proband method considers a family as many times as the number of probands it contains. In other words, for a family with b probands and r affected offspring out of s offspring, each of the b probands contributes $r - 1$ to R and $s - 1$ to S, so that the total contributions of the family to R is $b(r - 1)$ and the total contribution to S is $b(s - 1)$. The proband method estimate of the segregation ratio p for an entire dataset of n families, where family i has b_i probands, r_i affected offspring and s_i offspring, is therefore

$$\tilde{p} = \frac{\sum b_i(r_i - 1)}{\sum b_i(s_i - 1)} \tag{2.29}$$

where the summations are taken over all n families. In essence, an affected offspring who is a sibling of b probands is counted b times in both the numerator and the denominator, while an unaffected offspring with the same number of proband siblings is not counted in the numerator but counted b times in the denominator.

The proband method can also be used to obtain an estimator of the ascertainment probability π. The estimate takes the form of a ratio B/R, where B is an adjusted number of offspring who are probands, and R is an adjusted number of offspring who are affected. A family that has b probands and r affected offspring contributes $b(b - 1)$ to B, and $b(r - 1)$ to R. The proband method estimate of the ascertainment probability π for an entire dataset of n families, where family i has b_i probands, r_i affected offspring and s_i offspring, is therefore

$$\tilde{\pi} = \frac{\sum b_i(b_i - 1)}{\sum b_i(r_i - 1)} \tag{2.30}$$

where the summations are again taken over all n families.

Example 2.9

The application of the proband method for Fisher's data is set out as follows:

r = Number of affected offspring per family

T = Total number of probands in such families

S = Total number of siblings of the probands, i.e. sT

R = Total number of affected siblings of the probands, i.e. $(r - 1)T$

B = Total number of proband siblings of the probands.

r	T	S	R	B
1	140	560	0	0
2	184	736	184	104
3	80	320	160	66
4	26	104	78	38
5	2	8	8	2
Total	432	1728	430	210

Hence $\bar{p} = 430/1728 = 0.2488$, $\tilde{\pi} = 210/430 = 0.488$. These estimates would suggest that disorder is recessive and that ascertainment is incomplete.

The singles method   The principle of the singles method is similar to that of the proband method, except in its treatment of families with multiple probands. The method takes as 'effective observations' all offspring except those who are the only proband in the family, so that R is defined as the total number of affected offspring minus the number of families with only one proband, and S the total number of offspring minus the number of families with only one proband. The rationale is that an offspring can be considered an 'effective observation' only if there is a proband in the rest of the family. In other words, only those offspring whose ascertainment did not depend on their own affection status are considered 'effective observations'. An offspring who is the sole proband in a family must be affected in order to be included in the sample, and is therefore not considered an 'effective observation'. Such probands are called 'singles'.

Let the number of 'singles' in a sample of n families be d, then the singles method estimator of the segregation ratio p is simply

$$\bar{p} = \frac{\sum r_i - d}{\sum s_i - d} \tag{2.31}$$

where r_i is the number of affected offspring, and s_i the total number of offspring, in family i, for $i = 1, \ldots, n$. In other words, family i contributes 0 to R and $s_i - 1$ to S if it contains 1 proband, but r_i to R and s_i to S if it contains more than 1 proband.

The same principle can also be used to obtain an estimate of the ascertainment probability π. The singles method estimate of π is given by

$$\tilde{\pi} = \frac{\sum b_i - d}{\sum r_i - d} \tag{2.32}$$

where b_i is the number of probands in family i.

Example 2.10
For Fisher's data, the total number of offspring is 1700, the total number of affected offspring is 623, the total number of probands is 434, and the number

of families with only one proband is 259. The singles method estimates for p and π are therefore

$$\bar{p} = (623 - 259)/(1700 - 259) = 0.2526$$

$$\bar{\pi} = (434 - 259)/(623 - 259) = 0.481$$

These estimates are very close to those obtained using the proband method.

Standard errors for the proband and singles methods Although both the proband method and the singles method estimators of the segregation ratio are conceptually appealing and mathematically simple (both being a quotient of 2 variables), their standard errors are more complicated. The variance of a quotient of two random variables, R/S, is approximately

$$V\left(\frac{R}{S}\right) = \left(E\left(\frac{R}{S}\right)\right)^2 \left(\frac{V(R)}{[E(R)]^2} + \frac{V(S)}{[E(S)]^2} - \frac{2C(R,S)}{E(R)E(S)}\right) \tag{2.33}$$

where the expectation $E(R/S)$ is approximately

$$E\left(\frac{R}{S}\right) = \frac{E(R)}{E(S)} - \frac{C(R,S)}{[E(R^2)]} + \frac{E(R)V(S)}{[E(S)]^2} \tag{2.34}$$

The variances of the two estimators can be found by obtaining the appropriate expressions for $E(R)$, $E(S)$, $V(R)$, $V(S)$, $C(R,S)$ and substituting into the above formula, where R and S are, of course, defined differently for the proband and singles methods. Omitting mathematical details (see Fisher, 1934; Davie, 1979), the variance of the proband method estimator of the segregation ratio p is

$$V(\bar{p}) = \frac{(1-p)\sum\left(\dfrac{s(s-1)n_s(1 + \pi + p\pi(s-3))}{1 - g_0}\right)}{\pi\sum\left(\dfrac{s(s-1)n_s}{1 - g_0}\right)^2} \tag{2.35}$$

and the variance for the singles method estimator of p is

$$V(\bar{p}) = \frac{p(1-p)\sum\left(\dfrac{sn_s[(1 - g_1 + (s-1)p(1-p)\pi^2 g_2]}{1 - g_0}\right)}{\sum\left(\dfrac{sn_s(1 - g_1)}{1 - g_0}\right)^2} \tag{2.36}$$

where $g_j = (1 - p\pi)^{s-j}$ and n_s is the number of ascertained sibships of size s, and the summations are over s. Davie found that the variance of the singles method estimator is less than the that of the proband method estimator (except under single ascertainment when the two methods are equivalent) because the latter method puts too much weight on sibships with multiple probands.

Example 2.11

Substituting the estimates of π, $p = 0.25$, $s = 5$ and $n_s = 340$ into the variance formulae for the proband method and singles method, we find for the proband method,

$$\text{Var}(\tilde{p}) = 0.000187$$

$$\text{SE}(\tilde{p}) = 0.0137$$

and for the singles method

$$\text{Var}(\bar{p}) = 0.000168$$

$$\text{SE}(\bar{p}) = 0.0130$$

For both methods the estimate for the segregation ratio p is well within two standard errors of 0.25. The data can therefore be considered compatible with the hypothesis of recessive transmission. The discrepancy between these results and that obtained by assuming complete ascertainment emphasizes the importance of recording the number of probands in each family.

The likelihood method   We now present a likelihood method for segregation analysis for a putative recessive disorder under the assumption of incomplete ascertainment. The treatment here is similar to those of Bailey (1951a,b) and Morton (1958, 1959).

We require the likelihood of observing r affected offspring in an ascertained family with s offspring. First, we consider the probability that a segregating family (i.e. a family that is potentially able to produce an affected offspring) with s offspring is ascertained. In order to become a proband, an offspring in a segregating family must first be affected and then be selected. The probability of an offspring in a segregating family becoming a proband is therefore πp. A segregating family with s offspring is ascertained if any of the offspring is a proband; the probability of ascertainment is therefore $1 - (1 - \pi p)^s$.

Let the number of probands in a family be B. When the individual probands cannot be identified and so the precise value of B is unknown, the likelihood function for a family with r affected offspring out of s offspring is

$$\left. \begin{aligned} P(X = r \,|\, B > 0; s, \pi, p) &= \frac{P(B > 0 \,|\, X = r; \pi)\, P(X = r; s, p)}{P(B > 0; s, \pi, p)} \\[2mm] &= \frac{[1 - (1 - \pi)^r]\binom{s}{r} p^r (1 - p)^{s-r}}{1 - (1 - \pi p)^s} \end{aligned} \right\} \tag{2.37}$$

for $r = 1, \ldots, s$. Incidentally, in the case of complete ascertainment, $\pi = 1$, this likelihood function simplifies to

$$P(X = r \,|\, B > 0; s, \pi = 1, p) = \frac{\binom{s}{r} p^r (1 - p)^{s-r}}{1 - (1 - p)^s} \tag{2.38}$$

and in the case of single ascertainment, $\pi = 0$, this likelihood function simplifies to

$$P(X = r \mid B > 0; s, \pi = 0, p) = \left. \frac{r\pi \binom{s}{r} p^r (1-p)^{s-r}}{s\pi p} \right\}$$

$$= \binom{s-1}{r-1} p^{r-1} (1-p)^{s-r} \right\} \tag{2.39}$$

When the probands are individually identified and so the value of B is known $(B = b)$, then this additional information can be incorporated into the likelihood function

$$P(X = r, B = b \mid B > 0; s, \pi, p) = \left. \frac{P(B = b \mid X = r; \pi) P(X = r; s, p)}{P(B > 0; s, \pi, p)} \right\}$$

$$= \frac{\binom{r}{b} \pi^b (1-\pi)^{r-b} \binom{s}{r} p^r (1-p)^{s-r}}{1 - (1-\pi p)^s} \right\} \tag{2.40}$$

for $r = 1, \ldots, s$; $b = 1, \ldots, r$. We can therefore write down the log-likelihood of each individual family, regardless of whether the number of probands is precisely known or not. Since the families represent independent observations, the overall log-likelihood is simply the sum of the log-likelihoods of the individual families. The maximization of the log-likelihood function with respect to p and π can be achieved by Fisher's method of scoring. This method has the advantage that the score and information can be calculated separately for each independent subset of data, and the total score and information can be obtained by summing over these contributions.

For a family with r affected and $s - r$ normal offspring and an unknown number of probands, the score functions obtained by partial differentiation of the log-likelihood function with respect to p and π are

$$S(p) = \left. \frac{r}{p} - \frac{s-r}{1-p} - \frac{\pi s (1-\pi p)^{s-1}}{1 - (1-\pi p)^s} \right\}$$

$$S(\pi) = \frac{r(1-\pi)^{r-1}}{1 - (1-\pi)^r} - \frac{ps(1-\pi p)^{s-1}}{1 - (1-\pi p)^s} \right\} \tag{2.41}$$

Similarly, for a family with r affected and $s - r$ normal offspring and b probands, the score functions are

$$S(p) = \left. \frac{r}{p} - \frac{s-r}{1-p} - \frac{\pi s (1-\pi p)^{s-1}}{1 - (1-\pi p)^s} \right\}$$

$$S(\pi) = \frac{b}{\pi} - \frac{r-b}{1-\pi} - \frac{ps(1-\pi p)^{s-1}}{1 - (1-\pi p)^s} \right\} \tag{2.42}$$

In both cases, each family contributes the following elements to the information matrix

$$
\left.
\begin{aligned}
I(p,p) &= E[S(p)]^2 \\
I(\pi, \pi) &= E[S(\pi)]^2 \\
I(\pi, p) &= I(p, \pi) = E[S(\pi)][S(p)]
\end{aligned}
\right\}
\tag{2.43}
$$

Although algebraically cumbersome, these elements are easy to calculate with a computer for any values of p and π. The increments d_p and d_π that are used to revise the estimates of p and π at iteration j of the scoring algorithm are then given by the solutions of the simultaneous linear equations

$$
\left.
\begin{aligned}
I_j(p,p)d_p + I_j(p, \pi)d_\pi &= S_j(p) \\
I_j(\pi,p)d_p + I_j(\pi,\pi)d_\pi &= S_j(\pi)
\end{aligned}
\right\}
\tag{2.44}
$$

The implementation of this algorithm for families in which the number of probands is unknown is demonstrated using Fisher's data as follows.

Example 2.12
The following calculations are those involved in one iteration of the scoring algorithm for the likelihood method applied to Fisher's segregation data when probands are unknown

$$r = \text{number of affected offspring}$$

$$l = \text{probability (likelihood) of family}$$

$$s(p) = \text{score for } p \text{ due to family}$$

$$s(\pi) = \text{score for } \pi \text{ due to family}$$

$$\ln(l) = \text{log-likelihood due to family}$$

$$n = \text{number of families}$$

Starting values $p_0 = 0.36$, $\pi_0 = 0.99$

r	l	$s(p)$	$s(\pi)$	$s(p)^2l$	$s(p)^2l$	$s(p)s(\pi)l$	$\ln(l)$	n
1	0.336	−4.426	0.6629	6.5865	0.1476	−0.986	−1.090	140
2	0.381	−0.086	−0.327	0.0028	0.0408	0.0108	−0.962	132
3	0.214	4.2535	−0.346	3.8868	0.0258	−0.316	−1.537	54
4	0.060	8.5938	−0.347	4.4622	0.0072	−0.180	−2.806	13
5	0.006	12.934	−0.347	1.1371	0.0008	−0.030	−4.991	1
Sum				16.075	0.2225	−1.503		340

$$S(p) = 140(-4.426) + 132(-0.086) + 54(4.2535)$$
$$+ 13(8.5938) + 1(12.934) = -276.870$$

$$S(\pi) = 140(0.6629) + 132(-0.327) + 54(-0.346)$$
$$+ 13(-0.347) + 1(-0.347) = 26.029$$

$I(p,p) = 340(16.075) = 5465.729$

$I(\pi,\pi) = 340(0.2225) = 75.659$

$I(\pi,p) = 340(-1.503) = -511.102$

$\ln L = 140(-1.090) + 132(-0.962) + 54(-1.537)$
$$+ 13(-2.806) + 1(-4.991) = -404.250$$

The increments for p and π can then be calculated as $d_p = -0.0502$ and $d_\pi = 0.0050$. The revised values for p and π are therefore $p_1 = 0.3098$ and $\pi_1 = 0.9950$.

The ability to maximize the likelihood over both p and π allows hypotheses about these parameters to be tested by comparing likelihoods of *nested models*. In the most general model, both p and π are unrestricted in the maximization. The hypothesis of complete ascertainment corresponds to a model where p is unrestricted but π is set to 1. The hypothesis of recessive inheritance corresponds to a model where π is unrestricted but p is set to 0.25. The hypothesis of complete ascertainment and recessive inheritance corresponds to a model where π is set to 1 and p is set to 0.25. The parameter estimates of these three models, and their log-likelihoods, are shown as follows.

Example 2.13
The results of a likelihood analysis of Fisher's segregation data when probands are unknown are as follows.

Model	$\hat{p}$	$\hat{\pi}$	2 ln L	χ^2	df	P-value
General	0.2989	0.9069	−793.65	0	0	—
Complete ascertainment	0.3085	(1)	−793.85	0.20	1	0.65
Recessive inheritance	(0.25)	0.4707	−794.95	1.30	1	0.25
$\pi = 1$ and $p = 0.25$	(0.25)	(1)	−813.73	20.08	2	0.00004

These results indicate that neither the hypothesis of complete ascertainment nor the hypothesis of recessive inheritance can be rejected. However, the results are incompatible with the joint hypothesis of complete ascertainment and recessive inheritance. Standard errors of the parameter estimates of the general model can be obtained by inverting the final information matrix and taking the square roots of the appropriate diagonal elements (i.e. the variances). This yields the standard errors $SE(\hat{p}) = 0.0286$ and $SE(\tilde{\pi}) = 0.2400$. The large standard error of $\tilde{\pi}$ is because, without knowledge of the number of probands in each family, the data contain little information on the value of π.

The same scoring algorithm can be used to maximize the likelihood for the case where the number of probands in each family is known. Since in this case the likelihood of a family depends on both the number of affected offspring and the number of probands, there are $1 + 2 + 3 + 4 + 5 = 15$ types of families to be considered, instead of the five types of families in Example 2.12.

Omitting computational details, the results of the likelihood analysis on the complete Fisher segregation data are shown as follows.

Example 2.14
Results of a likelihood analysis of Fisher's segregation data when probands are known.

Model	$\hat{p}$	$\hat{\pi}$	2 ln L	χ^2	df	p
General	0.2526	0.4753	−1116.71	0	0	—
Complete ascertainment	0.3085	(1)	−12853.4	11736	1	0
Recessive inheritance	(0.25)	0.4707	−1116.75	0.04	1	0.84

These results support the hypothesis of recessive inheritance but reject the hypothesis of complete ascertainment. For the general model, the parameter estimates are $\hat{p} = 0.2526$ and $\hat{\pi} = 0.4753$, with standard errors $SE(\hat{p}) = 0.0129$ and $SE(\hat{\pi}) = 0.0310$. These standard errors are smaller than those obtained using the likelihood method without knowledge of the number of probands in each family. Evidently, knowledge of the number of probands in each family has contributed much information on the values of p and π. Incidentally, the maximum likelihood estimate of p and its standard error are in close agreement to the values obtained by the proband and singles methods.

We have analysed Fisher's data twice, first assuming that the number of probands is unknown for all families, and then assuming that the number of probands is known for all families. It is possible to perform a similar analysis when the number of probands is known in some families but not in others. All that is necessary for the method of scoring is the ability to write down the log-likelihood, score, and information functions of each family.

2.5   Interpreting deviations from Mendelian segregation ratios

The confirmation that the segregation ratios of a trait conforms to Mendelian values provides strong evidence that the trait is determined by the alleles at a single locus, because there are few alternative explanations for precise ratios such as 1:1 and 1:3. However, there are many possible explanations for why segregation ratios might not conform to Mendelian values.

The most obvious interpretation of a significant deviation from Mendelian segregation is that the trait is not governed by the alleles at a single locus. However, before reaching this conclusion, potential confounding factors should be excluded. One possible confounding factor is the failure to take proper allowance for the methods by which the families were ascertained. We have already seen in Example 2.8 how the assumption of complete ascertainment, when in reality ascertainment was incomplete, led to grossly misleading estimates of segregation ratios. In general, segregation analysis is very sensitive to misspecification of the method of ascertainment. As a result, a segregation analysis is usually only worthwhile on family material for which the method of ascertainment is systematic and accurately known.

Another possible explanation of a significant deviation from Mendelian segregation is *differential survival*. It is possible that gametes with certain haplotypes have a decreased probability of undergoing fertilization, and that zygotes with certain genotypes have a decreased probability of developing into viable fetuses. This preferential loss of certain genotypes can lead to an apparent distortion of the segregation ratio, and therefore the inappropriate rejection of a Mendelian basis for the trait.

Another reason for a significant deviation from Mendelian segregation is the presence of *phenocopies*, which are sporadic cases of the disease due to environmental factors. In other words, there may be a mixture of genetic and environmental cases in the population. The proportion of cases that are phenocopies is called the phenocopy rate. It is possible to incorporate the phenocopy rate, denoted as α, in the statistical analysis. For a suspected dominant disorder, for example, a proportion α of families with one affected and one unaffected parent will have a segregation ratio of almost 0, while the rest (proportion $1 - \alpha$) of such families will have a segregation ratio of $1/2$. It is therefore possible to test for Mendelian segregation under this model. Similarly, a phenocopy rate can be incorporated into the segregation analysis of a suspected recessive condition.

Yet another reason for a significant deviation from Mendelian segregation is the *incomplete penetrance* of the disease gene. Incomplete penetrance refers to the presence of some individuals who possess the disease genotype (individuals with two copies of the disease allele for a recessive condition, and individuals with one or two copies of the disease allele for a dominant condition) but do not develop the disease. In general, incomplete penetrance will lead to a decrease in the phenotypic segregation ratio. It is possible in principle to incorporate a penetrance parameter as well as a segregation ratio in the statistical analysis, but in practice these two parameters will often be highly confounded with each other if only sibship data are available. In other words, the two parameters can, to some extent, compensate for each other, so that there are many combinations of the two parameters that can explain the same data equally well. The incorporation of incomplete penetrance into segregation analysis generally requires the consideration of larger family units and more sophisticated statistical methods. These methods will be described briefly in Chapter 5.

2.6 Population frequencies: Hardy–Weinberg equilibrium

Mendelian segregation leads to simple and predictable segregation ratios in the offspring of specific mating types. Since a population consists of the offspring of a mixture of different mating types, the ratios of the different genotypes in a population are weighted averages of the segregation ratios of the different mating types, the weights being the relative frequencies of the different mating types. When the mating type frequencies arise from random mating, the ratios of the different genotypes follow a mathematical result established independently by the English mathematician Hardy (Hardy, 1908) and the German physician Weinberg (Weinberg, 1908). Hardy published his famous result in the journal *Science*, because he thought it was too trivial for his fellow mathematicians. Consider a bialleic locus with alleles A and a. Let the frequencies of the three genotypes AA, Aa and aa in a large population be P, $2Q$, and R, such that $P + 2Q + R = 1$. Hardy's result was that, if individuals in the population mated with each other at random, these frequencies would be such that

$$Q^2 = PR \tag{2.45}$$

To show how this elegant result follows from random mating, we consider the possible mating types in the population, the frequencies at which these occur, and the distribution of genotypes among the offspring. The necessary information is summarized in Table 2.2.

Table 2.2 A biallelic locus under random mating

			Offspring		
Father	Mother	Frequency	AA	Aa	aa
AA	AA	(P)(P)	1	0	0
AA	Aa	(P)(2Q)	0.5	0.5	0
AA	aa	(P)(R)	0	1	0
Aa	AA	(2Q)(P)	0.5	0.5	0
Aa	Aa	(2Q)(2Q)	0.25	0.5	0.25
Aa	aa	(2Q)(R)	0	0.5	0.5
aa	AA	(R)(P)	0	1	0
aa	Aa	(R)(2Q)	0	0.5	0.5
aa	aa	(R)(R)	0	0	1

The frequency of a genotype in the entire population of offspring is a weighted average of the frequencies in the offspring of different mating types, the weight attached to a mating type being its frequency in the population. Let the frequency of genotype AA among the offspring of the population be P_1 (the subscript 1 indicating generation 1),

$$\left.\begin{aligned} P_1 &= (1)P^2 + \left(\frac{1}{2}\right)2PQ + \left(\frac{1}{2}\right)2PQ + \left(\frac{1}{4}\right)4Q^2 \\ &= P^2 + 2PQ + Q^2 \\ &= (P + Q)^2 \end{aligned}\right\} \tag{2.46}$$

Similarly, it can be shown that the frequencies of genotypes Aa ($2Q_1$) and aa (R_1) among the offspring are

$$\left.\begin{aligned} 2Q_1 &= 2(P + Q)(R + Q) \\ R_1 &= (R + Q)^2 \end{aligned}\right\} \tag{2.47}$$

The proportions of the three genotypes among the population of offspring therefore satisfy the relation $Q_1^2 = P_1 R_1$. Moreover, if these offspring are mated at random, then the proportions of the three genotypes in the next generation are

$$
\left.\begin{aligned}
P_2 &= (P_1 + Q_1)^2 = P_1 \\
2Q_2 &= 2(P_1 + Q_1)(R_1 + Q_1) = 2Q_1 \\
R_2 &= (R_1 + Q_1)^2 = R_1
\end{aligned}\right\} \tag{2.48}
$$

In other words, the relative frequencies of the genotypes will remain unchanged after a second generation of random mating. It follows that these frequencies will continue to be in the *Hardy–Weinberg* ratio $Q^2 = PR$ as long as matings in the population are random with respect to the locus. It is in this sense that this ratio of frequencies represents an *equilibrium*.

Perhaps a simpler way of stating the Hardy–Weinberg equilibrium is to relate genotype frequencies to allele frequencies. If the frequencies of alleles A and a are p and q, respectively, then, in the absence of differential fertility, the frequencies of gametes with alleles A and a will be p and q. Under random mating, paternal gametes are combined with maternal gametes at random (*panmixia*). The frequencies of genotype AA, Aa and aa are therefore p^2, $2pq$, and q^2, regardless of the genotype frequencies in the parental generation. Since the allele frequencies corresponding to these genotype frequencies remain unchanged at p and q, the same genotype frequencies will be maintained in subsequent generations as long as random mating applies in the population. The same principle can be applied to a locus with more than two alleles. Let the alleles be A_1, A_2, ..., A_m, with frequencies p_1, p_2, ..., p_m. Under Hardy–Weinberg equilibrium, the frequency of a homozygous genotype such as A_iA_i is p_i^2, and the frequency of a heterozygous genotype such as A_iA_j $(i \neq j)$ is $2p_ip_j$.

The Hardy–Weinberg equilibrium has many important applications. Since there are few (if any) alternative explanations of the characteristic ratios, the demonstration of such ratios constitutes strong evidence for a genetic basis for a trait. This is particularly useful if a family study involving parents and offspring is not feasible.

Example 2.15
In a study in Iceland, the frequencies of MM, MN and NN blood groups in a random sample of the population were found to be 233, 385 and 129, respectively (Mourant, 1954). Are these data consistent with the Hardy–Weinberg equilibrium? This question can be addressed with the Pearson chi-squared test or the likelihood ratio chi-squared test. For the Pearson chi-squared test, it is necessary to calculate the expected frequencies of the three blood groups, under the null hypothesis of the Hardy–Weinberg equilibrium. To do this, we first estimate the allele frequencies. In a total of $233 + 385 + 129 = 747$ individuals there is a total of $2 \times 747 = 1494$ genes at the locus, in which allele M occurs $(2 \times 233) + 385 = 851$ times. The sample frequency of allele M is therefore $851/1494 = 0.5696$. Similarly, the sample frequency of allele N is 0.4304. The expected frequencies of the genotypes MM, MN and NN are therefore $(0.5696)^2 = 0.3245$, $2(0.5696)(0.4304) = 0.4903$ and $(0.4304)^2 = 0.1852$. These frequencies can be multiplied by the

number of individuals (747) to obtain the expected numbers of the different blood groups in the sample, under the hypothesis of Hardy–Weinberg equilibrium. It is convenient to tabulate the calculation of the Pearson chi-squared statistic, as follows.

	MM	MN	NN	Total
Observed (O)	233	385	129	747
Expected (E)	242.37	366.26	138.37	747
$(O-E)^2/E$	0.3622	0.9588	0.6345	1.9555

The overall chi-squared statistic of 1.9555 with one degree of freedom gives a P-value of 0.1620. The number of degrees of freedom is one (rather than two) because the calculation of the expected numbers involved estimating, from the data, the frequency of one of the alleles (and thus fixing the frequency of the other allele because the two allele frequencies must sum to 1). The test result indicates that the observed genotype frequencies are consistent with the hypothesis of Hardy–Weinberg equilibrium, supporting a Mendelian genetic basis for MN blood group. The likelihood ratio chi-squared test requires the calculation of two likelihoods. One of these is the maximum likelihood over all possible values of the population proportions of the three groups, and the other is the maximum likelihood over all sets of population proportions consistent with Hardy–Weinberg equilibrium. The maximum likelihood estimates of the population proportions can be found by standard methods (involving differentiation of the log-likelihood function) to be simply the sample proportions, i.e. $233/747 = 0.3119$, $385/747 = 0.5154$ and $129/747 = 0.1727$. The maximum likelihood is therefore $(0.3119)^{233}$ $(0.5154)^{385}$ $(0.1727)^{129}$. The maximum likelihood estimates of the proportions, constrained by Hardy–Weinberg equilibrium, have been shown to be 0.3245, 0.4903 and 0.1852, so that the likelihood under this hypothesis is $(0.3245)^{233}$ $(0.4903)^{385}$ $(0.1852)^{129}$. The likelihood ratio chi-squared test can be set out as follows.

Model	Parameter values	2 ln(likelihood)
General	0.3119, 0.5154, 0.1727	−1506.38
Hardy–Weinberg	0.3245, 0.4903, 0.1852	−1508.34

The chi-squared statistic of 1.9592 with 1 degree of freedom gives a P-value of 0.1616. These results are in excellent agreement with those obtained by the Pearson chi-squared test.

Example 2.16
The locus for red cell phosphatase has three alleles A, B and C. Spencer *et al.* (1964) collected data on the frequencies of the six possible genotypes for red cell acid phosphatase in a random sample of 178 individuals. The frequencies of the genotypes AA, AB, AC, BB, BC and CC were 17, 86, 5, 61, 9 and 0 respectively. Are these data consistent with Hardy–Weinberg equilibrium?

The sample frequency of allele A is $[(2 \times 17) + 86 + 5] \ /356 = 0.3511$. Similarly, the sample frequencies of alleles B and C are 0.6096 and 0.0393. The expected frequency of AA in a sample of 178 individuals is therefore $178 \times (0.3511)^2 = 21.9$. The expected frequencies of the other genotypes are similarly calculated. The Pearson chi-squared analysis can be set out as follows.

	AA	AB	AC	BB	BC	CC	Total
Observed (O)	17	86	5	61	9	0	178
Expected (E)	21.9	76.2	4.9	66.1	8.5	0.3	178
$(O - E)^2/E$	1.11	1.26	0.00	0.40	0.03	0.28	3.08

The overall chi-squared statistic of 3.08 can be referred to a chi-squared distribution with three degrees of freedom to give a P-value of 0.38. The number of degrees of freedom is three rather than five because of the estimation from the data of two allele frequencies for the calculation of expected genotype frequencies.

The likelihood ratio chi-squared test is also applicable for multiallele loci. For the above data, the likelihood ratio chi-squared statistic with three degrees of freedom works out to be 3.41, which gives a P-value of 0.33.

2.6.1 Estimation of allele frequencies for non-codominant loci

The Hardy–Weinberg equilibrium can also be used to estimate gene frequencies for Mendelian dominant and recessive diseases from the prevalence of the disease, if the assumption of random mating is reasonable. Unlike codominant traits, for which the maximum likelihood estimate of the population frequency of an allele is simply the sample proportion of the allele, non-codominant traits are complicated by the fact that not all genotypes are distinguishable from each other, so that it may be impossible to count the number of an allele in a sample. In this situation, the Hardy–Weinberg equilibrium often provides a reasonable assumption that allows the estimation of allele frequencies.

Example 2.17
Phenylketonuria is a recessive condition in which heterozygous individuals with one copy of the disease allele are not distinguishable from homozygous normal individuals. Suppose that five cases of phenylketonuria are present in a random sample of 55 715 babies (Raine *et al.*, 1972), what is a good estimate of the frequency of the disease gene?

Since the number of disease alleles in a sample therefore cannot be counted directly, some assumption must be made concerning the ratio of heterozygous to homozygous genotypes among phenotypically normal individuals. The Hardy–Weinberg equilibrium is such an assumption that is usually an accurate approximation to the true situation. Let the disease and normal alleles at the phenylketonuria locus be D and d, with frequencies p and $1 - p$, and the three genotypes be DD, Dd and dd, with frequencies q_{11}, q_{12} and q_{22} in a sample. The fact that the phenylketonuria is recessive means that the genotypes Dd and dd are phenotypically normal and hence indistinguishable from each other, so that we do not know q_{12} and q_{13} separately, but only the total $q_{12} + q_{13}$. Since q_{11} is expected to be the square of p, a reasonable estimate of p is the square root of q_{11}. In fact, this turns out to be the maximum likelihood estimate of p. To show this, let the number of affected and unaffected individuals in a random sample be n_1 and n_2, then the log-likelihood under Hardy–Weinberg equilibrium is

$$\ln L(p) = n_1 \ln(p^2) + n_2 \ln(1 - p^2)$$

Setting the derivative of this log-likelihood function to 0 leads to

$$\frac{2\hat{p}n_1}{\hat{p}^2} - \frac{2\hat{p}n_2}{1 - \hat{p}^2} = 0$$

which gives

$$\hat{p} = \left(\frac{n_1}{n_1 + n_2} \right)^{1/2}$$

For the phenylketonuria data, the maximum likelihood estimate of the disease gene frequency is therefore $(5/55\ 715)^{1/2}$, or 0.009473. To find the standard error of this estimate, we use the result that, if the log-likelihood function is $L(p)$, then the sampling variance of the maximum likelihood estimate of $\hat{p}$ is

$$\text{Var}(\hat{p}) = \frac{-1}{E\left(\dfrac{d^2 \ln L(p)}{dp^2} \right)}$$

Omitting the mathematical details, the sampling variance of $\hat{p}$ works out to be

$$\text{Var}(\hat{p}) = \frac{1 - p^2}{4n\left(1 - \dfrac{p}{2}\right)}$$

where $n = n_1 + n_2$, is the sample size and p is the true value of the allele frequency. An estimate of the standard error of p is therefore

$$\text{SE}(\hat{p}) = \left(\frac{1 - \hat{p}^2}{4n\left(1 - \dfrac{\hat{p}}{2}\right)} \right)^{1/2}$$

For the phenylketonuria data, this gives a standard error of 0.002123 for the maximum likelihood estimate of the disease gene frequency. A 95% confidence interval for the disease gene frequency is therefore $(0.0052, 0.0136)$.

Example 2.18
Another similar situation that involves more than two alleles is the ABO blood group system, which has three alleles, A, B and O. Of the six possible

genotypes, only four are phenotypically distinguishable. The distinguishable phenotypes are blood group A (genotypes AA and AO), blood group B (genotypes BB and BO), blood group AB (genotype AB), and blood group O (genotype OO). We wish to estimate the frequencies of the alleles in Berlin, using the frequencies of the four blood groups A, B, AB and O (9123, 2987, 1269 and 7725, respectively) in a large random sample (Bernstein, 1925; quoted by Vogel and Motulsky, 1986).

Let the frequencies of alleles A, B and O be p, q and $1 - p - q$, and the counts of the phenotypes A, B, AB and O in a random sample be n_A, n_B, n_{AB} and n_0, with total sample size n. Under Hardy–Weinberg disequilibrium, the expected frequencies of these four phenotypes are $p^2 + 2p(1 - p - q)$, $q^2 + 2q(1 - p - q)$, $2pq$ and $(1 - p - q)^2$. The log-likelihood of the data is therefore

$$\ln(L(p,q)) = n_A \ln[p^2 + 2p(1 - p - q)] + n_B \ln[q^2 + 2q(1 - p - q)]$$
$$+ n_{AB} \ln(2pq) + n_0 \ln[1 - p - q)^2]$$

The maximization of this log-likelihood function with respect to p and q can be attempted by setting the partial derivatives of the function with respect to p and q to zero and solving the resulting simultaneous equations. However, this is laborious, and Bernstein (1925) has given an approximate solution. The method is based on the probabilities of certain groupings of phenotypes.

$$P(A,O) = p^2 + 2p(1 - p - q) + (1 - p - q)^2$$
$$= (p + 1 - p - q)^2$$
$$= (1 - q)^2$$
$$P(B,O) = q^2 + 2q(1 - p - q) + (1 - p - q)^2$$
$$= (q + 1 - p - q)^2$$
$$= (1 - p)^2$$

These give rise to the following estimates

$$\tilde{p} = 1 - \left(\frac{n_B}{n} + \frac{n_0}{n} \right)^{1/2}$$

$$\tilde{q} = 1 - \left(\frac{n_A}{n} + \frac{n_0}{n} \right)^{1/2}$$

For the Berlin data, these formulae give the estimates $\tilde{p} = 0.28755$ and $\tilde{q} = 0.10651$. Substituting these estimates into the log-likelihood function gives a value of -24822.7575.

The EM algorithm can be used to obtain more accurate maximum likelihood estimates of the allele frequencies, since the difficulty in the estimation arises from the *incomplete data*, i.e. the uncertainty about how many of the n_A individuals with blood group A have genotype AA, and about how many of the n_B individuals with blood group B have genotype BB.

Let the counts of the genotypes AA, AO, BB, BO, AB, OO (i.e. the complete data) be n_{AA}, n_{AO}, n_{BB}, n_{BO}, n_{AB}, n_{OO}, then $n_A = n_{AA} + n_{AO}$,

$n_B = n_{BB} + n_{BO}$. Given the initial parameter values p_0 and q_0 and the observed value n_A, the expected values of n_{AA} and n_{AO} are

$$E(n_{AA}) = \frac{p^2}{p^2 + 2p(1-p-q)} n_A$$

$$E(n_{AO}) = \frac{2p(1-p-q)}{p^2 + 2p(1-p-q)} n_A$$

The expected values of n_{BB} and n_{BO} can be calculated similarly. Given these four expected counts and the two observed counts n_{AB}, n_{OO}, the revised allele frequencies are simply the sample proportions of the alleles, i.e.

$$p_1 = \frac{2E(n_{AA}) + E(n_{AO}) + n_{AB}}{2n}$$

$$q_1 = \frac{2E(n_{BB}) + E(n_{BO}) + n_{AB}}{2n}$$

These revised values of the allele frequencies are used as the input to the next iteration, to produce a new set of complete data and a new set of revised allele frequencies. The application of this iterative procedure to the ABO data, using the allele frequency estimates from the Bernstein method as starting values, produced rapid convergence.

Iteration (i)	p_i	q_i
0	0.28755345	0.10650869
1	0.28765996	0.10655098
2	0.28768093	0.10655454
3	0.28768473	0.10655493
4	0.28768541	0.10655498
5	0.28768553	0.10655499
6	0.28768555	0.10655499
7	0.28768555	0.10655499

The maximum likelihood estimates of p and q are therefore 0.28769 and 0.10655, extremely close to the estimates obtained by the Bernstein method. The value of the log-likelihood function at these allele frequencies (i.e. the maximum log-likelihood) works out to be -24822.7551, only slightly higher than the value of the log-likelihood at the allele frequencies of the Bernstein method.

2.6.2   Testing Hardy–Weinberg equilibrium for codominant loci

For a dominant or recessive biallelic trait, the Hardy–Weinberg equilibrium cannot be tested because only two categories of individuals are distinguishable. This allows the allele frequency to be estimated under the assumption of

Hardy–Weinberg equilibrium, but leaves no additional degree of freedom for testing the assumption itself. The situation is different for loci with three or more alleles.

Example 2.19
For the ABO data, the assumption of Hardy–Weinberg equilibrium can be tested because an unrestricted model of the data would involve three parameters (i.e. four phenotype frequencies which sum to 1), while the Hardy–Weinberg model would involve only two parameters (i.e. three allele frequencies which sum to 1), leaving one degree of freedom for testing the adequacy of the Hardy–Weinberg model in relation to the unrestricted model. The log-likelihood of the ABO data under the unrestricted model is obtained by substituting the sample proportions of the phenotypes into the log-likelihood function, i.e.

$$\ln L = 9123\ln\frac{9123}{21104} + 2987\ln\frac{2987}{21104} + 1269\ln\frac{1269}{21104} + 7725\ln\frac{7725}{21104}$$

This works out to be -24822.3785. The maximum likelihood under Hardy–Weinberg equilibrium has been found in Example 2.10 to be -24822.7551, so that the likelihood ratio chi-squared statistic, which is twice the difference between these log-likelihoods, is 0.7531, which with 1 degree of freedom corresponds to a P-value of 0.3855. The data are therefore consistent with the hypothesis that ABO blood groups are determined by a triallelic locus in Hardy–Weinberg equilibrium.

2.6.3 Testing Hardy–Weinberg equilibrium for multi-allele loci

When the number of alleles at the locus is large relative to the sample size, the Pearson chi-squared test, which relies on an asymptotic sampling distribution, may be inaccurate. This problem is similar to that of ordinary contingency tables, for which the usual (Cochran's) rules for the validity of the chi-squared test require that no expected cell count is less than 1, and no more than 20% of the expected cell counts are less than 5. Translating these rules to the chi-squared test for Hardy–Weinberg equilibrium leads to the requirement that no expected genotype frequency is less than 1, and that no more than 20% of the expected genotype frequencies are less than 5.

When these requirements are violated by a particular data set, then the P-value associated with the Pearson chi-squared statistic calculated from the data set cannot be reliably obtained from the usual asymptotic distribution. The exact P-value can be obtained by calculating the probability distribution of the Pearson chi-squared statistic. This involves going through all possible samples of genotype counts consistent with the observed allele counts and, for each sample of possible genotype counts, calculating the Pearson chi-squared statistic and the probability of the sample under the hypothesis of Hardy–Weinberg equilibrium. For a locus with m alleles, the probability of obtaining a sample of size n with the $m(m+1)/2$ genotype counts $f_{11}, f_{21}, f_{22}, f_{31}, f_{32}, f_{33}, \ldots, f_{mm}$ (denoted as the vector f), conditional on the m allele counts $f_1, f_2, f_3, \ldots, f_m$, under the hypothesis of Hardy–Weinberg equilibrium, is given by the ratio (Levene, 1949)

$$P(f) = \frac{P_2}{P_1} 2^H \qquad (2.49)$$

where H is the total count of heterozygous genotypes, P_2 is the number of permutations of n objects (genotypes) with counts $f_{11}, f_{21}, f_{22}, ..., f_{mm}$ and P_1 is the number of permutations of $2n$ objects (alleles) with counts $f_1, f_2, ..., f_m$.

$$\left. \begin{aligned} H &= \sum_{i>j} f_{ij} \\ P_1 &= \frac{(2n)!}{f_1! f_2! \cdots f_m!} \\ P_2 &= \frac{n!}{f_{11}! f_{21}! f_{22}! \cdots f_{mm}!} \end{aligned} \right\} \qquad (2.50)$$

The exact P-value is the sum of the probabilities over the sets of expected genotype counts for which the Pearson chi-squared statistic is greater than or equal to the actual Pearson chi-squared statistic of the observed data.

When the sample size is large, exact calculation of the P-value becomes very laborious, and it is often sufficient to have a fairly accurate estimate of the P-value from Monte Carlo simulation. Instead of going through all possible samples of genotype counts, random samples of genotype counts are generated by Monte Carlo simulation, conditional on the observed allele counts and assuming Hardy–Weinberg equilibrium. An estimate of the P-value is the proportion of simulated samples for which the Pearson chi-squared statistic is greater than or equal to the actual Pearson chi-squared statistic of the observed data.

A very simple method of generating random samples of genotype counts, conditional on the observed alleles counts and assuming Hardy–Weinberg equilibrium is suggested by the equivalence between Hardy–Weinberg equilibrium and panmixia (Guo and Thompson, 1992). The $2n$ alleles in the sample can be randomly permuted to a certain order, and the n consecutive pairs of alleles taken as the n genotypes in a simulated random sample. Additional random permutations of the $2n$ alleles then give rise to further simulated random samples until the required number of replicates for the estimation of the P-value is obtained.

2.7   Interpreting significant deviations from Hardy–Weinberg equilibrium

There are many possible explanations for a significant deviation from Hardy–Weinberg equilibrium. One possible reason is that the genetic basis of the trait has been misspecified. For example, if one were unable to distinguish blood group O from blood group AB, then it might be tempting to hypothesize that the three distinguishable categories A, B and the combined group of AB and O are determined by a codominant biallelic locus. The Berlin data would then have given the frequencies 9123, 2987 and 8994, which are inconsistent with Hardy–Weinberg equilibrium.

Another reason for deviation from the Hardy–Weinberg equilibrium is non-random mating in the population. One form of non-random mating is population stratification, where matings between individuals from different strata are less likely to occur than matings between individuals of the same stratum. In this situation, Hardy–Weinberg disequilibrium may apply to the separate strata but not to the population as a whole. Another form of non-random mating is assortative mating, where the probability of mating between two individuals is related to their phenotypic similarity. An extreme example of assortative mating is selection by sex, since only opposite-sex pairs can produce offspring. Non-random matings may also arise from prohibition against or encouragement for matings between certain classes of relatives. For example, sibling marriage is almost universally prohibited, but marriages between cousins are encouraged in some cultures.

Deviation from the Hardy–Weinberg equilibrium can arise even when matings do occur at random within a population, if there are differences in the death rates of individuals with different genotypes. For example, some mutations are lethal in the homozygous form. Differential survival causes deviations from Hardy–Weinberg equilibrium for two reasons. The first reason is that it distorts the relative frequencies of the possible mating types, and consequently the distribution of genotypes among the offspring. The second reason is that the preferential loss of individuals with certain genotypes has a direct effect on the distribution of genotypes in the surviving population.

Another cause for deviation from the Hardy–Weinberg equilibrium is the preferential selection for individuals with certain genotypes in the sampling process. For example, if a sample is selected to contain only individuals with a Mendelian dominant disorder, then no homozygous normal individuals will be included, so that the sample will clearly deviate from Hardy–Weinberg equilibrium.

2.8 Conclusions

The law of segregation has many important consequences for the patterns of distribution of genotypes in families and in populations. When a discrete phenotypic trait is determined by the genotype at a single locus, the consequences of Mendelian segregation can be observed directly in the patterns of distribution of the trait in families and in populations. The statistical methods described in this chapter can be used to assess the evidence in favour or against the operation of Mendelian inheritance for a trait, by testing the hypothesis of Mendelian segregation ratios in sibships or Hardy–Weinberg proportions in populations. However, great caution is needed in the interpretation of the results from these analyses, because a true underlying Mendelian ratio can be distorted for many reasons, including sampling artefacts. In other words, these tests are quite specific in terms of detecting single gene action, but are not robust to the influence of potential confounders.

In the course of this chapter, we have also introduced some statistical concepts and tools that will be used in subsequent chapters. We emphasized the importance of taking appropriate account of the method of sample selection in statistical analysis. We described briefly various hypothesis testing and parameter estimation procedures (including likelihood ratio tests and maximum likelihood estimation). We also outlined the EM algorithm and the method of scoring for obtaining maximum likelihood estimates.

3

The Analysis of Genetic Linkage

The law of segregation is concerned with the transmission of alleles at a single locus. The law of assortment, on the other hand, was formulated to describe the simultaneous transmission of alleles at two or more loci. Unfortunately, because the loci of the traits studied by Mendel were all located on separate chromosomes, it was originally proposed that alleles at different loci were transmitted independently of each other. Subsequent experiments have shown, however, that independent assortment was applicable only to loci on separate chromosomes. In contrast, alleles at loci on the same chromosome can display a phenomenon known as *linkage*. This phenomenon is the basis of an important method in genetic research called linkage analysis, the aim of which is to infer the relative positions of two or more loci by examining the patterns of allele-transmission from parent to offspring, or the patterns of allele-sharing by relatives.

Linkage analysis is an important tool for the mapping of genetic loci. As a method for mapping disease loci, it has the advantage that no knowledge of the pathophysiological mechanisms of the disease is required. With the availability of numerous DNA markers throughout the human genome, linkage analysis has succeeded in mapping the mutations responsible for hundreds of Mendelian diseases. The current challenge is to use linkage analysis to map susceptibility loci for common diseases with complex genetic and environmental determinants.

3.1 Definition of linkage

The genotype of an individual at loci $A, B, C, \ldots$, written as $A_{(f)}A_{(m)}B_{(f)}B_{(m)}C_{(f)}C_{(m)}D_{(f)}D_{(m)}\ldots$, is formed by the haplotypes of two gametes, $A_{(f)}B_{(f)}C_{(f)}D_{(f)}\ldots$ inherited from the father, and $A_{(m)}B_{(m)}C_{(m)}D_{(m)}\ldots$ inherited from the mother. The haplotype of a gamete produced by the individual will consist of a mixture of paternal and maternal alleles, e.g. $A_{(f)}B_{(m)}C_{(m)}D_{(f)}\ldots$. When the number of loci considered is large, this haplotype will almost certainly constitute a new combination of alleles, different from both the paternal and the maternal haplotypes.

When only two loci are considered, a gamete may contain two alleles from the same parental gamete, i.e. $A_{(f)}B_{(f)}$ or $A_{(m)}B_{(m)}$, or one allele from each parental gamete, i.e. $A_{(m)}B_{(f)}$ or $A_{(f)}B_{(m)}$. In the first case, the haplotype of the gamete is the same as the haplotype of one of the parental gametes, as far as these two loci are concerned. Such gametes are defined as parental types or non-recombinants with respect to the two loci. In the second case, however, the haplotype of the gamete constitutes a new combination of alleles different from either parental haplotype. Such gametes are defined as non-parental types or recombinants with respect to the two loci. The recombination fraction (usually denoted as θ) between the two loci is defined as the probability that a gamete is recombinant, i.e. $A_{(m)}B_{(f)}$ or $A_{(f)}B_{(m)}$, with respect to the loci.

Loci on the same chromosome are said to be syntenic, and those on different chromosomes are said to be non-syntenic. For two non-syntenic loci, the independent segregation of chromosomes during meiosis ensures that recombinant and non-recombinant gametes are equally likely to occur. The recombination fraction is therefore $1/2$. For two syntenic loci, however, separation of the two paternal alleles or the two maternal alleles requires the occurrence of a crossover between the two loci. The closer the two loci, the less likely that a crossover will occur between them in meiosis, and the more likely that the two paternal alleles or the two maternal alleles will be transmitted together to an offspring. This relative excess of non-recombinant over recombinant gametes means that the recombination fraction between the two loci will be less than $1/2$. Two loci with a recombination fraction of less than $1/2$ are said to be in linkage. The smaller the recombination fraction, the more tightly linked are the two loci.

3.2   Crossing over and map distance

In order to understand the relationship between recombination fraction and physical distance, it is necessary to examine the process of crossing over in meiosis, which is responsible for the generation of recombinant haplotypes at two syntenic loci. At an early stage of meiosis, each of the 46 chromosomes becomes duplicated to form two sister strands *(chromatids)* connected to each other at a region called the centromere. The homologous chromosomes (and the sex chromosomes) then form pairs, so that each resulting complex consists of four chromatids known as a *tetrad* (Figure 3.1). At this stage the non-sister chromatids adhere to each other in a semi-random fashion at regions called *chiasmata*. Each chiasma represents a point where crossing over between two non-sister chromatids can occur. Chiasmata do not occur entirely at random, as they are more likely further away from the centromere, and it is unusual to find two chiasmata in very close proximity to each other. Observations on meioses suggest that each chromosome (i.e. each pair of sister chromatids) must have at least one chiasma, resulting in an *obligatory crossover*. Some chromosomes have an obligatory crossover on each side of the centromere (i.e. each chromosome arm). The average number of chiasmata for a chromosome

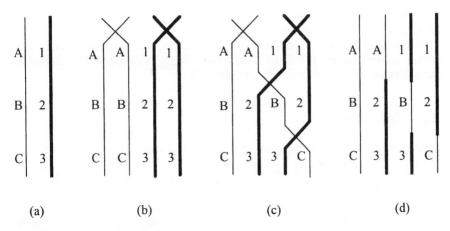

Figure 3.1 Crossover in meiosis.

depends on the length of the chromosome, ranging from just over 1 for chromosome 21 (the shortest) to nearly 4 for chromosome 1 (the longest). On average, there are more chiasmata in female than in male meioses.

Each gamete receives one chromatid from a tetrad to make up the haploid complement of 23 chromosomes. Each chromosome consists of a number of segments from the two parental chromosomes; the number of segments is determined by the number of crossovers that occurred in the formation of the chromatid that became the chromosome. If no crossover occurred, then the chromosome will be a replicate of an entire parental chromosome. If one crossover occurred, then the chromosome will consist of two segments, one from each parental chromosome. If two crossovers occurred, then the chromosome will consist of three segments, two segments from one parental chromosome and one segment from the other parental chromosome. The two segments from the same parental chromosome must occupy the two ends of the chromosome, separated from each other in between by the segment from the other parental chromosome. In general, the chromosome will consist of alternating segments from the two parental chromosomes, each switch from one parental chromosome to the other being the result of a crossover in meiosis.

The genetic map distance (in units of Morgans) between two loci is defined as the expected number of crossovers occurring between them on a single chromatid during meiosis. Since each chromosome consists of a tetrad, and each crossover involves two chromatids, the genetic map distance between two loci is also equal to half the average number of crossovers between them for the tetrad as a whole. The genetic map length of an entire chromosome is equal to half the average number of crossovers that occur in the tetrad in a meiosis. As noted above, the average number of chiasmata in a tetrad in a meiosis varies according to the length of the chromosome, being just over 1 for chromosome 21 and just under 4 for chromosome 1. The map lengths of these chromosomes are therefore approximately 0.5 and 2 Morgans, respectively. There are on average about 53 chiasmata over all the autosomes in a male meiosis, giving a total autosomal map length of approximately 26.5 Morgans. The average number of chiasmata is greater in female meioses, giving a female map length of approximately 39 Morgans.

Another commonly used unit of map distance is the centiMorgan (cM), which is defined as $1/100$ of a Morgan. One centiMorgan corresponds to approximately 1 000 000 base pairs (1000 kB).

3.3 Map functions

A mathematical relationship that converts map distance (m) to recombination fraction (θ) is called a *map function*. The map length of a chromosomal interval is defined as the average number of crossovers in the interval of a single chromatid, whereas the recombination fraction between the loci at the two ends of the interval is the probability that the two alleles at these two loci are derived from different parental chromosomes (i.e. recombinant). The two ends of the interval will be derived from the same parental chromosome if no crossover or an even number of crossovers occurs in the interval, and from the different parental chromosomes if an odd number of crossovers occurs in the interval. Mather (1938) deduced that the recombination fraction between two loci is half the probability of no chiasma (i.e. crossover) occurring in all four strands of the tetrad between the loci. Since all crossovers occur between non-sister chromatids, the sum of the numbers of crossovers in an interval experienced by the two members of each pair of sister chromatids must be equal to the total number of chiasmata in the four strands. If there is no chiasma in the tetrad, then all four daughter strands will be non-recombinant. If the number of chiasmata is odd, then for each pair of sister chromatids, one member must have an odd number of crossovers and the other an even number, so that the proportion of recombinant strands is $1/2$. If the number of chiasma is even, then either both members of a pair of sister chromatids have an even number of crossovers, or both members have an odd number of crossovers, and these two possibilities are equally likely. The average proportion of recombinant strands is therefore $1/2$. The probability of obtaining a recombinant strand is therefore $1/2$ as long as there is at least one chiasma between the two loci. In other words, if the probability of no chiasma between two loci is p_0, then the recombination fraction is

$$\theta = \frac{1 - p_0}{2} \tag{3.1}$$

The simplest map function, known as the Morgan map function, assumes that chromosomal segments can have at most one crossover, and that the probability of a crossover occurring in a segment is proportional to the map length of the segment. The probability of a chiasma occurring in a distance of m map units is therefore $2m$, which gives

$$\theta = \frac{1 - p_0}{2} = \frac{1 - (1 - 2m)}{2} = m \tag{3.2}$$

This function is admissible for $0 \leqslant m \leqslant 1/2$, since for $m > 1/2$ it leads to recombination fractions of greater than $1/2$. It may therefore serve as a reasonable approximation for short distances, but is not applicable for long segments of chromosomes.

The second simplest map function is the Haldane function, which assumes that crossovers occur at random independently of each other. Under this assumption, the occurrence of crossovers between two loci on a chromosome is a Poisson process (i.e. they are equally probable at any point between the loci), so that the number of crossovers between the loci follows a Poisson distribution. Since map distance, m, is defined as the average number of crossovers per chromatid in a given interval, the average number of crossovers for the tetrad as a whole is $2m$. The assumption of a Poisson process implies that the probability of no chiasma in the interval, p_0, is e^{-2m}. Using Mather's formula, this gives the Haldane map function

$$\theta = \frac{1 - p_0}{2} = \frac{1 - e^{-2m}}{2} \qquad (3.3)$$

whose inverse is

$$m = -\frac{1}{2}\ln(1 - 2\theta) \qquad (3.4)$$

Another way of deriving the Haldane function is to note that map distances, being expectations, are additive, but recombination fractions are not. Consider the loci A, B and C. A gamete is a recombinant with respect to A and C if and only if it is a recombinant with respect to A and B but not B and C, or if it is a recombinant with respect to B and C but not A and B. Therefore, denoting the recombination fractions between these loci as θ_{AC}, θ_{AB} and θ_{BC}, the independence assumption implies the relationship

$$\theta_{AC} = \theta_{AB}(1 - \theta_{BC}) + \theta_{BC}(1 - \theta_{AB}) = \theta_{AB} + \theta_{BC} - 2\,\theta_{AB}\theta_{BC} \qquad (3.5)$$

This can be rewritten as

$$1 - 2\theta_{AC} = 1 - 2\theta_{AB} - 2\theta_{BC} + 4\theta_{AB}\theta_{BC} = (1 - 2\theta_{AB})(1 - 2\theta_{BC}) \qquad (3.6)$$

An additive relationship is then obtained by taking logarithms.

$$\ln(1 - 2\theta_{AC}) = \ln(1 - 2\theta_{AB}) + \ln(1 - 2\theta_{BC}) \qquad (3.7)$$

This suggests using $\ln(1 - 2\theta)$ as a map function, but since the derivative of this is $-2/(1 - 2\theta)$, multiplication by a factor $-1/2$ is desirable in order to obtain a derivative of 1 for small values of θ (so that θ becomes approximately equal to m at small distances). This gives the Haldane map function $m = -(1/2)\ln(1 - 2\theta)$.

In reality, the Haldane map function does not appear to be accurate at small distances. Empirical observations show that the probability of having two crossovers occurring in close proximity to each other is often less than that predicted by the Haldane map function. This is a phenomenon known as *interference*. At very short distances, interference appears to be complete so that, assuming that locus B is between loci A and C, recombination between A and B implies non-recombination between B and C, and vice versa. Recombination fractions therefore become approximately additive at short distances

$$\theta_{AC} = \theta_{AB} + \theta_{BC} \tag{3.8}$$

whereas at very long distances interference becomes negligible and the relationship

$$\theta_{AC} = \theta_{AB} + \theta_{BC} - 2\theta_{AB}\theta_{BC} \tag{3.9}$$

is more accurate. At some intermediate distance the relationship might be described as

$$\theta_{AC} = \theta_{AB} + \theta_{BC} - 2c\theta_{AB}\theta_{BC} \tag{3.10}$$

where c is a value between 0 and 1 defined as the *coincidence* ($1 - c$ is defined as the *interference*), and is a property of the intervals AB and BC. Let $\theta = f(m)$ be a map function consistent with this relationship, which allows for interference, then

$$f(m + d) = f(m) + f(d) - 2cf(m)f(d)$$

$$\frac{f(m + d) - f(m)}{d} = \frac{f(d)}{d} - \frac{2cf(m)f(d)}{d} \tag{3.11}$$

If we require that at short distances $\theta = f(m) = m$, then as d tends to 0, $f(d)/d$ tends to 1, and we have the derivative

$$f'(m) = 1 - 2c_0 f(m) = 1 - 2c_0\theta \tag{3.12}$$

where c_0 is known as a marginal coincidence, distinguished from c because it is the limit as one of the two intervals approaches 0. When c_0 is a non-zero constant, this differential equation yields the solution

$$m = \int \frac{1}{1 - 2c_0\theta} \, d\theta = \frac{-1}{2c_0} \ln(1 - 2c_0\theta) \tag{3.13}$$

which is the Haldane map function when $c_0 = 1$. However, interference suggests that smaller values of c_0 are appropriate for smaller values of θ. This would lead to an infinite number of map functions, but Kosambi (1944) noted that if c_0 were allowed to be an appropriate function of θ, then a single mapping function could be derived. The simplest function of θ that increases in the interval $0 < \theta < 1/2$ and takes the value 0 at $\theta = 0$ and the value 1 when $\theta = 1/2$ is $c_0 = 2\theta$. Then the differential equation becomes

$$f'(m) = 1 - 2c_0\theta = 1 - 4\theta^2 \tag{3.14}$$

Integration then yields the function

$$m = \frac{1}{4} \ln \frac{1 + 2\theta}{1 - 2\theta} \tag{3.15}$$

with inverse

$$\theta = \frac{1}{2} \frac{e^{4m} - 1}{e^{4m} + 1} \tag{3.16}$$

This is known as the Kosambi map function. There are, of course, functions of θ other than 2θ that have the property of being 0 when $\theta = 0$ and being 1 when $\theta = 1/2$. The Carter–Falconer map function is defined as the solution of the differential equation when $c_0 = (2\theta)^3$, i.e.

$$f'(m) = 1 - 2c_0\theta = 1 - 16\theta^4 \tag{3.17}$$

The Felsenstein map function is obtained by assuming that when $\theta = 0$, the coincidence c_0 is not necessarily 0 and may take an arbitrarily small value, say K. The function of θ required should therefore be K when $\theta = 0$ and 1 when $\theta = 0$. The function $c_0 = K - 2\theta(K - 1)$ satisfies this requirement and yields $c_0 = 2\theta$ (assumed by the Kosambi function) as a special case. The Felsenstein map function for a given value of K is obtained by solving the differential equation

$$f'(m) = 1 - 2c_0\theta = 1 - 2\theta[K - 2\theta(K - 1)] \tag{3.18}$$

This family of map functions based on substituting different definitions of c_0 into the differential equation $f'(m) = 1 - 2c_0\theta$ may appear somewhat arbitrary. A different map function based on observed patterns of chiasmata in human meioses has been proposed by Sturt (1976). This map function is based on the empirical observation that, with the exceptions of the short arms of the acrocentric chromosomes (i.e. 13–15, 21–22), the variance of the number of chiasmata per chromosome arm of an entire tetrad is always approximately equal to its mean minus 1 (McDermott, 1973). If chiasmata were randomly distributed as a Poisson process, then the mean and variance of the number of chiasmata in any chromosomal segment should be equal. The observation that the mean exceeds the variance by 1 for most chromosome arms suggests that one chiasma is obligatory for these chromosome arms. Sturt's model is that there is always one chiasma occurring in a random position among the four strands of such a chromosome arm, and that additional chiasmata also occur at random along the arm with no interference.

Let the length of a chromosome arm containing an obligate crossover be L map units, so that the average number of chiasmata in the tetrad is $2L$. The average number of non-obligate crossovers in the entire arm is therefore $2L - 1$, so that the average number in a segment of map distance m is $2m[(2L - 1)/(2L)] = m(2L - 1)/L$. The probability of the obligate crossover occurring in an interval of m map units is m/L, so that the probability of an obligate crossover not occurring in an interval is $1 - m/L$. Since additional crossovers occur as a Poisson process with mean $m(2L - 1)/L$, the probability of no additional crossover occurring in the interval of length m is $e^{-m(2L-1)/L}$. The overall probability of no crossover occurring in a segment of m map units is thus

$$p_0 = \left(1 - \frac{m}{L}\right) e^{-m(2L - 1)/L} \tag{3.19}$$

so that application of Mather's formula yields the Sturt map function

$$\theta = \frac{1 - p_0}{2} = \frac{1}{2}\left(1 - \left(1 - \frac{m}{L}\right) e^{-m(2L - 1)/L}\right) \tag{3.20}$$

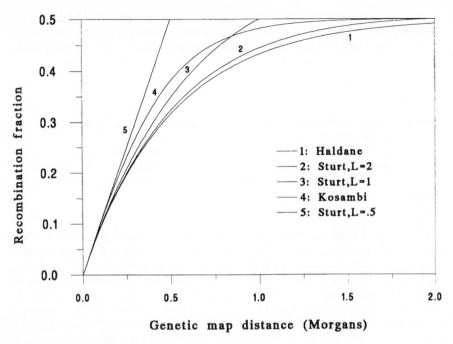

Figure 3.2 Map functions.

This function implies that the shorter the chromosome arm, the stronger the interference. When $L = 1/2$ (map units), $\theta = m$, and interference is complete. As L increases to above 2 map units, interference becomes almost negligible.

Karlin and Liberman (1978) and Risch and Lange (1979) have generalized the Sturt map function to a family of map functions where the assumption is that the number of chiasmata for an entire chromosome arm follows some discrete probability distribution. The Haldane map function is obtained by assuming that the number of chiasmata is distributed as a Poisson random variable, and the Sturt map function is obtained by assuming that the number of chiasmata is distributed as a Poisson random variable plus a unit constant. Although there are other map functions in this family, the Sturt map function is based on empirical observations, and is supported by a recent comparative study of several map functions using multilocus pedigree data (Weeks *et al.*, 1993).

Conversion of m to θ or vice versa using a number of different map functions can be performed interactively using the MAPFUN computer program. Figure 3.2 shows the shapes of several map functions.

3.4   Genetic markers for linkage studies

In order for a polymorphism to be useful as a genetic marker, it should be easily and reliably detectable and highly variable (so that unrelated individuals are likely to have different alleles).

It is possible to obtain the sequence of base pairs at a specific locus, thus allowing detection of any allele. However, this process of DNA *sequencing* is time consuming, and the information obtained is often more detailed than is necessary for linkage analysis. Fortunately, there are several types of genetic polymorphisms for which convenient methods of measurement are available.

3.4.1   Classical markers

If the transmission of a phenotypic trait is Mendelian, then it is possible to infer the underlying genotype (i.e. the alleles present at the locus) from the phenotypic trait with a high degree of certainty. The trait can therefore be used as an indicator of the underlying genotype. Examples of such classical genetic markers include ABO blood groups, HLA (Human Leucocyte Antigens), colour blindness and G6PD deficiency.

These classical markers have a number of disadvantages. Polymorphisms that produce variation in the organism are relatively rare because evolutionary pressures often favour one allele so that the others tend to become rare or extinct. Classical markers are therefore rare, and when they do occur, the number of different alleles is usually small. The only classical markers that are highly polymorphic in humans are those in the HLA system.

Another problem with classical markers is that they do not always allow all genotypes to be discriminated. If one allele is dominant and the other recessives, studying the phenotype will not provide any information to distinguish heterozygous subjects from those who are homozygous for the dominant allele.

3.4.2   RFLP markers

Bacterial restriction endonucleases, which cleave DNA at sequence-specific sites, break down a very long DNA molecule into small fragments. If the variation in DNA sequence at a particular locus is such that one of the variants is cleaved by a restriction enzyme and the other is not, then the variant that is not cleaved at that locus will be associated with a longer fragment of DNA. This kind of sequence variation is known as restriction fragment length polymorphism (RFLP) or simply restriction polymorphism.

The laboratory method of detecting RFLP involves breaking down a sample of DNA with a restriction enzyme, separating the fragments according to size by electrophoresis, and using radiolabelled oligonucleotides (probes) to identify and locate the specific complementary fragments. RFLP markers can be found in non-coding as well as coding DNA. However, they are usually biallelic.

3.4.3   Hypervariable markers

At certain loci in the genome the variation between individuals occurs in the form of a variable number of repeats of a particular sequence of base pairs. The number of repeats may vary from one to several hundred, and each of these possible numbers of repeats then represents a different allele. The number of different alleles at such loci is therefore potentially very large, making them ideal markers for linkage analysis.

The terms *variable number of tandem repeats* (VNTR) and *minisatellite* are sometimes used to describe markers based on such loci. When the repeated sequence is very short (2 to 4 base pairs), however, the terms *short tandem repeats* (STR) and *microsatellite* are usually used. The most commonly used repeats are CA-repeats, consisting of cytosine and adenosine nucleotide, sometimes written (CA)n. Of course, since the complementary bases on the other strand are guanine and thymine, these could equally well be referred to as GT-repeats. STR markers are particularly useful because of their abundance in the genome and the ease and reliability of their detection.

The main method for detecting STR is based on the *polymerase chain reaction* (PCR), which amplifies a segment of DNA flanked by two specific sequences. The selective amplification of the segment depends on the availability of two oligonucleotide primers that are complementary to the two specific sequences flanking the segment. Almost any segment, including an STR, can be amplified, because oligonucleotides of any sequence can be manufactured.

PCR involves the repetition of a cycle of three steps. First, the sample DNA containing the target segment is heated to a high temperature so that the two strands of DNA separate. When the temperature is reduced, the oligonucleotide primers cross-hybridize with the sample DNA at the sites where the sequence is complementary. One of the primers hybridizes to one strand of the sample DNA at one end of the segment to be amplified, and the other hybridizes to the other strand, at the opposite end of the segment to be amplified. Starting at the point where a primer has hybridized to a strand of sample DNA, the enzyme polymerase uses the sample DNA as a template to build a new strand of complementary DNA by adding one nucleotide at a time to extend the primer. Thereafter, the cycle is repeated, and the newly formed strand of DNA is separated from the sample DNA by heating. Provided the newly formed strand has extended past the second primer site, the second primer will be able to hybridize to it and then the new strand can itself be used as a template, creating further copies of the sequence between the two primer sites.

The number of copies of the target segment produced by a PCR increases exponentially with the number of cycles which are carried out. Because each stage of the cycle proceeds at a different temperature, PCR can be conveniently carried out by mixing together all of the necessary reagents and then repeatedly heating and cooling the mixture. If some of the primers or nucleotides are radiolabelled then the new copies of the test segment can be measured by autoradiography. Different alleles can be distinguished from each other by electrophoresis, as segments of different sizes (i.e. numbers of repeats) travel at different speeds in an electric field (electrophoresis).

3.4.4   Indices of marker informativeness

To be useful as a marker for linkage analysis, a locus should be highly polymorphic so that alleles inherited from different sources are likely to be distinguishable from each other. An ideal index for marker informativeness should therefore measure not only the number of possible alleles occurring at the locus, but also the frequencies of these alleles. Two such indices are commonly used. The first index is simply the probability that a randomly selected individual from the population under random mating is heterozygous at the locus. This index, called *heterozygosity* and denoted as H, is defined as follows

$$H = 1 - \sum_{i=1}^{n} p_i^2 \qquad (3.21)$$

where p_i is the frequency of the ith allele at the locus, and n is the total number of alleles. Another popular index, called *polymorphism information content* and denoted as PIC, is defined as

$$PIC = 1 - \sum_{i=1}^{n} p_i^2 - \sum_{i=1}^{n-1} \sum_{j=i+1}^{n} 2p_i^2 p_j^2 \qquad (3.22)$$

The rationale of the last term in the definition of PIC is that, if a parental mating is $A_i A_j \times A_i A_j$ (where $i \neq j$), then there is a probability $1/2$ that the parental origins of the alleles transmitted to an offspring can be traced (i.e. when the offspring genotype is $A_i A_i$ or $A_j A_j$), and probability $1/2$ that the parental origins of the alleles transmitted to an offspring cannot be traced (i.e. when the offspring genotype is $A_i A_j$). Since the probability of the parental mating type in a randomly mating population is $4p_i^2 p_j^2$, multiplication by a factor of $1/2$ yields the contribution of $2p_i^2 p_j^2$ in the definition of PIC (Botstein *et al.*, 1980).

3.5   Linkage analysis using fully informative gametes

The aim of linkage analysis is to make inferences about the relative positions of two or more loci. In the simple case of two loci, the problem reduces to the testing of the hypothesis of linkage (versus the hypothesis of no linkage) and the estimation of the recombination fraction between the loci. If the number of recombinant and non-recombinant gametes in a random sample of gametes can be counted, then an estimate of the recombination fraction is simply the proportion of gametes that are recombinant, and a test of linkage is simply a test of whether this proportion is equal to $1/2$ (the null hypothesis of no linkage) or less than $1/2$ (the alternative hypothesis of linkage).

The conditions under which the numbers of recombinant and non-recombinant gametes can be counted directly are easy to achieve in experimental organisms but are rarely realized in humans. Although linkage analysis is primarily concerned with the haplotypes of gametes, direct data are available usually on genotypes of individuals. It is therefore necessary to make inferences about the two underlying gametic haplotypes of an individual from the genotypes of the individual and of the parents. Furthermore, since recombinants and non-recombinants are defined in terms of the haplotypes of one gametic generation in relation to the haplotypes in the previous gametic generation, the unambiguous identification of recombinants and non-recombinants usually requires genotypic data from three generations of individuals.

Example 3.1
Consider the three-generation pedigree

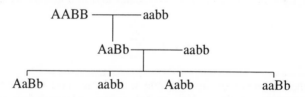

This pedigree consists of eight individuals and therefore potentially 16 gametes. In generation 1 (the grandparents) the haplotypes of the individuals can be deduced (AB/AB in the grandfather and ab/ab in the grandmother), but it is not possible to deduce whether they are recombinant or not, since the haplotypes of the previous generation are not known. In generation 2 (the parents), the haplotypes can also be deduced (AB/ab in the father and ab/ab in the mother), but again it is not possible to deduce whether they are recombinant or not. In the father this is because the haplotypes of his parents are AB/AB and ab/ab, which implies that, regardless of recombination, the haplotypes AB/ab must be transmitted. In the mother, the inability to infer the recombination status of the haplotypes is simply due to lack of knowledge of the haplotypes of her parents.

In generation 3 (the children), the four gametes contributed by the mother must all have the ab haplotype, and are therefore not informative with regard to recombination status, for the same reasons that the haplotypes of the father are not informative. The four remaining gametes, contributed by the father, are therefore AB, ab, Ab and aB. We have already deduced that the father's haplotypes are AB/ab. It is therefore apparent that the first two offspring haplotypes contributed by the father (AB and ab) are non-recombinants, and the other two (Ab and aB) are recombinants.

In summary, of the 16 gametic haplotypes contained in this pedigree of eight individuals, 12 have entirely unknown recombination status, and are therefore said to be uninformative for linkage. The remaining four are said to be fully informative because their recombination status can be deduced with certainty. Among these fully informative gametes are two recombinants and two non-recombinants.

This example illustrates some of the conditions necessary in order for the recombination status of a haplotype to be determined, in other words, for the haplotype to be fully informative for linkage. These conditions are, firstly, that the person's genotype can be determined with certainty from a trait that can be measured (the phenotype). Secondly, the genotypes of the two parents must be known in sufficient detail for the haplotype present in the individual to be determined. Thirdly, the genotypes of the grandparents must be known in sufficient detail for the haplotypes present in the parents to be determined. The haplotype information on a parent is known as the *phase* of the parent's meioses. Fourthly, it is necessary that the parent transmitting the haplotype is heterozygous for both loci concerned (i.e. doubly heterozygous), so that the four gametic haplotype classes can be distinguished from each other.

The simplest form of linkage analysis is to collect a random sample of three generation pedigrees. Suppose that in such a sample there are N fully informative gametes of which R are recombinants, how do we test for linkage and estimate the recombination fraction?

The maximum likelihood estimate of the recombination fraction is simply the proportion of fully informative gametes that are recombinant

$$\hat{\theta} = \frac{R}{N} \qquad (3.23)$$

when $R < (N/2)$, and

$$\hat{\theta} = \frac{1}{2} \qquad (3.24)$$

when $R > (N/2)$, since recombination fractions greater than $1/2$ are inadmissible on biological grounds. When $R < (N/2)$, the estimate $\hat{\theta} = R/N$ has an approximate standard error of $(\hat{\theta}(1 - \hat{\theta})/N)^{1/2}$. Since the expected values of the number of recombinants and non-recombinants are both $N/2$ under the null hypothesis, the Pearson chi-squared statistic

$$T = \frac{(R - N/2)^2}{N/2} + \frac{(N - R - N/2)^2}{N/2} = \frac{(N - 2R)^2}{N} \qquad (3.25)$$

provides a one-tailed test for linkage, with one degree of freedom. Thus, if $R > (N/2)$, the value of T is reassigned to 0 and the test considered non-significant. If $R \leqslant (N/2)$, then the P-value is half the probability that the value of T is exceeded by a chi-squared random variable with one degree of freedom.

The likelihood ratio test is an alternative to the Pearson chi-squared test. Since each gamete has probability θ of being a recombinant and probability $1 - \theta$ of being a non-recombinant, the likelihood function is

$$L(\theta) = \theta^R (1 - \theta)^{N-R} \qquad (3.26)$$

The log-likelihood function is therefore

$$\ln L = R \ln \theta + (N - R)\ln(1 - \theta) \qquad (3.27)$$

The null hypothesis of non-linkage implies $\theta = 1/2$, so that the value of the log-likelihood function is

$$\ln L_0 = N \ln\left(\frac{1}{2}\right) \qquad (3.28)$$

Under the alternative hypothesis of linkage $(\theta < 1/2)$, the maximum log-likelihood is

$$\ln L_1 = R \ln\left(\frac{R}{N}\right) + (N - R) \ln\left(1 - \frac{R}{N}\right) \qquad (3.29)$$

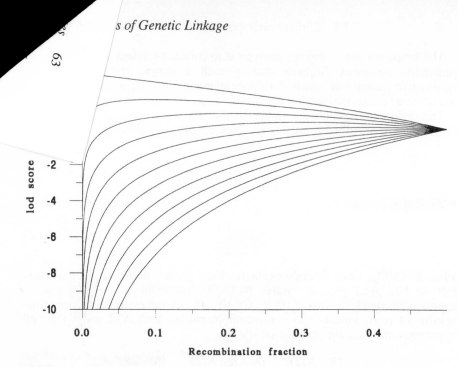

Figure 3.3 Possible lod score functions for ten fully informative gametes.

when $R \leqslant (N/2)$, and

$$\ln L_1 = \ln L_0 \tag{3.30}$$

when $R > (N/2)$. The likelihood ratio statistic $2(\ln L_1 - \ln L_0)$ is an asymptotically 50:50 mixture of a point probability mass at 0 and a chi-squared distribution with one degree of freedom. It therefore provides a one-tailed test for linkage, in the same way as the Pearson chi-squared statistic.

In linkage analysis, it is customary to take the common (base 10) logarithm of the likelihood function, and then define the difference between the log-likelihood at a certain value of θ and the log-likelihood at $\theta = 1/2$ to be the 'lod score' at that value of θ. The lod score is therefore a function of θ in the range $0 \leqslant \theta \leqslant 1/2$ that always has value 0 at $\theta = 1/2$. The maximum of the lod score function occurs at the maximum likelihood estimate of θ, and its value is equal to the likelihood ratio statistic $2(\ln L_1 - \ln L_0)$ divided by a factor of $2 \ln 10$ (approximately 4.6). It is customary to plot lod score against recombination fraction in order to obtain a visual impression of the relative support for different values of recombination fraction. Figure 3.3 shows some examples of lod score curves for data consisting of ten fully informative gametes.

3.6 Linkage analysis of phase-unknown meioses

It is often possible to obtain linkage information from a family even when the recombinants and non-recombinants in the family cannot be individually identified. One situation when this occurs is when genotype data are available for two generations of a family. The unavailability of the grandparental genotypes implies that in a doubly heterozygous parent, the haplotypes present, i e. the phase of the meiosis, cannot be determined. This prevents the offspring haplotypes from being classified unambiguously into recombinants and non-recombinants.

Example 3.2
Consider the pedigree in Example 3.1 but with the grandparents missing

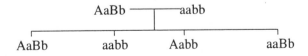

As before, the parental haplotypes themselves and the offspring haplotypes contributed by the mother are entirely uninformative for linkage. The four paternally transmitted haplotypes AB, ab, Ab, aB are potentially informative, but this time we do not know whether the haplotypes present in the father are AB/ab or Ab/aB (i.e. we do not know the phase of the paternal meioses). If the haplotypes present in the father were AB/ab, then AB and ab would be non-recombinants and Ab and aB recombinants. On the other hand, if the haplotypes present in the father were Ab/aB, then Ab and aB would be non-recombinants and AB and ab recombinants. The offspring haplotypes can therefore be classified into two groups (AB and ab versus Ab and aB), where one group is recombinant and the other is non-recombinant, but it is not possible to decide which is which.

This example shows that with a phase unknown, doubly heterozygous meiosis, the offspring haplotypes can be classified into two groups, where one group is non-recombinant and the other group is recombinant, but which is which depends on the unknown phase of the parental meiosis. The analysis of such data is therefore more complicated than those from three-generation families.

Consider first the case of multiple offspring haplotypes from the same doubly heterozygous phase-unknown parent. Suppose that there are X offspring haplotypes classified into one group and Y offspring haplotypes classified into the other. Let $N = X + Y$, then the Pearson chi-squared statistic

$$T = \frac{(X - Y)^2}{N} \tag{3.31}$$

has exactly the same form as that in the case of fully informative gametes. The only difference is that in this case the test is two-tailed. A large discrepancy between X and Y is taken as evidence for linkage, regardless of whether $X > Y$ or $Y > X$. The variables X and Y are interchangeable without affecting the value of the test statistic T.

Since the two possible parental phases are equally likely, the likelihood function is

$$L(\theta) = \frac{1}{2}\theta^X(1 - \theta)^Y + \frac{1}{2}\theta^X(1 - \theta)^Y \tag{3.32}$$

Again, X and Y can be interchanged without affecting the likelihood function $L(\theta)$. The maximum of this function has no simple analytic form, but can be obtained numerically, for example, by the method of scoring. If the log-likelihood maximized over $0 \leq \theta \leq 1/2$ is denoted as $\ln L_1$ and the log-likelihood at $\theta = 1/2$ is denoted as $\ln L_0$, then the likelihood ratio statistic $2(\ln L_1 - \ln L_0)$ might be thought to provide a one-tailed chi-squared test with one degree of freedom, of the null hypothesis $\theta = 1/2$ against the alternative hypothesis $\theta < 1/2$.

However, it can be shown that the asymptotic distribution of $2(\ln L_1 - \ln L_0)$ is not a 50:50 mixture of a point probability mass at 0 and a chi-squared distribution with one degree of freedom (Sham *et al.*, 1996). Taking the first and second derivatives of the log-likelihood function and evaluating them at $\theta = 1/2$ shows that the log-likelihood function will have a maximum at $\theta = 1/2$ when $(X - Y)^2/N < 1$. When $\theta = 1/2$, $(X - Y)^2/N$ is asymptotically chi-squared with one degree of freedom, so that $P[(X - Y)^2/N < 1] \approx 0.68$. The asymptotic distribution of the likelihood ratio statistic $2(\ln L_1 - \ln L_0)$ is therefore 0 with probability 0.68, and some other distribution with probability 0.32. The unusual distribution of $2(\ln L_1 - \ln L_0)$ makes it less convenient than $(X - Y)^2/N$ as a test statistic for linkage. However, this does not preclude the use of $2(\ln L_1 - \ln L_0)$ entirely because its exact distribution can be found numerically for any value of N. It can be shown, for example, that as N increases, the mean and variance of $2(\ln L_1 - \ln L_0)$ converges to approximately 0.4 and 1.16 (the respective limits for phase-known families are 0.5 and 1.25). In practice, however, a single parent will seldom contribute sufficient offspring haplotypes to warrant a formal test of linkage. It is therefore necessary to have a method for combining data on the offspring haplotypes contributed by several parents.

In the case of fully informative gametes, information from several parents can be combined by simply summing up the numbers of recombinant and non-recombinant gametes produced by the parents. This produces the total counts of recombinant and non-recombinant gametes which can then be subjected to a binomial, normal, or chi-squared test of whether the underlying proportion is 1:1. This simple counting procedure, however, is not possible in the case of phase-unknown meioses, because we do not know which of the two groups of haplotypes produced by a parent represents recombinants and which represents non-recombinants. This situation is therefore more conveniently dealt with using the likelihood ratio approach than the Pearson chi-squared approach.

When the contributions from all phase-unknown parents are independent, an extension of the Pearson chi-squared test might be as follows. Suppose that, of the N_i offspring haplotypes of the ith phase-unknown parent, X_i are classified into one group and Y_i into the other such that $X_i \leq Y_i$. In other words, X_i represents the smaller and Y_i the larger of the two groups of offspring haplotypes. The mean (M_i) and variance (V_i) of X_i can be easily obtained by reference to a binomial random variable R_i with parameters N_i and $1/2$, since $X_i = R_i$ when $R_i < N_i/2$ and $X_i = N_i - R_i$ when $R_i \geq N_i/2$. The test statistic

$$T = \frac{\left(\sum X_i - \sum M_i \right)^2}{\sum V_i} \tag{3.33}$$

has asymptotically a chi-squared distribution with one degree of freedom, and provides a one-tailed test for linkage. In other words, if $(\sum X_i - \sum M_i) > 0$, then

T is reassigned a value of 0, and the test considered non-significant, but if $(\Sigma\ X_i - \Sigma\ M_i) \leqslant 0$, then the P-value is half the probability that the value of T is exceeded by a chi-squared random variable with one degree of freedom.

The likelihood approach is convenient because of the additivity of the log-likelihood functions from independent observations. Letting the numbers of gametes in the two groups from the ith phase-unknown parent be X_i and Y_i, the overall log-likelihood function is

$$\ln L = \sum \ln \left[\frac{1}{2}\ \theta^{X_i}(1 - \theta)^{Y_i} + \frac{1}{2}\ \theta^{X_i}(1 - \theta)^{Y_i} \right] \qquad (3.34)$$

This log-likelihood function can be maximized numerically over θ to obtain an estimate of θ, and to obtain a likelihood ratio test statistic $2(\ln L_1 - \ln L_0)$, where $\ln L_1$ is the maximum value of $\ln L$ over $0 \leqslant \theta \leqslant 1/2$, and $\ln L_0$ is the value of $\ln L$ at $\theta = 1/2$. It can be shown that, if the number of independent contributions to $\ln L$ is I, then the probability that $\ln L$ maximizes at $\theta = 1/2$ is asymptotically equal to the probability that a chi-squared random variable with I degrees of freedom will exceed I. Since this probability approaches $1/2$ as I becomes large, the distribution of the overall likelihood ratio statistic $2(\ln L_1 - \ln L_0)$ approaches a 50:50 mixture of a probability mass at 0 and a chi-squared distribution with one degree of freedom. (This explains why a one-tailed chi-squared test is appropriate for the overall likelihood ratio statistic of a large number of families, regardless of whether the constituent observations are phase-known or phase-unknown, or a mixture of both.)

3.7 Linkage analysis of general pedigrees

In practice, many families encountered in human linkage studies, especially in those involving a hypothetical disease locus, do not simply consist of one or more phase-known or phase-unknown parents and their offspring. Families may range in size and structure from pairs of relatives to multi-generational pedigrees consisting of tens or hundreds of individuals, with missing information in some family members. Because of this variability, the likelihood approach is attractive because the overall log-likelihood function is simply the sum of the log-likelihood functions of the families. This enables maximum likelihood estimation and likelihood ratio tests to proceed as usual. In contrast, it is much more difficult to construct a Pearson chi-squared statistic that is able to summarize information from families of different sizes and structures.

Example 3.3
Consider the pedigree in Example 3.1 but with only the offspring generation available for study

$$\text{AaBb} \qquad \text{aabb} \qquad \text{Aabb} \qquad \text{aaBb}$$

The analysis of this family is now complicated by not knowing the parental mating type. However, a likelihood approach is still possible by considering all possible parental mating types. The second offspring requires that the two parents must each have an allele a and an allele b. The first offspring requires that the two parents also to have an allele A and an allele B between them. The possible parental mating types (including phase) are therefore (AB/ab)×(AB/ab), (AB/ab)×(Ab/aB), (Ab/aB)×(Ab/aB), (AB/ab)×(Ab/ab), (Ab/aB)×(Ab/ab), (AB/ab)×(aB/ab), (Ab/aB)×(aB/ab), (AB/ab)×(ab/ab), (Ab/aB)×(ab/ab), (Ab/ab)×(aB/ab). For each of these possible parental mating types, the probability of each offspring genotype can be derived. For example, if the parental mating type is (AB/ab)×(AB/ab), then without recombination in either meiosis, each parent contributes either AB or ab, so that the offspring genotypes are AABB, AaBb, aabb, with probabilities 1/4, 1/2, 1/4. With recombination in one meiosis but not the other, one parent contributes AB or ab while the other contributes Ab or aB, so that the offspring genotypes are AABb, AaBB, Aabb, aaBb, each with probability 1/4. With recombination in both meioses, each parents contributes either Ab or aB, so that the offspring genotypes are AAbb, AaBb, aaBB with probabilities 1/4, 1/2, 1/4. The probabilities of these three situations, as a function of θ, are $(1 - \theta)^2$, $2\theta(1 - \theta)$ and θ^2. The probability of each offspring genotype given the parental mating type is a weighted sum of the conditional probabilities of the offspring genotype in the three situations, each situation being weighted by its probability. For example, the probability of offspring genotype AABB given the parental mating type (AB/ab)×(AB/ab) is $(1/4)$ $(1 - \theta)^2 + (0)$ $[2\theta(1 - \theta)] + (0)$ $(\theta^2) = (1 - \theta)^2/4$. Similarly, the conditional probabilities of the observed offspring genotypes AaBb, aabb, Aabb, aaBb given parental mating type (AB/ab)×(AB/ab) are $[(1 - \theta)^2 + \theta^2]/2$, $(1 - \theta)^2/4$, $\theta(1 - \theta)/2$, $\theta(1 - \theta)/2$. Since the offspring genotypes are conditionally independent given a parental mating type, the conditional probability of a set of offspring genotypes given a parental mating type is simply the products of the conditional probabilities of the individual offspring genotypes given the parental mating type. For example, the conditional probability of the set of offspring genotypes AaBb, aabb, Aabb, aaBb given the parental mating type (AB/ab)×(AB/ab) is $[(1 - \theta)^2 + \theta^2]$ $(1 - \theta)^4\theta^2/32$. The unconditional probability of a set of offspring genotypes is then a weighted sum of the conditional probabilities of the offspring genotypes under all possible parental mating types, each parental mating type being weighted by its probability. If reasonable assumptions can be made regarding the probabilities of the possible parental mating types, then the probability of a set of offspring genotypes becomes simply a function of θ, and can be used as a likelihood function for θ. Assuming allele frequencies of p_1 and p_2 ($= 1 - p_1$) for A and a, and q_1 and q_2 ($= 1 - q_1$) for B and b, and assuming random mating, the contribution of the parental mating type (AB/ab)×(AB/ab) to the likelihood function of the set of offspring genotypes in the above pedigree is $(2p_1p_2q_1q_2)^2[(1 - \theta)^2 + \theta^2](1 - \theta)^4\theta^2/32$. The overall likelihood of the sibship data is the sum of all such contributions from all ten possible parental mating types.

This example illustrates that, in the presence of missing data, the log-likelihood function can become very complicated. Another possible complicating factor is that the phenotype of a locus may not allow the genotype of the locus to be inferred with certainty. This problem can be regarded as an example of incomplete data, in that what is observed captures only part of the true underlying situation. For a Mendelian recessive condition, for example, unaffected individuals may be heterozygous with one copy of the disease allele, or homozygous with zero copy of the disease allele. Furthermore, if penetrance of the homozygous disease genotype is incomplete, then even normal individuals can be homozygous with two copies of the disease allele. The likelihood function must therefore take account of all possible genotypes that are compatible with the observed phenotype of an individual. The inability to determine genotype from phenotype applies even to DNA markers, if phase information is regarded to be part of the genotype. This is because one can directly observe the alleles present in an individual (the phenotype), but not the paternal or maternal origins of the alleles.

The algebraic form of the overall log-likelihood function of a sample, being the sum of the log-likelihood functions of the constituent pedigrees, is usually not analytically tractable. Instead, the values of the log-likelihood function at various values of θ must be calculated using numerical algorithms implemented in a computer program. Numerical algorithms for evaluating likelihood functions of pedigrees are discussed in Section 3.10.

Although the log-likelihood function of a sample is usually time-consuming to evaluate, once obtained it can be used in the standard way to estimate θ, and to test for linkage. Thus, the value of θ that maximizes the log-likelihood function over $0 \leqslant \theta \leqslant 1/2$ is defined as the maximum likelihood estimate of θ, and the likelihood ratio statistic $2(\ln L_1 - \ln L_0)$, where $\ln L_1$ is the maximum value of the log-likelihood function over $0 \leqslant \theta \leqslant 1/2$, and $\ln L_0$ is the value of the log-likelihood function at $\theta = 1/2$, is asymptotically a $50:50$ mixture of 0 and chi-squared with one degree of freedom. This provides a test of the null hypothesis of non-linkage ($\theta = 1/2$) against the one-sided alternative ($\theta < 1/2$).

3.8 Linkage analysis of multiple loci

When only two loci are considered, linkage analysis is concerned with just one parameter, namely the recombination fraction, which reflects the relative frequencies of recombinant and non-recombinant haplotypes with respect to the two loci. Let the genotype of a parent be denoted by a paternal haplotype $A_{(f)}B_{(f)}$ and a maternal haplotype $A_{(m)}B_{(m)}$. A gametic haplotype is recombinant if it is $A_{(m)}B_{(f)}$ or $A_{(f)}B_{(m)}$ and non-recombinant if it is $A_{(m)}B_{(m)}$ or $A_{(f)}B_{(f)}$. This notation emphasizes that in linkage analysis, what matters is not the form of the allele but its parental origin. A gametic haplotype can be written as an ordered string of ms and fs, with an m signifying an allele from the parent's maternal haplotype, and an f signifying an allele from the parent's paternal haplotype. Furthermore, for the purpose of identifying recombinants and non-recombinants, it is sufficient to denote the gametic haplotype by a single digit which indicates whether the second allele is non-recombinant (0) or recombinant (1) with respect to the first allele.

The reason for introducing this notation is that it simplifies the representation of a multi-locus situation. A haplotype of k loci can be denoted by a $k - 1$ string of 0s and 1s, with the ith digit representing the recombination status of the $(i + 1)$th allele with respect to the first allele. This string of $k - 1$ digits specifies the recombination status between all $k(k-1)/2$ pairs of loci; pairs with different digits are recombinants while the others are non-recombinants. For example, in the case of three loci, A, B, C, there are four possible haplotype classes, 00, 01, 10, 11, each representing a unique combination of recombination states between the three possible pairs of loci (AB, BC, AC), as follows.

Haplotype ABC	Recombination status (interval)		
	AB	AC	BC
00	0	0	0
01	0	1	1
10	1	0	1
11	1	1	0

The frequency of a gametic haplotype is therefore equal to the joint probability of the co-occurrence of a set of recombination events. The recombination fraction between two loci is then a marginal probability that is equal to the sum of the frequencies of the haplotypes in which the two loci are recombinant. In the three-locus example, the loci A and B are recombinant in haplotypes 11 and 10, so that the recombination fraction of A and B is the sum of the haplotype frequencies of 11 and 10. For this three-locus system, the haplotype frequencies, denoted as $\gamma_{00}, \gamma_{01}, \gamma_{10}, \gamma_{11}$ and the recombination fractions, denoted as $\theta_{AB}, \theta_{BC}, \theta_{AC}$, are related as follows

$$\left.\begin{array}{l} \theta_{AB} = \gamma_{11} + \gamma_{10} \\ \theta_{BC} = \gamma_{01} + \gamma_{10} \\ \theta_{AC} = \gamma_{01} + \gamma_{11} \end{array}\right\} \tag{3.35}$$

These equations, together with the constraint

$$\gamma_{00} + \gamma_{01} + \gamma_{10} + \gamma_{11} = 1 \tag{3.36}$$

form a system of simultaneous linear equations that can be solved for the recombination fractions (i.e. marginal recombination probabilities) given the gametic frequencies (i.e. joint recombination probabilities), or vice versa. Because of this one-to-one correspondence, the likelihood function can be written in terms of either set of probabilities.

Example 3.4
Suppose that the loci A, B and C are syntenic in that order, with recombination fractions of 20% between A and B, and 20% between B and C. What are the probabilities of the four different haplotype classes given (1) the Morgan map function, (2) the Haldane map function, (3) the Kosambi map function, and (4) the Sturt map function with $L = 1$?
    The steps are the same for all map functions. First the recombination fractions between A and B and between B and C are transformed using the appropriate map function into genetic map units (Morgans). These are summed to give the length of the AC interval, which is then back transformed using the

appropriate inverse map function to give the recombination fraction between A and C. These three recombination fractions (θ_{AB}, θ_{BC}, θ_{AC}) are related to the haplotype probablities (γ_{00}, γ_{01}, γ_{10}, γ_{11}) by a set of simultanious linear equations.

(1) Morgan map function

$$\theta_{AB} = \theta_{BC} = 0.2$$

$$m_{AB} = m_{BC} = 0.2$$

$$m_{AC} = m_{AB} + m_{BC} = 0.4$$

$$\theta_{AC} = 0.4$$

$$\gamma_{11} + \gamma_{10} = \theta_{AB} = 0.2$$
$$\gamma_{01} + \gamma_{10} = \theta_{BC} = 0.2$$
$$\gamma_{01} + \gamma_{11} = \theta_{AC} = 0.4$$
$$\gamma_{00} + \gamma_{01} + \gamma_{10} + \gamma_{11} = 1$$

$$\gamma_{00} = 0.6$$
$$\gamma_{01} = 0.2$$
$$\gamma_{10} = 0.0$$
$$\gamma_{11} = 0.2$$

(2) Haldane map function

$$\theta_{AB} = \theta_{BC} = 0.2$$

$$m_{AB} = m_{BC} = 0.26$$

$$m_{AC} = m_{AB} + m_{BC} = 0.51$$

$$\theta_{AC} = 0.32$$

$$\gamma_{11} + \gamma_{10} = \theta_{AB} = 0.2$$
$$\gamma_{01} + \gamma_{10} = \theta_{BC} = 0.2$$
$$\gamma_{01} + \gamma_{11} = \theta_{AC} = 0.32$$
$$\gamma_{00} + \gamma_{01} + \gamma_{10} + \gamma_{11} = 1$$

$$\gamma_{00} = 0.64$$
$$\gamma_{01} = 0.16$$
$$\gamma_{10} = 0.04$$
$$\gamma_{11} = 0.16$$

Note that because the Haldane map function assumes independence of recombination events in different intervals, these gametic probabilities can be obtained more simply by

$$\gamma_{00} = \theta_{00} = (0.8)\,(0.8) = 0.64$$
$$\gamma_{01} = \theta_{01} = (0.8)\,(0.2) = 0.16$$
$$\gamma_{10} = \theta_{11} = (0.2)\,(0.2) = 0.04$$
$$\gamma_{11} = \theta_{10} = (0.2)\,(0.8) = 0.16$$

(3) Kosambi map function

$$\theta_{AB} = \theta_{BC} = 0.2$$
$$m_{AB} = m_{BC} = 0.21$$
$$m_{AC} = m_{AB} + m_{BC} = 0.42$$
$$\theta_{AC} = 0.34$$
$$\gamma_{11} + \gamma_{10} = \theta_{AB} = 0.2$$
$$\gamma_{01} + \gamma_{10} = \theta_{BC} = 0.2$$
$$\gamma_{01} + \gamma_{11} = \theta_{AC} = 0.34$$
$$\gamma_{00} + \gamma_{01} + \gamma_{10} + \gamma_{11} = 1$$
$$\gamma_{00} = 0.63$$
$$\gamma_{01} = 0.17$$
$$\gamma_{10} = 0.03$$
$$\gamma_{11} = 0.17$$

(4) Sturt $(L = 1)$ map function

$$\theta_{AB} = \theta_{BC} = 0.2$$
$$m_{AB} = m_{BC} = 0.24$$
$$m_{AC} = m_{AB} + m_{BC} = 0.48$$
$$\theta_{AC} = 0.34$$
$$\gamma_{11} + \gamma_{10} = \theta_{AB} = 0.2$$
$$\gamma_{01} + \gamma_{10} = \theta_{BC} = 0.2$$
$$\gamma_{01} + \gamma_{11} = \theta_{AC} = 0.34$$
$$\gamma_{00} + \gamma_{01} + \gamma_{10} + \gamma_{11} = 1$$
$$\gamma_{00} = 0.63$$
$$\gamma_{01} = 0.17$$
$$\gamma_{10} = 0.03$$
$$\gamma_{11} = 0.17$$

As in two-point linkage analysis, multipoint linkage analysis is simplest when gametic haplotypes can be classified unambiguously, which requires that the parent is heterozygous for all loci concerned, and that phase is known. In the ideal situation where all the gametes in a sample are fully informative, the data can be summarized simply as a set of gametic counts. The sample proportions of these counts are then the maximum likelihood estimates of the corresponding haplotype probabilities.

In a three-point analysis, for example, the estimates of the four gametic probabilities can be transformed to give estimates of the three recombination fractions. The relative magnitudes of the three recombination fractions give some indication of the *order* of the three loci, in that if θ_{AC} is larger than θ_{AB} and θ_{BC}, then the order ABC is suggested, with locus B being situated between loci A and C. In addition the estimates of θ_{AC}, θ_{AB}, θ_{BC} can be used to assess the extent of interference between recombination in the interval AB and recombination in the interval BC. The coefficient of *coincidence*, *c* (which is one minus the coefficient of *interference*), is defined by the relationship

$$\theta_{AC} = \theta_{AB} + \theta_{BC} - 2c\theta_{AB}\theta_{BC} \qquad (3.37)$$

which can be rearranged to give

$$c = \frac{\theta_{AB} + \theta_{BC} - \theta_{AC}}{2\theta_{AB}\theta_{BC}} \qquad (3.38)$$

For three-point analysis, the likelihood function can therefore be parameterized in terms of three gametic frequencies γ_{00}, γ_{01}, γ_{10} (the fourth gametic frequency $\gamma_{11} = 1 - \gamma_{00} - \gamma_{01} - \gamma_{10}$), or by three recombination fractions θ_{AB}, θ_{BC}, θ_{AC}, or by two recombination fractions plus the coefficient of coincidence θ_{AB}, θ_{BC}, *c*. A model that does not restrict any of these three parameters is said to be saturated. Restricting $c = 1$ corresponds to the hypothesis of no interference (when the Haldane map function applies), and this hypothesis can be assessed using a standard likelihood ratio test against the one-tailed alternative $c < 1$. If $\ln L_1$ is the log-likelihood maximized over $0 \leqslant c \leqslant 1$ and $\ln L_0$ is the log-likelihood at $c = 1$, then the test statistic $2(\ln L_1 - \ln L_0)$ provides a one-tailed chi-squared test with one degree of freedom for the presence of interference. Other map functions impose other values for *c*, and these too can be assessed by likelihood ratio tests. Three-point analysis can therefore be conducted by treating *c* as an independent parameter, or by imposing a particular map function.

When more than three loci are involved the situation becomes more complex. If *k* loci are involved, for example, then there are $k - 1$ intervals between adjacent loci, each of which can either have an even or an odd number of cross-overs. This produces 2^{k-1} classes of gametic haplotypes, and therefore $2^{k-1} - 1$ independent gametic frequencies (since the 2^{k-1} gametic frequencies must sum to 1). There are, however, only $k(k-1)/2$ recombination fractions between all pairs of loci. The $2^{k-1} - 1$ gametic frequencies are therefore not completely specified by the total set of $k(k-1)/2$ recombination fractions, for $k > 3$.

The concept of *recombination value* re-establishes the one-to-one relationship between recombination fractions and gametic frequencies for $k > 3$ (Liberman and Karlin, 1984). The recombination value of a set of intervals, which are not necessarily contiguous, is the probability of an odd number of crossovers occurring in the intervals. For a set of contiguous intervals, the recombination value is the recombination fraction of the two loci at the ends of the set of intervals. For a set of non-contiguous intervals, however, the recombination value is not a recombination fraction, but it is related to map distance in the same way that a recombination fraction is related to map distance, i.e. via a map function. Since each of the $k - 1$ intervals can be included or excluded in a set of intervals, there are $2^{k-1} - 1$ sets of intervals (ignoring the set with no interval) and hence $2^{k-1} - 1$ recombination values. There is a one-to-one relationship between these $2^{k-1} - 1$ recombination values and the $2^{k-1} - 1$ gametic frequencies, as specified by a set of simultaneous linear equations. This one-to-one correspondence allows the gametic frequencies to be calculated from a set of recombination fractions between adjacent loci under any map function.

Example 3.5

Suppose that the loci A, B, C and D are syntenic in that order, with recombination fractions of 20% between A and B, 20% between B and C, and 20% between C and D. What are the probabilities of the eight different haplotype classes given (1) the Haldane map function, (2) the Kosambi map function and (3) the Sturt map function with $L = 1$? The same principles as in Example 3.4 apply, except that the general concept of recombination values of sets of non-contiguous intervals is required. Let the inclusion or exclusion of the intervals AB, BC, CD be denoted by a vector of three 0s and 1s, where 0 indicates exclusion and 1 inclusion, then there are seven possible sets of intervals (001, 010, 011, 100, 101, 110, 111), excluding the set with no intervals. The relationship between gametic haplotype status (defined in terms of parental origin of alleles) and recombination values can then be represented as follows.

Haplotype ABCD	Recombination status (interval set)						
	001	010	011	100	101	110	111
000	0	0	0	0	0	0	0
001	1	0	1	0	1	0	1
010	1	1	0	0	1	1	0
011	0	1	1	0	0	1	1
100	0	1	1	1	1	0	0
101	1	1	0	1	0	0	1
110	1	0	1	1	0	1	0
111	0	0	0	1	1	1	1

This gives the set of simultaneous linear equations

$$\gamma_{001} + \gamma_{010} + \gamma_{101} + \gamma_{110} = \theta_{001} = \theta_{CD}$$
$$\gamma_{010} + \gamma_{011} + \gamma_{100} + \gamma_{101} = \theta_{010} = \theta_{BC}$$
$$\gamma_{001} + \gamma_{011} + \gamma_{100} + \gamma_{110} = \theta_{011} = \theta_{BD}$$
$$\gamma_{100} + \gamma_{101} + \gamma_{110} + \gamma_{111} = \theta_{100} = \theta_{AB}$$
$$\gamma_{001} + \gamma_{010} + \gamma_{100} + \gamma_{111} = \theta_{101} = \theta_{AB,CD}$$
$$\gamma_{010} + \gamma_{011} + \gamma_{110} + \gamma_{111} = \theta_{110} = \theta_{AC}$$
$$\gamma_{001} + \gamma_{011} + \gamma_{101} + \gamma_{111} = \theta_{111} = \theta_{AD}$$
$$\gamma_{001} + \gamma_{010} + \gamma_{101} + {}_{110} + \gamma_{001} + \gamma_{010} + \gamma_{101} + \gamma_{110} = 1$$

(1) Haldane map function

Because of the assumption of independence, the general method is unnecessary and the eight gametic probabilities are simply

$$\gamma_{000} = (0.8)\,(0.8)\,(0.8) = 0.512$$
$$\gamma_{001} = (0.8)\,(0.8)\,(0.2) = 0.128$$
$$\gamma_{010} = (0.8)\,(0.2)\,(0.2) = 0.032$$
$$\gamma_{011} = (0.8)\,(0.2)\,(0.8) = 0.128$$

$$\gamma_{100} = (0.2)\ (0.2)\ (0.8) = 0.032$$
$$\gamma_{101} = (0.2)\ (0.2)\ (0.2) = 0.008$$
$$\gamma_{110} = (0.2)\ (0.8)\ (0.2) = 0.032$$
$$\gamma_{111} = (0.2)\ (0.8)\ (0.8) = 0.128$$

(2) Kosambi map function

$$\theta_{AB} = \theta_{BC} = \theta_{CD} = 0.2$$
$$m_{AB} = m_{BC} = m_{CD} = 0.21$$

$$m_{001} = m_{CD} = 0.21$$
$$m_{010} = m_{BC} = 0.21$$
$$m_{011} = m_{BC} + m_{CD} = 0.42$$
$$m_{100} = m_{AB} = 0.21$$
$$m_{101} = m_{AB} + m_{CD} = 0.42$$
$$m_{110} = m_{AB} + m_{BC} = 0.42$$
$$m_{111} = m_{AB} + m_{BC} + m_{CD} = 0.64$$

$$\theta_{001} = \theta_{CD} = 0.2$$
$$\theta_{010} = \theta_{BC} = 0.2$$
$$\theta_{011} = \theta_{BD} = 0.34$$
$$\theta_{100} = \theta_{AB} = 0.2$$
$$\theta_{101} = \theta_{AB,CD} = 0.34$$
$$\theta_{110} = \theta_{AC} = 0.34$$
$$\theta_{111} = \theta_{AD} = 0.43$$

$$\gamma_{001} + \gamma_{010} + \gamma_{101} + \gamma_{110} = \theta_{001}$$
$$\gamma_{010} + \gamma_{011} + \gamma_{100} + \gamma_{101} = \theta_{010}$$
$$\gamma_{001} + \gamma_{011} + \gamma_{100} + \gamma_{110} = \theta_{011}$$
$$\gamma_{100} + \gamma_{101} + \gamma_{110} + \gamma_{111} = \theta_{100}$$
$$\gamma_{001} + \gamma_{010} + \gamma_{100} + \gamma_{111} = \theta_{101}$$
$$\gamma_{010} + \gamma_{011} + \gamma_{110} + \gamma_{111} = \theta_{110}$$
$$\gamma_{001} + \gamma_{011} + \gamma_{101} + \gamma_{111} = \theta_{111}$$
$$\gamma_{001} + \gamma_{010} + \gamma_{101} + \gamma_{110} + \gamma_{001} + \gamma_{010} + \gamma_{101} + \gamma_{110} = 1$$

$$\gamma_{000} = 0.48$$
$$\gamma_{001} = 0.14$$
$$\gamma_{010} = 0.03$$
$$\gamma_{011} = 0.14$$
$$\gamma_{100} = 0.03$$
$$\gamma_{101} = 0.00$$
$$\gamma_{110} = 0.03$$
$$\gamma_{111} = 0.14$$

(3) Sturt ($L = 1$) map function

$$\theta_{AB} = \theta_{BC} = \theta_{CD} = 0.2$$
$$m_{AB} = m_{BC} = m_{CD} = 0.24$$

$$m_{001} = m_{CD} = 0.24$$
$$m_{010} = m_{BC} = 0.24$$
$$m_{011} = m_{BC} + m_{CD} = 0.48$$
$$m_{100} = m_{AB} = 0.24$$
$$m_{101} = m_{AB} + m_{CD} = 0.24$$
$$m_{110} = m_{AB} + m_{BC} = 0.48$$
$$m_{111} = m_{AB} + m_{BC} + m_{CD} = 0.72$$

$$\theta_{001} = \theta_{CD} = 0.2$$
$$\theta_{010} = \theta_{BC} = 0.2$$
$$\theta_{011} = \theta_{BD} = 0.34$$
$$\theta_{100} = \theta_{AB} = 0.2$$
$$\theta_{101} = \theta_{AB,CD} = 0.34$$
$$\theta_{110} = \theta_{AC} = 0.34$$
$$\theta_{111} = \theta_{AD} = 0.43$$

$$\gamma_{001} + \gamma_{010} + \gamma_{101} + \gamma_{110} = \theta_{001}$$
$$\gamma_{010} + \gamma_{011} + \gamma_{100} + \gamma_{101} = \theta_{010}$$
$$\gamma_{001} + \gamma_{011} + \gamma_{100} + \gamma_{110} = \theta_{011}$$
$$\gamma_{100} + \gamma_{101} + \gamma_{110} + \gamma_{111} = \theta_{100}$$
$$\gamma_{001} + \gamma_{010} + \gamma_{100} + \gamma_{111} = \theta_{101}$$
$$\gamma_{010} + \gamma_{011} + \gamma_{110} + \gamma_{111} = \theta_{110}$$
$$\gamma_{001} + \gamma_{011} + \gamma_{101} + \gamma_{111} = \theta_{111}$$
$$\gamma_{001} + \gamma_{010} + \gamma_{101} + \gamma_{110} + \gamma_{001} + \gamma_{010} + \gamma_{101} + \gamma_{110} = 1$$

$$\gamma_{000} = 0.49$$
$$\gamma_{001} = 0.14$$
$$\gamma_{010} = 0.03$$
$$\gamma_{011} = 0.14$$
$$\gamma_{100} = 0.03$$
$$\gamma_{101} = 0.00$$
$$\gamma_{110} = 0.03$$
$$\gamma_{111} = 0.14$$

Just as the likelihood in a two-point linkage analysis function of a recombination fraction θ, the likelihood multi-point analysis is a function of a set of gametic frequencies or recombination values. It is possible to reparameterize the $2^{k-1} - 1$ gametic frequencies or the $2^{k-1} - 1$ recombination values in terms of the $k - 1$ recombination fractions between adjacent markers and a system of $2^{k-1} - k$ interference parameters (as shown above for the case of three loci). Submodels of the saturated model can be defined by setting various subsets of the interference parameters to specific values. In principle, multilocus data can be subjected to a likelihood analysis of a system of nested models in order to estimate the recombination fractions between adjacent loci and the levels of interference between recombination events in neighbouring intervals (Zhao *et al.*, 1990).

An alternative, more parsimonious approach to multilocus data is to assume a certain map function (with or without unknown parameters) which constrains all recombination values (and therefore gametic probabilities) as functions of the $k - 1$ recombination fractions between adjacent loci. Unfortunately, many map functions (e.g. the Kosambi, the Carter–Falconer, and the Felsenstein functions) are inappropriate for this purpose, as they can sometimes produce negative gametic frequencies for four or more loci (Liberman and Karlin, 1984). These map functions are therefore said to be *multilocus-infeasible*. The family of map functions proposed by Karlin and Liberman (1978) and Risch and Lange (1979) are multilocus feasible. The Morgan and Haldane map functions are the simplest members of this family. These two functions make the extreme assumptions of complete interference and no interference, respectively. The Sturt map function is the first member of this family that makes allowance for a variable degree of interference depending on the length of the chromosome arm. Although other map functions in this family have been proposed that also allow a variable degree of interference, the Sturt function was better supported than these other functions in a recent comparative study of several map functions in multilocus pedigree data (Weeks *et al.*, 1993). In practice, however, the Haldane function is usually used because of its computational simplicity, except when the chromosomal region considered is very small (much less than 0.5 map unit), in which case complete interference is sometimes assumed

There are two related aims for doing a linkage analysis involving multiple loci. The first purpose is map building, i.e. the construction of a map of a chromosomal region consisting of multiple marker loci. Map building involves ordering the loci and estimating the inter-loci distances. The second aim is disease mapping, i.e. the detection and localization of a disease locus using established maps of marker loci. The use of multiple markers in disease mapping increases the power of disease locus detection and the precision of localization.

3.8.1   Multipoint linkage analysis for map building

In principle, the problems of locus ordering and inter-loci distance estimation can be tackled simultaneously by comparing the likelihoods maximized over inter-loci distances for all possible locus orders. However, the number of possible orders, as well as the computer time and memory required for each multilocus likelihood calculation, increases rapidly with the number of loci. Even after taking into account the equivalence of two orders that are the reverse of each other, there are still $k!/2$ possible orders for k loci. Evaluation of the likelihoods of all possible orders rapidly becomes impractical as the number of loci increases ($2!/2 = 1$, $3!/2 = 3$, $4!/2 = 12$; $5!/2 = 60$, $6!/2 = 360$, $7!/2 = 2520$,

$8!/2 = 20\ 160$, $9!/2 = 181\ 440$, $10!/2 = 1\ 814\ 400$). It is therefore necessary to use preliminary methods to generate a small number of approximate orders, before proceeding to a formal likelihood analysis of these orders.

There are two main approaches to the generation of approximate orders. One approach is to start with a small number of markers whose order can be established by likelihood analysis, and then to proceed to place the remaining markers, one at a time, into one of the intervals between the markers already in the map. At each stage, the effect of placing the additional marker in each of the possible intervals on the likelihood is evaluated, and the placement that produces the highest likelihood is chosen. If one starts with two markers, for example, then the first additional marker can be placed in one of three intervals, and the next into one of four, and so on, so that the entire procedure will require only $3 + 4 + \ldots + k = (k-2)(k+3)/2$ likelihood evaluations. This type of approach is used in the BUILD option of the CRIMAP program.

The second approach for generating approximate orders is to analyse all pairs of loci using two-point linkage analysis, and then subject the $k(k-1)/2$ recombination fraction estimates (or maximum lod scores) to some method of seriation. The problem of converting a square matrix of dissimilarities (or distances) between objects into a set of coordinates that specify the relative positions of the objects is well known in multivariate exploratory analysis. The general class of methods for tackling this problem is known as multidimensional scaling. Any one of the several methods of multidimensional scaling can be applied to a k-by-k matrix of recombination fraction estimates to produce a two-dimensional representation of the k points. Except for a very short chromosomal segment, the k points will fall on a horseshoe-shaped curve rather than on a straight line, because the recombination fraction between the two furthest markers is at most $1/2$ but the sum of the recombination fractions between adjacent loci, arranged in any order, is likely to exceed $1/2$. Several variations of this approach have been proposed (Lalouel, 1977; Rao *et al.*, 1979; Curtis, 1994).

Once approximate orders have been generated, these can be subjected to formal multipoint likelihood analysis. The FLIPS option of the CRIMAP program systematically evaluates the effects of altering the order of neighbouring groups of loci in a preliminary map, in order to find an order that has a higher likelihood than the preliminary order.

3.8.2   Multipoint linkage analysis for disease mapping

The use of multipoint linkage analysis for disease mapping requires prior knowledge of the relative positions of several marker loci in the chromosomal region of interest. The positions of the markers can then be fixed, while the position of the disease locus is varied from one end of the region through all the inter-marker intervals to the other end of the region. A multilocus likelihood is calculated for each of these test positions, and also for a position that is unlinked to the group of markers. Denoting the log-likelihood at test position x by $\ln L_x$, and the log-likelihood at an unlinked position by $\ln L_\infty$, then the value $2(\ln L_x - \ln L_\infty)$ is defined as the *location score* at position x. Location scores can be divided by $2 \ln(10)$ (i.e. about 4.6) to give *multipoint lod scores*. It is customary to plot location score or multipoint lod score against map position in order to see if a disease gene can be localized to some interval in the region.

For a Mendelian disorder, recombination between a marker locus and the disease can often be inferred from the family data. The presence of even one recombinant gamete 'causes' the multipoint lod score at the marker to plunge to minus infinity, completely excluding the locus as the position of the disease gene. Since it is very unlikely (except in candidate gene studies) for a marker to be in complete linkage to the disease, multipoint lod score functions typically show a series of sharp dips to minus infinity at the positions of the markers, interspersed by more positive values between the markers. If the multipoint lod score in a region rises above the usual threshold of 3, then linkage to that region is declared.

There are two basic reasons why multiple markers are potentially more informative than a single marker for mapping disease loci. The first reason is that, since all markers are homozygous in a proportion of the population, it is inevitable that some gametes in a large sample will be uninformative for linkage, when only one marker is used. This loss of information can be reduced by using several nearby markers, so that it becomes unlikely for an individual not to have at least one heterozygous marker in the region.

The second reason why multiple markers are more informative than a single marker is that, unless the single marker is right on top of the disease locus ($\theta \approx 0$), it can only provide information about crossovers on one side of the disease locus. With two markers flanking the disease locus, information will be available on crossovers on both sides of the disease locus. The more closely spaced are the markers on the chromosomal segment containing the disease locus, the more precisely can one identify the positions of crossovers, and the more accurately can one localize the disease gene. This is reflected by a sharper peak of the multilocus likelihood function as the density of markers is increased. This continues until all the mapping (i.e. crossover) information in the sample has been extracted. This occurs when there is no crossover in the entire pedigree sample between the disease locus and the two nearest flanking markers. The entire interval between these two markers is then equally supported as the position of the disease gene. At this stage, adding additional markers to the same pedigree set will not help to localize the disease gene more precisely.

In the absence of interference, the occurrence of recombination events is a Poisson process with mean 1 in a chromosomal segment of 1 map unit (Morgan) long. It follows that the distance between the disease locus and the nearest recombination event on one side is exponentially distributed with a mean of 1 Morgan. When all recombination events in the n informative gametes in a pedigree set are considered, the mean (per Morgan) of the Poisson process becomes n, so that the expected distance between the disease gene and the nearest recombination event on one side is $1/n$. The disease gene is localized to the interval between the nearest recombination event on one side and the nearest recombination event on the other side. This interval, being the sum of two exponential random variables, has a gamma distribution with parameters $(2,n)$, which has a mean of $2/n$. This gives an approximate upper limit for the resolving power of a multipoint linkage analysis with n fully informative gametes. For example, if one wishes to narrow down the interval to an expected length of 1 cM, then a pedigree set containing 200 fully informative gametes is required (Kruglyak and Lander, 1995c).

The technical aspects and the potential advantages of using multipoint linkage analysis for mapping disease genes are discussed in greater detail in Lathrop *et al.* (1984 and 1985).

3.9 Model specification in linkage analysis

In linkage analysis, the parameter of primary interest is the recombination fraction θ in the case of a two-point analysis, or a set of recombination fractions (or map locations) in a multipoint analysis. These are the only parameters that appear in the log-likelihood function for simple pedigrees and simple codominant loci. However, in order to deal with more complex pedigrees and loci, it is helpful to introduce additional parameters in the framework of a general model. We now explain the rationale behind the general model, and some simplifying assumptions that are commonly made.

As a matter of definition, the general model makes a clear distinction between phenotype and genotype. The genotype of an individual is usually defined as the set of alleles present in the individual at the loci concerned. In linkage analysis, however, it is convenient to include phase information in the genotype. In other words, it is not sufficient to say that an individual's genotype is $A_1A_2B_1B_2$. It is necessary to specify whether the constituent haplotypes are A_1B_1 and A_2B_2, or A_1B_2 and A_2B_1. These two alternatives can be regarded as two different genotypes, denoted as A_1B_1/A_2B_2 and A_1B_2/A_2B_1, respectively. If parental origin is also taken into account and the paternal haplotype is placed first, then there are four possible genotypes, namely A_1B_1/A_2B_2, A_2B_2/A_1B_1, A_1B_2/A_2B_1 and A_2B_1/A_1B_2. Such genotypes are sometimes known as ordered genotypes. The phenotype of an individual is defined as the observed characteristics of the individual that are influenced by the loci concerned. The definition of the ordered genotype to include phase information implies that, even for a pair of codominant loci, the genotype is not uniquely determined by the phenotype if the subject is heterozygous at any locus. For instance, the observed phenotype may indicate that the alleles $A_1A_2B_1B_2$ are present in an individual, but this is consistent with the ordered genotypes A_1B_1/A_2B_2, A_2B_2/A_1B_1, A_1B_2/A_2B_1 and A_2B_1/A_1B_2. When the individual is homozygous at all loci, then there is a one-to-one correspondence between genotype and phenotype (for example the phenotype $A_1A_1B_1B_1$ must consist of the underlying genotype A_1B_1/A_1B_1) but even then it is convenient to consider genotype and phenotype as conceptually different.

The relationship between phenotype and genotype is specified by a set of parameters known as the *penetrance parameters*. In general, the phenotype consists of one or more variables, each of which can be discrete or continuous. The value of each variable in an individual is assumed to be a function of the individual's own genotype (and possibly other personal characteristics such as age and sex). In other words, the phenotype of an individual is assumed to be conditionally independent of the genotypes of other pedigree members, given the individual's own genotype. In general, the relationship between phenotype and genotype can be specified by defining a multivariate probability (or density) function over all possible values of the phenotypic variables for each of the possible multilocus genotypes. In practice, it is usual to simplify the situation by assuming one phenotypic variable for each locus. This simplification is appropriate for a marker locus, since the genotypes at such a locus are of no consequence other than for determining the alleles present at the locus. For a disease locus, the simplification is also often appropriate, although occasionally it may be useful to model a single phenotypic trait as a function of the genotypes at two or more loci (a *multilocus model*), or several phenotypic traits to be influenced by the genotype at a single locus (a *pleiotropic model*). In any case, the conditional independence assumption implies that, given the genotypes of all the individuals in a pedigree, the probability of the pedigree phenotypic data is simply the product of the conditional probabilities of phenotypes of the individuals. Denoting the genotype and phenotype of the ith individual in a pedigree by g^i and x^i, and the set of genotypes and phenotypes in the pedigree by the vectors g and x, the conditional probability of x given g can be written as

$$P(x \mid g) = \Pi P(x_i \mid g_i) \tag{3.39}$$

where the product is taken over all pedigree members. This probability can be modified to take account of other personal characteristics such as age and sex, denoted c, that also have an effect on x

$$P(x \mid g,c) = \Pi P(x_i \mid g_i,c_i) \tag{3.40}$$

Each of the conditional probabilities of a phenotype given a genotype, $P(x_i \mid g_i,c_i)$, is a function of the penetrance parameters. For instance, if an autosomal dominant disorder has disease allele D and normal allele d, then four penetrance parameters are required, namely the conditional probabilities of disease given the four possible ordered genotypes D/D, D/d, d/D, d/d. Since the disorder is dominant, these penetrance parameters take the values (1,1,1,0). If, however, the disorder is specific to men only, then eight penetrance parameters are required, which take the values (1,1,1,0) in men, and (0,0,0,0) in women. In linkage analysis, classes of individuals who differ in penetrance parameters are known technically as *liability classes*.

It is usual in linkage analysis to make the simplifying assumption that the phenotype of a locus depends only on the alleles present at that locus and not on the parental origins of the allele. Thus, an autosomal dominant disorder requires only three penetrance parameters for the three unordered genotypes DD, Dd, dd, with values 1, 1, 0. In general, however, penetrance parameters for ordered genotypes are necessary in order to deal with *genomic imprinting*, which is the phenomenon that some alleles have an effect on phenotype only when they are of paternal or maternal origin. In the autosomal dominant example, if the disease allele D has an effect only when it is paternally transmitted, then the appropriate values of the penetrance parameters of the genotypes DD, Dd, dD, dd are 1, 1, 0, 0, respectively.

Since pedigree genotypes g are not directly observed, the likelihood of a set of pedigree data is just the unconditional probability of the pedigree phenotypes x, and this can be expressed as the sum of the joint probabilities of x and g over all possible values of g, i.e.

$$P(x) = \Sigma P(x \mid g)P(g) \tag{3.41}$$

where the summation is taken over all possible values of **g**. The genotypes of individuals in a pedigree are interrelated to each other by genetic transmission from parent to offspring. This genetic transmission implies that, conditional on the genotypes of the two parents, the genotype of an offspring is independent of the genotypes of any other pedigree members or the genotype frequencies in the population. For example, if the father and mother of a child have genotypes A_1B_1/A_2B_2 and A_2B_2/A_2B_2, then the possible genotypes of the child are A_1B_1/A_2B_2, A_2B_2/A_2B_2, A_1B_2/A_2B_2, A_2B_1/A_2B_2, with probabilities $(1-\theta)/2$, $(1-\theta)/2$, $\theta/2$, $\theta/2$, where θ is the recombination fraction between loci A and B. Since θ determines the probabilities of haplotype transmission from parent to offspring and hence the probability distribution of offspring genotype conditional on parental genotypes, it is known as a *transmission parameter*. When more than two loci are involved, it is necessary to specify the recombination fractions between all pairs of adjacent loci (or, equivalently, the map positions of all the loci), together with some map function, in order to determine the probabilities of all possible gametic haplotypes. These recombination fractions or map positions are transmission parameters.

Individuals whose parents are not included in the pedigree are known as founders. The parameters that determine the probability distribution of genotypes in the founding members of a pedigree are known as *population parameters*. In the most general case, the population parameters consist of the frequencies of all possible ordered genotypes at the loci concerned. Thus, if the analysis concerns two loci, one with m_1 and the other with m_2 alleles, then the number of haplotypes is m_1m_2, and the number of possible ordered genotypes is $(m_1m_2)^2$. The number of independent genotype frequencies is therefore $(m_1m_2)^2 - 1$ (since the genotype frequencies must sum to 1), which increases rapidly with the number of alleles at the loci. At least one of two different levels of simplification is therefore usually made. The first level of simplification assumes that the ordered genotypes are the result of the random union of haplotypes, so that the genotype frequencies can be expressed in terms of haplotype frequencies. The population parameters therefore consist only of $m_1m_2 - 1$ independent haplotype frequencies. The second level of simplification assumes further that haplotypes are the result of a random combination of alleles, so that the genotype frequencies can be expressed in terms of allele frequencies. The population parameters are then reduced to just $m_1 + m_2 - 2$ independent allele frequencies. In practice, the second level of simplification is sufficiently realistic unless the two loci are extremely close to each other. It is therefore usual to specify allele frequencies rather than haplotype or genotype frequencies.

If the n members of a pedigree are ordered such that the f founders precede the $n - f$ non-founders, then the joint probability of the genotypes of all members in a pedigree can be written as a product as follows

$$
\left.
\begin{aligned}
P(\mathbf{g}) &= P(g_1)P(g_2|g_1)P(g_3|g_1, g_2) \\
&\quad \dots P(g_n|g_1, g_2, \dots, g_{n-1}) \\
&= P(g_1) \dots P(g_f)P(g_{f+1}|g_{f+1, \mathrm{f}} g_{f+1, \mathrm{m}}) \\
&\quad \dots P(g_n|g_{n, \mathrm{f}}, g_{n, \mathrm{m}})
\end{aligned}
\right\}
\tag{3.42}
$$

where $g_{j,f}$ and $g_{j,m}$ denote the genotypes of the father and mother of the jth (non-founding) member of the pedigree. The likelihood of a pedigree is a multiple summation of products each involving n penetrance parameters, f population genotype frequencies (for the f founders) and $n - f$ conditional transmission probabilities (for the $n - f$ non-founders) over all possible combinations of genotypes for the n individuals in the pedigree. Denoting the penetrance, population frequency, and the transmission probability of genotype g_i by $\text{pen}(x_i | g_i)$, $\text{pop}(g_i)$ and $\text{tran}(g_i | g_{i,f}, g_{i,m})$, respectively, this multiple summation can be written as

$$P = \sum_{G_1} \cdots \sum_{G_n} \prod_1^n \text{pen}(x_i | g_i) \prod_1^f \text{pop}(g_i) \prod_{f+1}^n \text{tran}(g_i | g_{i,f}, g_{i,m}) \qquad (3.43)$$

where G_1 represents all possible genotypes of individual 1, G_2, represents all possible genotypes of individual 2, and so on. For two loci with m_1 and m_2 alleles, each person can have $(m_1 m_2)^2$ possible ordered genotypes, so that there are $(m_1 m_2)^{2n}$ possible combinations of ordered genotypes for the entire pedigree of n individuals. The likelihood is then a sum of $(m_1 m_2)^{2n}$ terms, each term being a product of $2n$ probabilities. The number of terms in the summation increases rapidly with the number of loci and alleles included in the analysis. Considering all possible combinations of genotypes separately in the calculation of the likelihood function can therefore be prohibitively computer-intensive for large pedigrees and for multilocus analysis. Efficient algorithms are therefore necessary for multipoint linkage analysis of general pedigree data.

It may be noticed that the above likelihood formulation does not allow for *ascertainment*. In studies that aim to build maps with marker loci, ascertainment can be legitimately ignored because the pedigrees are usually selected from the population according to criteria that are entirely unrelated to the loci being considered. However, ascertainment is also ignored in many linkage studies of disease loci, even when there is deliberate selection of families with multiple affected members. Many of these studies do not use systematic methods of ascertainment, but merely identify families that contain more than a certain number of affected members from clinical populations. Fortunately, if the selection of pedigrees is based on phenotypic information of the disease locus but not the marker loci, the data can be analysed under the assumption of random sampling from the population without an inflation to the false positive rate of declaring linkage (for exceptions to this rule, see Section 3.14).

3.10 Algorithms for likelihood calculations of pedigree data

The formulation of the pedigree likelihood as a multiple summation of products between population, transmission and penetrance parameters, over all combinations of possible genotypes, was proposed by Elston and Stewart (1971), who also suggested a recursive algorithm that reduces the computational burden of the evaluation of the multiple sum. This so-called Elston–Stewart algorithm has since been extended to deal with complexities such as consanguineous matings (Ott, 1974; Lange and Elston, 1975; Cannings *et al.* 1978). Many time and memory saving devices have also been added to the basic algorithm, in order to speed up multilocus likelihood calculations. These techniques have been implemented in a number of widely used computer programs, including LIPED (Ott, 1976), LINKAGE (Lathrop *et al.*, 1984), MENDEL (Lange *et al.*, 1988) and FASTLINK (Cottingham *et al.*, 1993). The latest technique involves the coding of genotypes as 'transmitted and non-transmitted sets' and the use of 'fuzzy inheritance' (O'Connell and Weeks, 1995). Another general approach for calculating pedigree likelihoods, distinct from the Elston–Stewart algorithm, has also been developed (Lander and Green, 1987). This approach is particularly efficient for multipoint likelihood calculations, but is currently limited to pedigrees of up to about 10 non-founders (Kruglyak *et al.*, 1996).

3.10.1   The Elston–Stewart algorithm

The Elston–Stewart algorithm is based on a particular way of handling the pedigree likelihood function, which is expressed as a multiple sum of products of penetrance, population and transmission parameters over the all possible combinations of genotypes of the pedigree members

$$P = \sum_{G_1} \cdots \sum_{G_n} \prod_1^n \text{pen}(x_i \mid g_i) \prod_1^f \text{pop}(g_i) \prod_{f+1}^n \text{tran}(g_i \mid g_{i,\text{f}}, g_{i,\text{m}}) \quad (3.44)$$

Looking at this function purely from a mathematical point of view, it is clear that there are n summations, each indexed by the possible ordered genotypes of a pedigree member. The obvious way of evaluating this function is to run through all possible combinations of values of all the indices, calculate the product for each possible combination, and finally sum the products over all possible combinations. If each pedigree member has g possible ordered genotypes, then there are g^n possible combinations of ordered genotypes for a pedigree of size n. Each genotype combination is associated with a product which consists of n penetrance parameters and n population/transmission parameters The procedure therefore requires $g^n(2n-1)$ multiplications followed by $g^n - 1$ additions. These numbers are vast even for moderately large n and g.

Looking at the likelihood function more closely, however, it may become apparent that each factor in the product is indexed by the genotype of one individual or by the genotypes of three individuals: two parents and an offspring. The product can therefore be rearranged and factored into two parts such that the indices of some pedigree members are confined to the first part or to the second part, while others occur in both. For each combination of indices contained in the first part, the second part can be summed over the indices confined to it. Each such summation results in a factor indexed by pedigree members common to the two parts. The function therefore becomes a multiple sum indexed only by pedigree members contained in the first part of the original product. This multiple sum can be subjected to further 'partial summations' to eliminate other indices. This process can be repeated until all indices are eliminated, when a single number, the value of the likelihood function, is obtained.

Example 3.6
A non-genetic example is the multiple summation

$$S = \sum_{i=1}^{2} \sum_{j=1}^{2} \sum_{k=1}^{2} a_i b_{ij} c_{jk}$$

Evaluating this sum as it is, i.e.

$$S = a_1 b_{11} c_{11} + a_1 b_{11} c_{12} + a_1 b_{12} c_{21} + a_1 b_{12} c_{22} + a_2 b_{21} c_{11}$$
$$+ a_2 b_{21} c_{12} + a_2 b_{22} c_{21} + a_2 b_{22} c_{22}$$

requires $2^3 - 1 = 7$ additions and $2^3 2 = 16$ multiplications. However, if we rewrite it as

$$S = \sum_{i=1}^{2} a_i \sum_{j=1}^{2} b_{ij} \sum_{k=1}^{2} c_{jk}$$

then two additions are required to calculate $c_{1+} = c_{11} + c_{12}$, $c_{2+} = c_{21} + c_{22}$, four multiplications and two additions are required to calculate $b_{1+} = b_{11} c_{1+} + b_{12} c_{2+}$, $b_{2+} = b_{21} c_{1+} + b_{22} c_{2+}$, and finally two multiplications and one addition are required to calculate $S = a_1 b_{1+} + a_2 b_{2+}$. The entire calculation therefore involves $2 + 2 + 1 = 5$ additions and $4 + 2 = 6$ multiplications. This represents a saving of two additions and six multiplications.

This procedure is highly applicable to the problem of pedigree likelihood calculation for two reasons. The first reason is that each term in the product of penetrance, population and transmission parameters is indexed by at most three individuals (two parents and an offspring) so that there is no need to consider more than three sets of genotypes simultaneously. Thus, the likelihood function of a nuclear family with C children may be decomposed as

$$L = \sum_{G_f} \text{pen}(x_f|g_f)\text{pop}(g_f) \sum_{G_m} \text{pen}(x_m|g_m)\text{pop}(g_m)$$
$$\prod_{i=1}^{C} \sum_{G_i} \text{pen}(x_i|g_i)\text{tran}(g_i|g_f g_m)$$

(3.45)

The second reason is that a pedigree is essentially a number of nuclear families linked together by certain individuals. A simple three-generation pedigree may, for example, consist of two nuclear families in which an offspring in one family is a parent in the other. One can therefore sum the terms for members of one of the families to obtain the conditional probabilities of that family given each of the possible genotypes of the linking individual. The likelihood of the entire pedigree can then be obtained by summing over the terms for members of the other family, including the linking individual and the 'attached' conditional probabilities. This procedure, sometimes known as 'clipping' or 'peeling', can deal with large multi-generational pedigrees by considering one nuclear family at a time, until no summation remains and a single likelihood value is obtained. In essence, the Elston–Stewart algorithm reduces the number of arithmetic operations required for calculating a multiple summation of a product by shifting some of the summation signs into the product. This was an important advance, but the algorithm nevertheless requires all possible genotypes of each pedigree member to be considered in each summation, and this is an enormous number if several highly polymorphic loci are involved. The inadequacy of the basic Elston–Stewart algorithm for multipoint likelihood calculations has led to the development of methods of approximating the multipoint likelihood function by considering two-point likelihood functions between pairs of loci (Curtis and Gurling, 1993). However, the Elston–Stewart algorithm has recently been speeded up by techniques that reduce the number of possible genotypes for each pedigree member without altering the likelihood function. One technique is to eliminate from the likelihood calculations all genotypes that are incompatible with the observed phenotype of an individual. Another technique is to recode, for each locus, all alleles that are absent in the typed members of a pedigree into a single dummy allele, and to give to this dummy allele a population frequency equal to the sum of the frequencies of the absent alleles. Allele-recoding has been extended to the individual level in the VITESSE program (O'Connell and Weeks, 1995), which converts the full list of possible ordered genotypes of each pedigree member into a reduced list by lumping together all paternal and maternal alleles that are clearly not transmitted to any offspring into a paternal 'non-transmitted set' and a maternal 'non-transmitted set', respectively.

3.10.2   The Lander–Green algorithm

In some sense, by 'peeling off' one nuclear family at a time, the Elston–Stewart algorithm is designed to deal with large pedigrees but not with large numbers of loci. Lander and Green (1987) developed an alternative approach to calculating the pedigree likelihood that considers the entire pedigree one locus at a time, before proceeding to compute the multipoint likelihood by combining information from all loci. This so-called Lander–Green algorithm is therefore complementary to the Elston–Stewart algorithm in that it is more limited by the size of the pedigree than by the number of loci.

The Lander–Green algorithm is based on a hidden Markov formulation of the pattern of inheritance at several ordered loci. Recall that the linkage information of a haplotype can be summarized as a string of fs and ms, where an f indicates an allele derived from the parent's paternal haplotype and an m indicates an allele derived from the parent's maternal haplotype. At a single locus, the linkage information of each non-founding member can be summarized by just two binary digits, one for the status of the allele in the paternal haplotype, and one for the status of the allele in the maternal haplotype. A pedigree with $n - f$ non-founders contains $2(n - f)$ potentially informative gametes so that the pattern of inheritance at a single locus can be described by a vector of $2(n - f)$ elements. Each element of this *inheritance vector*, v, describes the parental status of the allele at the locus in one gamete: it is arbitrarily defined as 0 if the allele is paternal and 1 if the allele is maternal. There are therefore $2^{2(n-f)}$ possible inheritance vectors, each describing a different pattern of allele transmissions at the locus. For each possible inheritance vector at the locus, the probability of the phenotypic data relevant to the locus can be decomposed as a sum of products of probabilities of phenotypes (*x*) given genotypes (*g*) and th\ probabilities of genotypes (*g*) given the inheritance vector (*v*)

$$P(x|v) = \sum_{G} P(x|g)P(g|v)$$

where the summation is taken over all combinations of possible genotype (G) at the locus. This probability is therefore a function of the penetrance and population parameters of the locus. The $2^{2(n-f)}$ such probabilities, one for each possible inheritance vector, can be arranged as the diagonal elements of a square $2^{2(n-f)}$-by-$2^{2(n-f)}$ matrix, denoted as Q. Since all $2^{2(n-f)}$ possible inheritance vectors are equally likely prior to the consideration of the phenotypic data, the likelihood of the data at a single locus is proportional to the sum of these $2^{2(n-f)}$ probabilities. This can be written in matrix form as

$$P(x) \propto 1^{T}Q1 \tag{3.47}$$

where x represents the phenotypic data at the locus and 1 is a column vector with all $2^{2(n-f)}$ elements equal to 1. When k ordered loci are considered jointly in a multipoint analysis, the joint likelihood can be factorized as

$$P(x_1, x_2, .., x_k) = P(x_1)P(x_1 | x_2)P(x_3 | x_1, x_2)....$$
$$P(x_k | x_1, x_1, x_2, ..., x_{k-1}) \tag{3.48}$$

where x_1, x_2, ..., x_k represent phenotypic data at the k ordered loci. The necessity to condition on all preceding loci can be avoided by recognizing that, at each locus, the probability of the phenotypic data is a function of its own inheritance vector, which is conditionally independent of the inheritance vectors of all preceding loci given the inheritance vector of the immediate preceding locus. In other words, the k inheritance vectors of the k ordered loci constitute a hidden Markov chain. The conditional probability of an inheritance vector v_{i+1} at locus $i+1$, given an inheritance vector v_i at loci i, is $\theta_i^{j}(1 - \theta_i)^{2(n-f)-j}$, where θ_i is the recombination fraction between loci i and $i+1$, and j is the number of changes in the elements of the inheritance vector from v_i to v_{i+1}. There are $[2^{2(n-f)}]^2$ possible combinations of v_i and v_{i+1}, each associated with a characteristic conditional probability; so that there are $[2^{2(n-f)}]^2$ conditional probabilities that can be arranged in a square *transition matrix* T_i. The joint likelihood of the multilocus phenotype data is then given by

$$P(x_1, x_2, .., x_k) \propto 1^{T}Q_1T_1Q_2T_2...T_{k-1}Q_k1 \tag{3.49}$$

This is the basic form of the Lander–Green algorithm (Lander and Green, 1987) which, like the Elston–Stewart algorithm, has had various refinements added to reduce the number of necessary arithmetic operations. The algorithm and its various refinements have been implemented in CRIMAP (Lander *et al.*, 1987), MAPMAKER (Lander *et al.*, 1987; Kruglyak and Lander, 1995a,b; Kruglyak *et al.*, 1995) and GENEHUNTER (Kruglyak *et al.*, 1996).

With the development of VITESSE and GENEHUNTER, exact multipoint likelihood computations have become feasible for large pedigrees with a moderate number of marker loci, and for moderate size pedigrees with a large number of marker loci. The only situation not currently amenable to exact multipoint likelihood calculation is when the pedigree size and the number of marker loci are both large.

3.11 Incomplete penetrance, phenocopies and liability classes

For a classical Mendelian disorder, all individuals with a high risk genotype (DD in the case of a recessive disorder, Dd and DD in the case of the dominant disorder) will eventually develop the disorder if they live for long enough. In this situation, the disease gene (or the disease genotype) is said to have *complete penetrance*. If, however, there are individuals with a high risk genotype who do not develop the disease despite living through the age-range in which the disease occurs, then the penetrance of the disease gene (or the disease genotype) is said to be incomplete.

Another characteristic of a classical Mendelian disorder is that it is confined to individuals with a high risk genotype. If there are individuals without a high risk genotype who develop a disorder phenotypically indistinguishable from the genetic form, then such individuals are called *phenocopies*. The *phenocopy rate* is usually defined as the proportion of cases of the disorder in the population that are phenocopies, while the *sporadic risk* is defined as the probability of the disorder developing in individuals without a high risk genotype.

In the general linkage model of Section 3.9, incomplete penetrance and phenocopies are represented by penetrance parameters. Let the probabilities of disease in individuals with genotypes DD, Dd and dd be denoted by f_2, f_1 and f_0 (so that the subscript specifies the number of disease alleles in the genotype), then these probabilities are penetrance parameters for the disease locus. In other words, during the calculation of the likelihood, the conditional probabilities of disease phenotype given disease genotype take the values f_2, f_1, f_0 for individuals designated as affected, and $(1 - f_2)$, $(1 - f_1)$, $(1 - f_0)$ for individuals designated as unaffected. For a dominant disorder, incomplete penetrance is represented by setting a value for f_1 and f_2 that is less than 1, and phenocopies are represented by setting a value for f_0 that is greater than 0. Similarly, for a recessive disorder, incomplete penetrance is specified by setting a value of f_2 that is less than 1, and phenocopies are specified by setting a value for f_0 and f_1 that is greater than 0.

The ideal way of dealing with incomplete penetrance and phenocopies is to identify subclinical features that characterize non-penetrant carriers of the high risk genotype, and features that differentiate genetic from non-genetic forms of the disorder. These features may enable the phenotype to be redefined to have full penetrance and no phenocopy. Failing this, the next best approach for a disorder that is nearly Mendelian is to estimate the genotype-specific risks of the disease from the segregation ratios observed in family data. The penetrance parameters in the linkage analysis are then fixed at these estimated values.

Setting a single value for the penetrance of a genotype is equivalent to assuming that all individuals with the genotype have the same probability of having the disease. This is clearly unrealistic for diseases that have a variable age of onset in adult life, since the probability of having the disease increases with age among individuals with the high risk genotype. There may be other sources of variability, such as an earlier average age at onset in males than in females, or vice versa. It is therefore not sufficient to associate a single penetrance value with each genotype, but a penetrance function that depends on personal characteristics such as age and sex. In principle, this penetrance function may take any form, but in practice it is usual to divide individuals into classes such that any two individuals who share the same class as well as the same genotype will have approximately the same probability of being affected. It is therefore sufficient to set a single penetrance value for each genotype, within each class of individuals. Each of these classes therefore requires three penetrance values to be specified, so that the total number of penetrance values that need to be specified is three times the number of classes.

A *liability class* is defined as a group of individuals specified to have the same penetrance values. For c liability classes, there are $3c$ penetrances which can be denoted as $f_{2,1}, f_{1,1}, f_{0,1}, f_{2,2}, f_{1,2}, f_{0,2}, \ldots, f_{2,c}, f_{1,c}, f_{0,c}$ so that the first subscript specifies the number of disease alleles in the genotype and the second subscript specifies the liability class. Each individual is assigned into a single liability class, and this determines the penetrances that are applicable to the individual. An individual assigned to the ith liability class, for example, will have penetrance parameters that take the values $f_{2,i}, f_{1,i}, f_{0,i}$ if the individual is designated as affected, and $(1 - f_{2,i}), (1 - f_{1,i}), (1 - f_{0,i})$ if the individual is designated as unaffected.

When the phenotype is defined as the presence or absence of a single disease category, liability classes can be used to specify different penetrance values for the disease category (i.e. genotype-specific probabilities of being affected) to groups who differ in terms of other risk factors (e.g. age and sex). Used in this way, every individual is assigned to a liability class, and within each liability class individuals are designated as either affected or unaffected. Within the ith liability class, the values of the penetrance parameters are $f_{2,i}, f_{1,i}, f_{0,i}$ for individuals designated as affected, and $(1 - f_{2,i})$, $(1 - f_{1,i})$, $(1 - f_{0,i})$ for individuals designated as unaffected.

Liability classes can also be used to specify different penetrance values for multiple phenotypic categories, which may reflect the diverse manifestations of a disease gene (pleiotropy), various grades of disease severity, or various levels of diagnostic certainty. This involves creating a liability class for each phenotypic category, and setting the penetrance values of each liability class to be the conditional probabilities of the phenotypic category it represents, given the three genotypes at the disease locus. Since the assignment to a liability class implies the presence of the corresponding phenotype, every individual is designated as being 'affected'. As a result, all individuals assigned to the ith liability class will have penetrance parameters that take the values $f_{2,i}, f_{1,i}, f_{0,i}$.

Example 3.7
Suppose that an autosomal single-gene disorder is sex-limited such that it is dominant in males and recessive in females. How can this situation be modelled in terms of penetrance parameters?

Penetrance parameters are specified by both affection status and liability classes. One way of modelling the above situation is to code individuals with the disease as affected, and individuals without the disease as unaffected, and create one liability class for males and one liability class for females using penetrance values

Liability class	f_2	f_1	f_0
1 (males)	1	1	0
2 (females)	1	0	0

An alternative way of modelling the situation is to code every individual as affected, and create four liability classes for the four mutually exclusive and jointly exhaustive phenotypic categories of male with disease, male without disease, female with disease, and female without disease. Individuals with two copies of the disease alleles have probability $1/2$ of being a male with the disease and probability $1/2$ of being a female with the disease. Individuals with one copy of the disease allele have probability $1/2$ of being a male with the disease and probability $1/2$ of being a female without the disease. Individuals with zero copies of the disease allele have probability $1/2$ of being a male without the disease and probability $1/2$ of being a female without the disease. The appropriate penetrance values are therefore

Liability class	f_2	f_1	f_0
1 (males with disease)	0.5	0.5	0
2 (male without disease)	0	0	0.5
3 (female with disease)	0.5	0	0
4 (female without disease)	0	0.5	0.5

The penetrance values for each disease genotype sum to 1, since the liability classes represent mutually exclusive and exhaustive categories within each genotype. This, however, is not a strict requirement since multiplication of the penetrance values of any liability class by a constant will change all likelihoods by the same factor, so that all the ratios between likelihoods will remain unchanged. Multiplication of the above penetrance values by 2, for example, yields the equivalent (perhaps more natural) specification

Liability class	f_2	f_1	f_0
1 (males with disease)	1	1	0
2 (male without disease)	0	0	1
3 (female with disease)	1	0	0
4 (female without disease)	0	1	1

This example shows that the penetrance values of a liability class are best thought of as the *relative* probabilities of being designated as 'affected', for individuals in the liability class with the three different genotypes. This allows individuals whose disease status is unknown to be designated as being affected and to be assigned to a liability class where the three penetrance values are equal to any arbitrary positive number, provided that individuals with the three different disease genotypes are equally likely to have an unknown disease status.

3.12 Heterogeneity in recombination fraction

Another complexity that may arise in linkage analysis is that the recombination fraction may not appear to be the same for all meioses. This may be because of genuine differences in the rate of crossovers between the two loci. The most important example of this is the well documented higher average rate of crossovers in female as compared to male meioses. The recombination fraction between a disease locus and a marker locus may also appear to vary between families if the assumption of a single disease locus is violated. This occurs, for example, when the disorder is caused by an allele at one locus in some families, but a different allele at a separate locus in others.

Sex differences in recombination fraction can be modelled by defining sex-specific recombination fractions. The male recombination fraction θ_m and the female recombination fraction θ_f between two loci are then regarded as two separate parameters, and the log-likelihood function evaluated over the rectangular parameter space bounded by $0 \leqslant \theta_m \leqslant 1/2$ and $0 \leqslant \theta_f \leqslant 1/2$. Denoting the value of the log-likelihood function at $\theta_m = \pi_f = 0.5$ as $\ln L_0$, the maximum value of the log-likelihood function subject to the constraint of $\theta_m = \theta_f$ as $\ln L_1$, and the unconstrained maximum value of the log-likelihood function as $\ln L_2$, then a test of linkage allowing for unequal recombination fractions in males and females is provided by $2(\ln L_2 - \ln L_0)$ with two degrees of freedom, a test of linkage assuming equal recombination fractions in males and females is provided by $2(\ln L_1 - \ln L_0)$ with one degree of freedom, and a test of unequal recombination fractions in males and females is provided by $2(\ln L_2 - \ln L_1)$ with one degree of freedom.

For multipoint data, each interval between two adjacent loci can be parameterized by two recombination fractions, one for males and one for females, so that for k markers there are $2(k-1)$ sex-specific recombination fractions. A more parsimonious model can be obtained by assuming that the ratio of male map distance to female map distance is constant for all intervals, so that there are just $k-1$ male recombination fractions and one sex-ratio parameter. Restricting the sex-ratio parameter to one constrains male and female recombinations to be equal in all intervals. As in the case of two loci, nested models can be tested against each other by likelihood ratio tests.

When several markers are used to map a disease locus, some power can be gained by using correct sex-specific map distances rather than assuming an equal sex-ratio. However, since the gain is usually rather small, the convenient assumption of an equal sex-ratio is often made in practice.

Of greater importance to disease gene mapping are apparent variations in recombination fraction caused by multiple disease loci. These disease loci may occur in the same chromosomal region, but are more likely to be unlinked to each other (because of the size of the genome). A marker that is close to a particular disease locus will demonstrate linkage in families where the disease is caused by alleles at that locus. In other families, where the disease is caused by alleles at other loci, the marker will show no linkage with the disease. This apparent heterogeneity in recombination fraction due to multiple disease loci is known as *locus heterogeneity*.

Several methods have been proposed for the detection of locus heterogeneity and for the detection of linkage under the assumption of locus heterogeneity. The first method, proposed by Morton (1956), involves dividing the dataset into pre-defined subsets, each consisting of a single large pedigree or several families with similar ethnic backgrounds or clinical features. Three nested hypotheses are considered. The first hypothesis is that the recombination fraction is $1/2$ for all subsets. The relative support for this hypothesis is measured by the value of the log-likelihood function of the entire dataset evaluated at $\theta = 1/2$, which we denote as $\ln L_0$. The second hypothesis is that all subsets have the same value of θ which is not necessarily $1/2$. The relative support for this hypothesis is the maximum log-likelihood of the entire dataset over $0 \leq \theta \leq 1/2$, which we denote as $\ln L_1$. The third hypothesis is that the recombination fraction varies between subsets. The relative support for this hypothesis is obtained by maximizing the likelihood function over $0 \leq \theta \leq 1/2$, for each subset of families separately, and then summing the subset-specific maximum log-likelihoods. We denote the value of the log-likelihood maximized over subset-specific recombination fractions as $\ln L_2$.

Comparison of the first and second hypotheses using the likelihood ratio test statistic $2(\ln L_1 - \ln L_0)$ represents the usual test for linkage which assumes equal recombination fraction in all families. As discussed in Sections 3.4 and 3.5, this chi-squared test is one-tailed (i.e. $\theta = 1/2$ versus $\theta < 1/2$) and has one degree of freedom. Comparison of the second and third hypotheses using the likelihood ratio test statistic $2(\ln L_2 - \ln L_1)$ provides a test of heterogeneity in recombination fraction which is sometimes called the *M-test*. If there are s subsets and the true value of θ is neither 0 or $1/2$, then this statistic has asymptotically a chi-squared distribution with $s - 1$ degrees of freedom. This is an appropriate test when there is evidence for incomplete linkage in the overall sample and when there are prior reasons for dividing the data into a small number of large subsets. Comparison of the first and third hypotheses, using the likelihood ratio test statistic $2(\ln L_2 - \ln L_0)$, provides a test of linkage (sometimes called the *C-test*) that allows the recombination fraction to vary between subsets. This statistic is rarely used as it does not have a well-defined asymptotic distribution. However, for any given dataset, it is possible to estimate the significance level of the statistic by Monte Carlo simulation (MacLean *et al.*, 1992).

The second method, proposed by Smith (1959), assumes the presence of two disease loci that are unlinked to each other. A marker locus (or a set of marker loci in a single chromosomal region) can therefore be linked to at most one of these two loci. In the case of a single marker, this so-called *admixture model* assumes the marker is possibly linked to the disease locus in a proportion of the families, but is definitely unlinked in the rest. The proportion of families with possible linkage between the marker and the disease is defined as α, and the recombination fraction in these families is θ. The quantity α is therefore a new parameter that so far has been implicitly assumed to be 1. If the likelihood function of the ith family over $0 \leq \theta \leq 1/2$, assuming $\alpha = 1$, is $L_i(\theta)$, then the likelihood function of the family over the rectangular parameter space defined by $0 \leqslant \theta \leqslant 1/2$, $0 \leqslant \alpha \leqslant 1$ is

$$L_i(\theta, \alpha) = \alpha L_i(\theta) + (1 - \alpha)L_i(0.5) \tag{3.50}$$

The likelihood function of the entire dataset is then the product of these likelihood functions, point-by-point over the rectangular parameter space $0 \leqslant \theta \leqslant 1/2$, $0 \leqslant \alpha \leqslant 1$

$$L(\theta, \alpha) = T_i T L_i(\theta, \alpha) \tag{3.51}$$

Three nested hypotheses can be considered under the framework of this model. The null hypothesis is that there is no linkage at all in the families, which can be specified by either setting $\theta = 1/2$ or $\alpha = 0$. The next hypothesis is that all the families are linked, which can be specified by setting $\alpha = 1$. The last hypothesis is that a proportion of the families are linked, which does not involve any restriction on the two parameters. The relative support for these three competing hypotheses can be evaluated from the maximum values of the log-likelihood function over the regions in the rectangular parameter space $(0 \leqslant \theta \leqslant 1/2$, $0 \leqslant \alpha \leqslant 1)$ which are compatible with these hypotheses. An example of a log-likelihood surface over this rectangular parameter space is given in Figure 3.4.

The null hypothesis restricts the parameter space to the two lines $\theta = 1/2$ and $\alpha = 0$. The log-likelihood is constant for all points on these two lines, and so the relative support for this hypothesis is the value of the likelihood function on these lines, which we denote as $\ln L_0$. The hypothesis of linkage in all families restricts the parameter space to the line $\alpha = 1$, and so the relative support for this hypothesis is the maximum value of the log-likelihood function on this line, which we denote as $\ln L_1$. The hypothesis of linkage in a proportion of families does not impose any restriction, and so the relative support for this hypothesis is the maximum value of the log-likelihood function in the entire rectangle, which we denote as $\ln L_2$.

The usual test for linkage, which assumes that any linkage must apply to all families, is provided by the likelihood ratio statistic $2(\ln L_1 - \ln L_0)$. As discussed in Sections 3.4 and 3.5, this chi-squared test is one-tailed (i.e. $\theta = 1/2$ versus $\theta < 1/2$) and has one degree of freedom. The admixture model introduces two additional likelihood ratio statistics. The first additional statistic, $2(\ln L_2 - \ln L_1)$, provides a test of locus heterogeneity which is one-tailed ($\alpha = 1$ versus $\alpha < 1$) and has one degree of freedom. The second additional statistic, $2(\ln L_2 - \ln L_0)$, provides a test for linkage (sometimes called the *A-test*) that allows for some unlinked families. The asymptotic distribution of this statistic is not chi-squared because the two parameters θ and α are separate under the alternative hypothesis but are confounded under the null hypothesis, which can be specified by either $\theta = 1/2$ or $\alpha = 0$. A simple approximation to the asymptotic distribution of this statistic is that it is a $50 : 50$ mixture of a probability mass at 0 and the larger of two independent chi-squared random variables each with one degree of freedom (Faraway, 1993). Another approximation, based on a transformation of the parameters, expresses the distribution as a mixture of 0 with probability 0.42, chi-squared with one

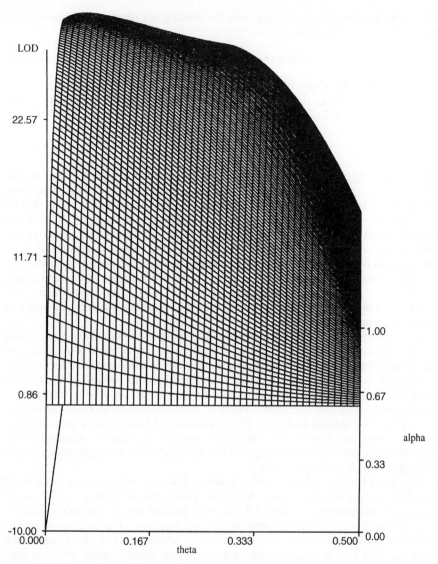

Figure 3.4 A log-likelihood surface under admixture model.

degree of freedom with probability 0.5, and chi-squared with two degrees of
freedom with probability 0.08 (Chiano and Yates, 1995).

In order to avoid the need to use an approximate asymptotic distribution
Liang (1993) proposed the statistic:

$$T = \sum_i \left(\frac{L(\hat{\theta})}{L\left(\frac{1}{2}\right)} - 1 \right) \tag{3.52}$$

where the sum is over all the pedigrees in the dataset, and the recombination fraction in the numerator is the maximum likelihood estimate of the recombination fraction for the dataset as a whole. The asymptotic distribution of this statistic is a $50:50$ mixture of 0 and a chi-squared random variable with one degree of freedom. However, this asymptotic distribution is likely to be accurate only when the number of pedigrees is fairly large.

3.13   Effects of model misspecification

The likelihood method of linkage analysis for gene mapping requires the specification of a precise statistical model, in which the parameter of primary interest is usually the recombination fraction between two loci, or the position of a locus relative to a set of fixed loci. Other parameters, such as allele frequencies and penetrances, are usually of secondary interest and considered as nuisance parameters. In linkage analysis, these nuisance parameters are not usually jointly estimated with the primary parameters, but are specified before the analysis according to prior knowledge of the loci. The analysis is 'optimal' when the model is correctly specified. Model misspecification of any form is expected to have detrimental effects, which may include an inflation of the false positive rate of declaring linkage, a reduction in the power to detect linkage, and biased estimates of the primary parameters.

The first concern of researchers with regard to model misspecification is that it may invalidate the statistical test of linkage, leading to an increased rate of false positive linkage findings. Fortunately, the likelihood ratio test (and the lod score method) is quite robust in this regard. By deriving the exact probability distribution of the lod score functions for nuclear family data, Clerget-Darpoux *et al.* (1986) found that misspecification of disease locus parameters (i.e. the frequency of the disease allele and the penetrances of the disease genotypes) did not inflate the false positive rate of the declaring linkage between the disease and marker loci. However, the test for linkage is not entirely robust to model misspecification. When pedigrees ascertained for a disease contain founders with unknown marker phenotypes, Ott (1992) showed that misspecification of the allele frequencies of the marker locus could lead to an increased rate of false positive linkage findings between the disease and the marker.

It turns out that the robustness of the test for linkage to model misspecification depends on the method of ascertaining the sample. The conditions in which an increased false positive rate of declaring linkage may occur have been investigated analytically and by simulation (Amos and Williamson, 1993; Williamson and Amos, 1995). If ascertainment is independent of both marker and disease loci, then the test is robust to misspecification of either the disease or the marker locus, but not both. If ascertainment is independent of the marker locus but not the disease locus (i.e. if there is selection with respect to the disease phenotype), then the test is robust to misspecification of the disease but not the marker locus. On the other hand, if ascertainment is independent of the disease locus but not the marker locus (an extremely rare situation), then the test is robust to misspecification of the marker but not the disease locus.

To help make sense of these conditions, recall the likelihood ratio statistic for linkage

$$T = \frac{\text{Max}_\theta\, P(M, D;\, \theta)}{P(M, D;\, \theta = 0.5)} \tag{3.53}$$

where M and D denote marker and disease phenotypic data respectively, and θ is the recombination fraction between the marker and disease loci. Not included in this formula but implicitly assumed are the genetic models specified for the disease and marker loci. Under the null hypothesis of $\theta = 0.5$, the marker and disease loci are independent, so that the likelihood ratio statistic can be written as

$$T = \frac{\text{Max}_\theta\, P(M\,|\,D;\, \theta)}{P(M\,|\,D;\, \theta = 0.5)} \tag{3.54}$$

This is a ratio of conditional likelihoods, where the disease locus is in the conditional part of the likelihood. The statistic therefore remains a valid test for linkage in samples selected for the disease, provided that the model for the marker locus is correctly specified (Hodge and Elston, 1994). Conversely, the likelihood ratio statistic can also be written as

$$T = \frac{\text{Max}_\theta\, P(D\,|\,M;\, \theta)}{P(D\,|\,M;\, \theta = 0.5)} \tag{3.55}$$

which is a ratio of conditional likelihoods, where the marker locus is in the conditional part of the likelihood. The statistic therefore remains a valid test for linkage in samples selected for the marker, provided that the model for the disease locus is correctly specified.

Since almost all pedigree samples used in linkage analysis of human diseases are selected on the basis of the disease phenotype, it is usually sufficient to obtain marker phenotypes for all founders and, failing this, to specify marker allele frequencies correctly in order to safeguard against an inflated rate of false positive linkage results. The remaining concern of researchers is then whether misspecification of the disease model may reduce the statistical power to detect linkage, leading to an increased rate of false negative results. The test of linkage is expected to be most powerful when the disease model is correctly specified (Maclean *et al.*, 1993a). All forms of model misspecification may result in a loss of power, but the extent of the loss depends on the nature and magnitude of the misspecification, as well as the characteristics and the marker set and the pedigree sample. For general pedigrees, the only practical way to quantify the reduction in power under a certain set of conditions is to simulate sets of the pedigree data under these conditions, and analyse the simulated datasets under the true and the misspecified models. The reduction in power is the proportion of simulated datasets in which linkage is detected with the true model, minus the proportion of simulated datasets in which linkage is detected with the misspecified model.

There are some general rules, however, that offer a rough guide to the likely reduction in power in various situations (Clerget-Darpoux *et al.*, 1986). Let the disease allele frequency be q and the penetrances f_0, f_1, f_2 be written as $f_0, f_0 + dt, f_0 + t$ (so that d represents the 'dominance' and t the 'effect size' of the disease allele). In a two-point analysis of a disease with a single marker, the reduction in power due to mild to moderate misspecification of q, f_0 and t is usually small, especially if the pedigrees are small (i.e. sibships or nuclear families). However, if d is specified as 1 when its true value is 0, or vice versa, then the reduction in power may be substantial, even for nuclear families. Two-point linkage analysis is therefore fairly insensitive to moderate misspecification of the disease model, provided that dominance is correctly specified.

This robustness of two-point linkage analysis to model misspecification is due to the confounding between recombination fraction and the other model parameters. In other words, the likelihood of the data is fairly constant over a wide range of different combinations of parameters values, such as a small recombination fraction (θ) with a large sporadic risk (f_0), or a larger θ with a smaller f_0. Often, if the disease locus is tightly linked to the marker, but the parameters of the disease locus are misspecified, then the lod scores at or near the marker (i.e. at small values of θ) are deflated, but the lod scores further away from the marker (i.e. at larger values of θ) are inflated. The over-estimation of θ is sometimes rationalized by the misinterpretation of phenocopies as recombinants although, in reality, the explanation must lie in the mathematical properties of the two-point likelihood function.

Multipoint linkage analysis, in contrast, is much more sensitive to misspecification of the disease model (Risch and Giuffra, 1992). The reduction in power due to the misspecification of any of the parameters q, f_0, t and d may be substantial. Often, if there is a disease locus in an interval spanned by several markers, but the parameters of the disease locus are misspecified, the lod score function is grossly deflated within the interval, and only becomes moderately positive outside the interval, beyond the two outermost markers. Intuitively, this is sometimes rationalized as the misinterpretation of phenocopies as recombinants everywhere in the interval. In reality, the explanation must lie in the mathematical properties of the multipoint likelihood function. In comparison to two-point analysis, there is less confounding between the position of the disease locus and the parameters of the disease model. This sensitivity of multipoint linkage analysis to model misspecification has led some researchers to favour two-point analysis when there are uncertainties about the true disease model. This is a somewhat negative view, as the situation with multipoint analysis can also be viewed in a positive light. The relative lack of confounding between the position and the other parameters of the disease locus means that multipoint data offer more information than two-point data for the joint estimation of these parameters, when the disease model is uncertain.

3.14 Linkage analysis of complex diseases

Complex diseases such as ischaemic heart disease, diabetes, and depression are not caused by a single gene, but by multiple genetic and environmental factors. A complete model of causation would include all these factors, their joint frequency distribution in the population, and their joint effect on the risk of illness in individuals. The elucidation of this causal system is the ultimate aim of aetiological research. In attempting to localize a disease gene by linkage analysis, however, we are focusing on just one component of the complex causal system. The hope is that the isolation of even a few components of the causal system may facilitate further progress in understanding pathophysiological mechanisms, leading to improved strategies of disease prevention and treatment.

The conventional disease model used in the linkage analysis of a Mendelian (or nearly Mendelian) disease, parameterized by a disease allele frequency q and three penetrances f_0, f_1, f_2, is clearly not an accurate representation of the causal system for complex diseases. How then, should linkage analysis be carried out for a complex disorder?

This question has no simple answer, as there are two different approaches to the problem, each having its own advocates. The first approach, initiated by Penrose (1935), is to abandon the so-called parametric method (in which θ, or map location, is the parameter of interest in a genetic model) of conventional linkage analysis, and to focus attention on the association between the sharing of disease status and the sharing of marker alleles by sets of relatives (usually sib-pairs). This approach is often called non-parametric or model-free. The other approach is to retain the parametric framework even though the conventional genetic model is only an approximation to reality. This approach relies on the robustness of the likelihood method to model misspecification, although the flexibility of the model can also be increased by treating parameters such as allele frequencies, penetrances, and admixture proportion as free rather than as fixed parameters.

3.14.1   Measures of allele-sharing by relatives

Allele-sharing is central to non-parametric methods of linkage analysis. There are two different definitions of allele-sharing, identity-by-state (IBS) or identity-by-descent (IBD). Two alleles of the same form (i.e. having the same DNA sequence) are said to be IBS. If, in addition to being IBS, two alleles are descended from (and are therefore replicates of) the same ancestral allele, then they are said to be IBD.

Example 3.8
Consider a nuclear family with the following genotypes at loci A and B, which are in extremely tight linkage

$$A_1A_2B_1B_1 \quad \overline{\top} \quad A_2A_2B_1B_2$$

$$A_1A_2B_1B_1 \qquad A_1A_2B_1B_2$$

How many alleles do the two siblings have that are shared (i) IBS and (ii) IBD, at locus A?

(i) The two siblings have identical genotypes (A_1A_2) at locus A, and are therefore IBS for both alleles at this locus.

(ii) The two A_1 alleles shared by the siblings must be descended from the same parental A_1 allele. These two alleles are therefore IBD. The two A_2 alleles shared by the siblings are descended from the other parent. Since this parent has two A_2 alleles, these are indistinguishable from each other, and it is impossible to determine whether two A_2 alleles shared by the siblings were descended from the same A_2 allele or not, using the information on locus A alone. However, the second parent transmitted B_1 to the first sibling and B_2 to the second sibling, and so the two A_2 alleles transmitted from the same parent to the two siblings could only be IBD if a recombination event had occurred between A and B in one of the two meioses. Since loci A and B are in extremely tight linkage, this is highly unlikely, and so the two siblings are IBD for only one allele (A_1) at locus A.

This example illustrates the distinction between IBD and IBS. In addition, it also hints at the existence of a close relationship between IBD status and recombination events. This close relationship implies that IBD is more directly relevant than IBS for linkage analysis.

There are many different IBD relationships between the alleles of a pair of relatives, say X and Y. At any autosomal locus, each member of a relative pair contains two alleles. Denoting the two alleles of X by X_1 and X_2, and the two alleles of Y by Y_1 and Y_2, then possible patterns of IBD sharing among these four alleles are:

$$S_1: \ X_1 = X_2 = Y_1 = Y_2$$
$$S_2: \ X_1 = X_2 \neq Y_1 = Y_2$$
$$S_3: \ X_1 = X_2 = Y_1 \neq Y_2$$
$$S_4: \ X_1 = X_2 \neq Y_1 \neq Y_2$$
$$S_5: \ X_1 \neq X_2 = Y_1 = Y_2$$
$$S_6: \ X_1 \neq X_2 \neq Y_1 = Y_2$$
$$S_7: \ X_1 = Y_1 \neq X_2 = Y_2$$
$$S_8: \ X_1 = Y_1 \neq X_2 \neq Y_2$$
$$S_9: \ X_1 \neq Y_1 \neq X_2 \neq Y_2$$

These patterns range from the situation where all four alleles are IBD from the same ancestral allele (S_1), to the scenario where none of the alleles is IBD with any of the other alleles (S_9). The probabilities of these nine patterns are called the 'coefficients of identity' (Jacquard, 1978). The values of these nine coefficients for two individuals are determined by the nature and the degree of the genetic relationship between the individuals.

The simplest genetic relationship is between a parent and an offspring, where the parent is non-inbred. One and only one allele at each autosomal locus in the parent is transmitted to an offspring, so that the two individuals will always share one allele IBD. There is therefore only one possible IBD pattern, namely S_8.

Another simple but important case is that of a pair of full siblings whose parents are non-inbred and genetically unrelated to each other. Since the parents are non-inbred and unrelated, the two alleles transmitted from different parents cannot be IBD with each other. This leaves just three possible IBD patterns (S_7, S_8, S_9). Let the variable D_f be 1 if the two siblings have received the same paternal allele, and 0 otherwise. Similarly, let the variable D_m be 1 if the two siblings have received the same maternal allele, and 0 otherwise. Both D_f and D_m are binomial random variables with parameters $(1, 1/2)$. The total IBD value of the sib-pair, D, is defined as the sum of D_f and D_m and is therefore a binomial random variable with parameters $(2, 1/2)$. In other words, the possible values of D are $0, 1, 2$, with probabilities $1/4, 1/2, 1/4$. The mean and variance of D are therefore 1 and $1/2$, respectively.

The usefulness of IBD values for linkage analysis is based on the fact that IBD values are independent for non-syntenic loci, but are positively correlated for syntenic loci. The closer the two loci, the greater is the correlation between their IBD values. Consider again the case of a full sibling pair. Let the total IBD values at loci A and B, with recombination fraction θ, be denoted as D_A and D_B. The marginal distributions of D_A and D_B are both binomial with parameters $(2, 1/2)$, but the conditional distribution of D_B given D_A is dependent on θ. For the two haplotypes transmitted from one parent, the IBD status at B is the same as the IBD status at locus A if and only if both haplotypes are non-recombinant with respect to A and B, or both haplotypes are recombinant with respect to A and B. The probability that locus B will have the same IBD status as locus A is therefore $\theta^2 + (1 - \theta)^2$, which is abbreviated as Ψ for convenience. The same considerations apply to the haplotypes transmitted from the other parent. Since the contributions from the two parents are independent, the conditional probabilities for the total IBD value at locus B (D_B) given the total IBD value at locus A (D_A) can be written as in Table 3.1.

Table 3.1 Conditional IBD distribution at locus B given IBD status at locus A

	$P(D_B \mid D_A)$		
	$D_B = 0$	$D_B = 1$	$D_B = 2$
$D_A = 0$	Ψ^2	$2\Psi(1 - \Psi)$	$(1 - \Psi)^2$
$D_A = 1$	$\Psi(1 - \Psi)$	$1 - 2\Psi(1 - \Psi)$	$\Psi(1 - \Psi)$
$D_A = 2$	$(1 - \Psi)^2$	$2\Psi(1 - \Psi)$	Ψ^2

The covariance between D_A and D_B is

$$\mathrm{Cov}(D_A, D_B) = E(D_A D_B) - E(D_A)E(D_B)$$
$$= \Psi - \frac{1}{2} \tag{3.56}$$

Since the variances of D_A and D_B are both $1/2$, the correlation between D_A and D_B is $2\Psi - 1$. This correlation ranges from the value of 0 when $\theta = 1/2$, to the value of 1 when $\theta = 0$, in accordance with intuition.

The concept of IBD sharing can be extended to a set of relatives. For a pedigree with f founders and $n - f$ non-founders where the founders are genetically unrelated, there are $2f$ distinct founder alleles at each locus. Each of these founder alleles may be present in a subset of the non-founders. All family members who share a founder allele are IBD for this particular allele. The combined pattern of IBD sharing of all $2f$ founder alleles in a family is called the IBD configuration of the family. If the founder alleles are labelled numerically, then the IBD configuration of a family can be expressed as a vector with two elements per family member, that is $\boldsymbol{u} = (u_{11}, u_{12}, u_{21}, u_{22}, \ldots, u_{n1}, u_{n2})$, where u_{ij} is the numerical label of the jth allele of family member i (Whittemore and Halpern, 1994a). This notation is illustrated by the following example.

Example 3.9
Consider a non-inbred nuclear family with two offspring where the four members, labelled as a, b, c and d, have the following genotypes at locus A

$$\text{a:}A_1A_2 \; \rule[0.5ex]{0.5cm}{0.4pt}\!\!\top\!\!\rule[0.5ex]{0.5cm}{0.4pt} \; \text{b:}A_3A_4$$

$$\text{c:}A_1A_3 \qquad \text{d:}A_1A_4$$

If the founder alleles are labelled as 1, 2, 3 and 4, then the IBD configuration is described by the vector $(1, 2, 3, 4, 1, 3, 1, 4)$. Given this configuration, the numbers of alleles IBD between all possible pairs of the family members can be expressed in matrix form as follows

	a	b	c	d
a	2	0	1	1
b	0	2	1	1
c	1	1	2	1
d	1	1	1	2

This example shows that the IBD configuration determines the matrix of pairwise IBD sharing. The reverse is not true, as the IBD configurations $(1, 2, 1, 3, 1, 4)$ and $(1, 2, 1, 3, 2, 3)$ are different from each other but both correspond to a pairwise IBD matrix in which all the off-diagonal elements are 1. The IBD configuration is therefore potentially more informative than the pairwise IBD matrix.

If the IBD configuration $\boldsymbol{u}$ at a particular test locus of the affected members of a pedigree is known, then the extent of IBD sharing at that locus among the affected members can be measured by some function of the configuration $S(\boldsymbol{u})$. A pairwise approach would suggest taking the average number of alleles IBD between all possible pairs of affected members. We denote this 'IBD-sharing' function, which is simply the average value of the off-diagonal elements in the pairwise IBD matrix, by $S_p(\boldsymbol{u})$.

An alternative 'IBD-sharing' function, which places more weight of the sharing of a single allele by multiple affected members, can be obtained as follows. Consider the 2^a vectors which can be formed by taking one allele from each of the a affected members, and label these vectors by $1, 2, 3, \ldots, 2^a$. For each of these 2^a vectors, calculate the number of permutations of the a

elements that would leave the vector unchanged. If there are $2f$ ancestral alleles which are labelled $1, 2, ..., 2f$, and the number of times that allele i occurs in vector h is denoted by $b_i(h)$, then the number of permutations of the elements in h that would leave h unchanged is

$$r(h) = \prod_{i=1}^{2f} b_i(h)! \tag{3.57}$$

A function that measures the extent of IBD sharing in an IBD configuration u is then the average value of $r(h)$ over all 2^a possible vectors h that can be formed from u.

$$S_w(u) = \frac{\sum_{h=1}^{2^a} r(h)}{2^a} \tag{3.58}$$

The 'IBD-sharing' functions $S_p(u)$ and $S_w(u)$ can be used in non-parametric methods of linkage analysis of families containing multiple affected members.

3.14.2 The distribution of IBD values of affected sib-pairs

Broadly speaking, non-parametric methods of linkage analysis are based on the excess of allele-sharing between related individuals with similar phenotypes, or the deficit in allele-sharing between individuals with dissimilar phenotypes. The simplest, and the most popular, family unit for non-parametric linkage analysis is an affected sib-pair, with or without parents. The popularity of using affected sib-pairs is partly because affected sib-pairs are often far more informative than unaffected sib-pairs, or sib-pairs with one affected and one unaffected member, under many plausible models of complex inheritance. This makes sense intuitively, since non-penetrant carriers are usually more frequent than phenocopies, so that the presence of disease is more indicative of the presence of the disease gene than the absence of the disease is indicative of the absence of the disease gene. Moreover, if the disease gene is rare, then it is absent in most parents whose offspring are all unaffected. Most families with two unaffected offspring are therefore uninformative for linkage.

The conditional distribution of IBD values of a sib-pair, given the disease status of the members of the pair, can be derived under a variety of models. The simplest situation is that a single disease locus is entirely responsible for the familial influence on the disease. Let this disease locus be denoted as A. It is assumed that locus A is biallelic with alleles A and a occurring at frequencies p and q, and that the penetrances of the three genotypes AA, Aa, aa are f_2, f_1 and f_0.

The IBD distribution at the disease locus A for a sib-pair conditional on the number of affected siblings (0, 1 or 2), under this simplistic set of assumptions, was derived by Suarez et al. (1978). These results were generalized by Risch (1989) to other classes of relatives (e.g. uncle–nephew, first cousins) and to more realistic multilocus models. The treatment by Risch was based on the recurrence risks of the disease in different classes of relatives of an affected proband. The recurrence risk of the disease in a relative of class R is denoted as K_R and the ratio of this risk to the population risk is denoted as λ_R. The subscript R may take the values M (monozygotic twin), S (sibling), O (offspring). The quantities K_R and λ_R are determined by the parameters of the underlying genetic model (i.e. p, f_0, f_1, f_2), as described in Chapter 5.

Denoting the population risk of the disease by K and the number of affected members in a sib-pair by X, the probability that both members of a sib-pair are affected (i.e. $X = 2$) is

$$P(X = 2) = KK_S \tag{3.59}$$

Because of the assumption that the only familial influence on the disease comes from locus A, two sibs that do not have any allele IBD at the disease locus are no different from two unrelated individuals from the population, as far as the disease is concerned. The probability that both members of a sib-pair are affected, given that they have no allele IBD at the disease locus, is therefore simply

$$P(X = 2 \mid D_A = 0) = K^2 \tag{3.60}$$

Similarly, the probability that both members of a sib-pair are affected, given that they have both alleles IBD at the disease locus, is

$$P(X = 2 \mid D_A = 2) = KK_M \tag{3.61}$$

and the probability that both members of a sib-pair are affected, given that they have one allele IBD at the disease locus, is

$$P(X = 2 \mid D_A = 1) = KK_O \tag{3.62}$$

By symmetry, the conditional IBD distribution given that neither member of the sib-pair is affected (i.e. $X = 0$) is given by the same formulae, with K (the population risk of being affected by the disease) being substituted by Q (the population risk of being unaffected, i.e. $1 - K$), and K_R (the recurrence risk of the disease in a relative of class R of an affected proband) being substituted by Q_R (the recurrence risk of being unaffected in a relative of class R of an unaffected proband). The conditional IBD distribution given that $X = 1$ can then be obtained by subtraction, using the equation

$$P(D_A) = \sum_{X=0}^{2} P(D_A \mid X) P(X) \tag{3.63}$$

Finally, the conditional IBD distribution at the marker locus B given the affection status of the sib-pair, $P(D_B \mid X)$, can now be derived from the conditional IBD distribution at the disease locus A given the affection status of the sib-pair, $P(D_A \mid X)$, by the following equation

$$P(D_B \mid X) = \sum_{D_A=0}^{2} P(D_B \mid D_A) P(D_A \mid X) \tag{3.64}$$

where the conditional distribution of the IBD status at locus B, given the IBD status at locus A, is given in Table 3.1. The IBD distribution at the marker locus (B) is equal to the IBD distribution at the disease locus (A) when θ (the recombination fraction) between the two loci is 0, and is equal to the 'null' IBD distribution (i.e. the probabilities of 0, 1 and 2 alleles IBD being 1/4, 1/2, 1/4 regardless of the value of X) when θ is 1/2. This 'distortion' of the IBD distribution at a marker locus as a function of its distance from the disease locus is the basis of sib-pair methods of linkage analysis.

Example 3.10

Suppose that a monogenic disease model has disease gene (locus A) frequency $p = 0.1$ and penetrances $f_0 = 0.01$, $f_1 = 0.1$, $f_2 = 0.5$. What are the IBD probabilities at a marker locus (B) at 5% recombination fraction from the disease locus (A), for sib-pairs with 0, 1 or 2 affected members, assuming that the population is under random rating?

We first calculate the following quantities from the given values of the parameters p, f_0, f_1, f_2, θ (and $q = 1 - p$) using the following formulae (derived in Chapter 5)

$$V_A = 2pq[p(f_1 - f_0) + q(f_2 - f_1)]^2$$
$$V_D = p^2q^2(f_0 - 2f_1 + f_2)^2$$
$$C_M = V_A + V_D$$
$$C_S = 0.5V_A + 0.25V_D$$
$$C_O = 0.5V_A$$
$$K = p^2f_2 + 2pqf_1 + q^2f_0$$
$$Q = 1 - K$$
$$K_M = K + C_M K^{-1}$$
$$K_S = K + C_S K^{-1}$$
$$K_O = K + C_O K^{-1}$$
$$Q_M = Q + C_M Q^{-1}$$
$$Q_S = Q + C_S Q^{-1}$$
$$Q_O = Q + C_O Q^{-1}$$
$$\Psi = \theta^2 + (1 - \theta)^2$$

The conditional IBD distribution given X (the number of affected siblings) is then calculated as

Number of affected sibs	IBD probabilities		
	$D_B = 0$	$D_B = 1$	$D_B = 2$
$X = 0$	0.248	0.500	0.252
$X = 1$	0.368	0.503	0.128
$X = 2$	0.063	0.495	0.442

The 'distortion' of IBD probabilities (from the 'null' values $0.25, 0.5, 0.25$) is therefore greatest for sib-pairs with two affected members.

This example illustrates the calculations involved in obtaining the conditional IBD distribution of a sib-pair given the affection status of the sib-pair, under a single locus model. The most complicated part of the calculation is concerned with obtaining the recurrence risks in relatives (K_M, K_S, K_O, K) given the disease model parameters (p, f_0, f_1, f_2). For complex disorders, however, the values of parameters (p, f_0, f_1, f_2) are typically unknown, but empirical estimates of the recurrence risks (K_M, K_S, K_O, K) are often available. If one starts with empirical values of (K_M, K_S, K_O, K), then some steps in the calculations are bypassed, and it is easy to obtain the IBD distribution at a marker locus of an affected sib-pair, for a given value of θ, under the assumption of a single disease locus.

The generalization of this method of obtaining the IBD distribution of an affected sib-pair to a multilocus model is straightforward, particularly if the effects of the alleles on the risk of disease are multiplicative. Under a multiplicative model involving n disease loci, the recurrence risk in a relative of class R of an affected proband can be written as a product of n terms

$$K_R = \prod_{i=1}^{n} K_{iR} \qquad (3.65)$$

where K_{iR} is the contribution of locus i. Risch (1990a) showed that the conditional IBD distribution for a marker locus linked to disease locus i can be obtained simply by substituting the values of K_{iR} into equations (3.59) to (3.64). Since the values of K_{iR} are almost never known at the beginning of an investigation, it is reasonable to let them be nth root of K_R (i.e. $(K_R)^{1/n}$, where n is the researcher's best guess of the number of loci that make an important contribution to the risk of the disease. In practice, a value of 3, or thereabout, is usually chosen.

Example 3.11
Suppose that the empirical relative risks of a disease in monozygotic cotwins, siblings and offspring of affected probands are 45, 10 and 10, and that the 'relative risks' of all contributory loci are identical. What are the IBD probabilities at the contributory loci for an affected sib-pair? If complete IBD information at such a locus is available, what is the sample size required to detect the excess of affected sib-pairs sharing two alleles IBD, at the 0.0001 significance level and 80% power?

Let there be k contributory loci, with 'relative risks' λ_{iM}, λ_{is}, λ_{io} for $i = 1$, ..., k. Since the contributions of the k loci are equal, the overall relative risks are $\lambda_M = \lambda_{iM}^k = 45$, $\lambda_S = \lambda_{iS}^k = 10$, $\lambda_O = \lambda_{iO}^k = 10$. The IBD probabilities at locus i are $z_{i0} = (1/4)(1/\lambda_{iS})$, $z_{i1} = (1/2)(\lambda_{iO}/\lambda_{iS})$, $z_{i2} = (1/4)(\lambda_{iM}/\lambda_{iS})$. These IBD probabilities must sum to 1, so that the number of loci, k, must satisfy the relationship $\lambda_{iM} = 4\lambda_{iS} - 2\lambda_{iO} - 1$, i.e. $40^{1/k} = 4(10^{1/k}) - 2(10)^{1/k} - 1$. The solution of this equation yields $k = 4.4$, when λ_{iM}, λ_{iS} and λ_{iO} are 2.375, 1.688 and 1.688 for each constituent locus. Under these 'relative risks', affected sib-pairs have a probability distribution of $z_0 = 0.148$, $z_1 = 0.5$ and $z_2 = 0.352$ for sharing 0, 1 and 2 alleles IBD, at each constituent locus. If a simple test of proportion of $z_2 = 0.25$ against $z_2 > 0.25$ is adopted, then the expected value of z_2 (0.352) would indicate that a sample size of 420 affected sib-pairs is required for 80% power to detect linkage at a significance level of 0.0001.

3.14.3   Non-parametric linkage analysis based on affected sib-pairs

The original sib-pair method proposed by Penrose (1935) was based on the idea that, if a large number of sib-pairs are collected and the disease and marker phenotypes of all members examined, then in the absence of linkage there should be no association between whether a sib-pair is alike or unlike with respect to the disease and whether it is alike or unlike with respect to the marker. Linkage is therefore supported if sib-pairs with two affected or two unaffected members are significantly more alike in terms of marker phenotypes compared with sib-pairs with just one affected member.

This sib-pair test was subsequently refined to give rise to the currently popular *affected sib-pair* (ASP) method. The first refinement was concerned with the definition of allele sharing as *identity-by-descent* (IBD) rather than merely *identity-by-state* (IBS). The second refinement was to focus attention exclusively on sib-pairs where both members are affected, since such pairs usually show greater 'distortions' of IBD values than sib-pairs with 0 or 1 affected member, as shown in the previous section. The superiority of IBD over IBS is obvious from the following simple example.

Example 3.12

Suppose that a family consists of two parents of unknown disease status and two affected offspring, and that the genotypes of all four individuals are A_1A_1. Since this family is entirely uninformative for linkage as far as this marker is concerned, it should be discarded by any reasonable method of linkage analysis. If allele-sharing is measured according to IBD, then the analysis will conclude that the IBD status for the sib-pair cannot be inferred. The sib-pair will therefore be appropriately discarded. If, however, allele-sharing is measured according to IBS, then the analysis will conclude that the two sibs share both alleles IBS. The sib-pair will therefore contribute, inappropriately, to the evidence of increased allele-sharing.

The ASP method is based on comparing the observed IBD distribution of affected sib-pairs to the expected distribution of $(1/4, 1/2, 1/4)$ under the null hypothesis of non-linkage. There is a large number of variations of this method in the literature, which can be broadly classified into those based on (or closely related to) Pearson chi-squared statistics (counting the numbers of sib-pairs sharing 0, 1, and 2 alleles IBD and comparing these numbers with their expectations) and those based on likelihood ratio statistics (treating IBD probabilities as unknown parameters).

In early versions of the counting methods, families are retained only if the parental genotypes always allow the IBD status of the sib-pair to be fully determined. The necessary conditions for this are that both parents must be heterozygous and that the two parents must not have the same genotype. Let the total number of affected sib-pairs in such families be n, and the numbers of pairs with IBD values of 0, 1 and 2 be n_0, n_1, and n_2 ($n = n_0 + n_1 + n_2$). Several simple test statistics have been proposed to assess whether these numbers deviate from the expected proportions of $(1/4, 1/2, 1/4)$. The simplest of these is the ordinary Pearson chi-squared statistic

$$S_1 = \sum_i \frac{(n_i - e_i)^2}{e_i} \tag{3.66}$$

where e_0, e_1 and e_2 are $n/4$, $n/2$ and $n/4$, respectively. This statistic can be referred to a chi-squared distribution with two degrees of freedom for a test of linkage.

Another family of test statistics are linear combinations of the form $vn_1 + n_2$ (Knapp *et al.*, 1995a). Among these statistics, the most popular is the so-called 'mean test', which is obtained by setting $v = 1/2$. Since the mean and variance of $(1/2)n_1 + n_2$ under the null hypothesis are $n/2$ and $n/8$, respectively, the test statistic

$$S_2 = \frac{\left(\frac{1}{2}n_1 + n_2\right) - \frac{n}{2}}{\left(\frac{n}{8}\right)^{1/2}} \tag{3.67}$$

has asymptotically a standard normal distribution under the null hypothesis of non-linkage. This is simply a test of whether the proportion of alleles IBD is $1/2$. Since the alternative hypothesis of linkage implies $[(1/2)n_1 + n_2] - n/2 > 0$, the test is one-tailed. This test can be shown to be locally most powerful (i.e. for θ close to $1/2$) under all possible single locus models of inheritance, and to be uniformly most powerful for all values of θ when $f_1^2 = f_0 f_2$ (Knapp *et al.*, 1995a). In simulation studies, the mean test appears to perform adequately under a wide range of conditions (Suarez and Van Eerdewegh, 1984; Blackwelder and Elston, 1985).

The restriction of the classical ASP method to 'fully informative' families can result in some loss of information. In some families, for example, those with parental genotypes $A_1 A_2 \times A_3 A_3$, IBD status can be deduced for the alleles transmitted from the $A_1 A_2$ parent but not the $A_3 A_3$ parent. In other families, the genotype of an individual (for example, a parent) may be unavailable, but the available genotypes in other family members may allow the probability distribution of the missing genotype to be calculated. An extension of the classical ASP method to make use of such partial information was developed by Sandkuijl (1989), and implemented in the ESPA program. For each affected sib-pair, the program attempts a probabilistic reconstruction of missing parental or sibling genotypes from the known genotypes of the family members. In practice, this involves calculating the probabilities of the possible genotype configurations, given the known genotypes in the pedigree, using the MLINK program. For each possible configuration, the number of alleles IBD, the number of alleles non-IBD, and the number of alleles whose IBD status is unknown, are counted. We denote these three counts, for configuration i, by n_{i1}, n_{i0} and $(2 - n_{i1} - n_{i0})$. The 'estimated' counts of alleles IBD and alleles non-IBD in the sib-pair is then the weighted sums $\sum_i p_i n_{i1}$, and $\sum_i p_i n_{i0}$, where p_i is the probability of configuration i. These counts are then aggregated across all the affected sib-pairs in the sample, to obtain the total 'estimated' counts of alleles IBD and alleles non-IBD. If these counts are denoted as N_1 and N_0, then ESPA computes the statistic $(N_1 - N_0)^2/(N_1 + N_0)$ and interprets it as a one-tailed chi-squared test for the hypothesis of linkage.

Example 3.13
To illustrate how ESPA deals with extended pedigrees, consider the following pedigree consisting of eight individuals (labelled I_1 to I_8) of whom three are affected (labelled A) and five are unaffected (labelled U). The genotypes at a marker locus are given after the affection status, with 0 indicating an unknown allele. The marker locus has four equally frequent alleles in the population.

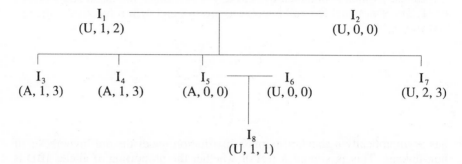

There are three affected sib-pairs in this pedigree, namely (I_3,I_4), (I_3,I_5) and (I_4,I_5). All three affected sib-pairs have a parent with missing genotype. In addition, two of them (I_3,I_5) and (I_4,I_5) have a sibling, namely I_5, with missing genotype. However, since the offspring of I_5 (i.e. I_8) has genotype (1,1), I_5 can be deduced to have genotype (1,0). There is no possibility of deducing the IBD status of the missing allele of I_5 with the alleles of the other two affected siblings. This allele is considered lost whatever the genotype of the missing parent I_2.

It is now necessary to consider the possible genotypes of the missing parent, I_2, the probabilities of these genotypes, and the associated IBD distributions of the three affected sib-pairs. Considering that allele 3 is present in the offspring I_3, I_4 and I_7, but absent in the partner I_1, the possible genotypes of I_2 are 31, 32, 33 and 34. A table of probabilities can then be constructed as follows:

I_2	$L(I_2)$	$L(I_3, I_4, I_5, I_8 \mid I_2)$	$L(I_3, I_4, I_5, I_8, I_2)$	$P(I_2 \mid I_3, I_4, I_5, I_8)$
31	$(1/2)^3$	$(1/2)^4$	$(1/2)^7$	$(1/2)^2$
32	$(1/2)^3$	$(1/2)^5$	$(1/2)^8$	$(1/2)^3$
33	$(1/2)^4$	$(1/2)^2$	$(1/2)^6$	$(1/2)$
34	$(1/2)^3$	$(1/2)^5$	$(1/2)^8$	$(1/2)^3$

and a corresponding tables of IBD status can be constructed as follows (with n_1, n_0 and L representing the number of alleles shared, not shared and lost, respectively).

	(I_3, I_4)			(I_3, I_5)			(I_4, I_5)		
I_2	n_1	n_0	L	n_1	n_0	L	n_1	n_0	L
31	2	0	0	0	0	2	0	0	2
32	2	0	0	1	0	1	1	0	1
33	1	0	1	1	0	1	1	0	1
34	2	0	0	1	0	1	1	0	1

The estimated number of alleles shared, not shared and lost for the three affected sib-pairs are obtained as the weighted sums over the possible genotypes of I_2.

	N_1	N_0	L
(I_3, I_4)	1.5	0	0.5
(I_3, I_5)	0.75	0	1.25
(I_4, I_5)	0.75	0	1.25

The estimated total number of alleles shared and not shared is therefore 3 and 0, and these are compared with the expected numbers of 1.5 and 1.5. The Pearson chi-squared statistic is thus 3. By referring this to a chi-squared distribution with one degree of freedom, ESPA outputs a P-value of 0.04, although a more exact P-value based on a binomial distribution is 0.125. The sample size of this illustrative example is obviously too small for a test of significance to be useful.

The ESPA program has many attractive features. The final counts N_1 and N_0 and the test statistic $(N_1 - N_0)^2/(N_1 + N_0)$ are easy to interpret, and the program handles pedigree data with multiple affected sib-pairs and missing genotypes. However, it is unclear whether the statistic $(N_1 - N_0)^2/(N_1 + N_0)$ is asymptotically chi-squared, as the counts N_1 and N_0 are estimates rather than observations. Moreover, multiple affected sib-pairs in the same family, which may not constitute independent observations, are included in the calculation of N_1 and N_0. This non-independence may distort the distribution of the test statistic. Also, the reconstruction of missing parental genotypes from the observed genotypes of the affected sib-pair may cause the test to be biased in favour of the null hypothesis. This is because the reconstruction of parental genotypes is easier for sib-pairs who are non-IBD for both alleles, than for sib-pairs who are IBD for both alleles. Thus, an affected sib-pair with four distinct alleles (e.g. A_1A_2, A_3A_4) will 'force' the two parents to have these four alleles even if parental genotypes are unavailable, so that the sib-pair will be given full weight in the analysis. On the other hand, an affected sib-pair who are both homozygous with the same allele (e.g. A_1A_1, A_1A_1) may be IBD for both alleles, but whether this is so will be uncertain unless the parental genotypes are available. The weights given to such sib-pairs will therefore be incomplete. The net effect of this bias is a spurious excess of non-IBD alleles. This problem can be avoided by ignoring the genotypes of the affected sib-pair when reconstructing the genotypes of the parents. However, this may result in some loss of information, which may be even more detrimental than the bias in favour of the null hypothesis, especially if the marker is highly polymorphic.

Likelihood methods of ASP analysis were introduced to provide a more satisfactory way of dealing with the problem of incomplete data (Risch, 1990b; Holmans, 1993). The statistical model is that each affected sib-pair has probabilities z_0, z_1 and z_2 of having 0, 1 and 2 alleles IBD. These probabilities, written as the vector z, are defined as the parameters of the model. The likelihood of a set of genotypic data x can be written as a function of z (and the allele frequencies at the marker locus, which are either known or estimated from the data). For a family containing one affected sib-pair, the likelihood can be decomposed as follows

$$L(z) = \sum_{i=0}^{2} z_i P(x\,|\,IBD = i) \tag{3.68}$$

which is a linear combination of z_0, z_1 and z_2. If the log-likelihood maximized with respect to z is denoted as $\ln L_1$ and the log-likelihood at the null hypothesis ($z_0 = 0.25$, $z_1 = 0.5$ $z_2 = 0.25$) is denoted as $\ln L_0$, then the likelihood ratio statistic $2(\ln L_1 - \ln L_0)$ is asymptotically chi-squared with two degrees of freedom and provides a test for linkage. There are only two free parameters because of the obvious constraint $z_0 + z_1 + z_2 = 1$

Holmans (1993) and Faraway (1993) showed that a single locus disease model constrains the parameters z_1 and z_2 to a triangular region defined by $2z_1 \leqslant 1$, $(z_1 + z_2) \leqslant 1$ and $(3z_1/2 + z_2) \geqslant 1$ (Figure 3.5). A more powerful test of linkage can be obtained by restricting the alternative hypothesis to this region, if the assumptions underlying the restrictions are valid. Let the maximum log-likelihood within this region be $\ln L_1^*$, then a likelihood ratio test statistic for linkage is $2(\ln L_1^* - \ln L_0)$. Using the method of Self and Liang (1987), the asymptotic distribution of this statistic was shown to be a mixture of chi-squared distributions with 0, 1 and 2 degrees of freedom (a chi-squared with 0 degree of freedom is defined as 0). The mixing proportions depend on marker allele frequencies, but are approximately $0.41, 0.50, 0.09$. This method has been implemented in the SPLINK program.

Example 3.14
Using SPLINK on the pedigree in Example 3.13, the estimated IBD probabilities are $z_0 = 0$, $z_1 = 0$ and $z_2 = 1$. The likelihood ratio chi-squared statistic is given as 1.848885, with an associated P-value of 0.147355. The program also gives an equivalent lod score of 0.401480.

In essence, this method expresses the likelihood of the marker data in terms of the two parameters z_1 and z_2 instead of the usual parameters p, f_0, f_1, f_2, θ. When the pedigree structure is an affected sib-pair (and other pedigree members with unknown affection status) the likelihood function depends on the traditional parameters p, f_0, f_1, f_2 and θ only through the two parameters z_1 and z_2. In other words, the parameters p, f_0, f_1, f_2 and θ are confounded with each other in such a way that all combinations of parameter values which

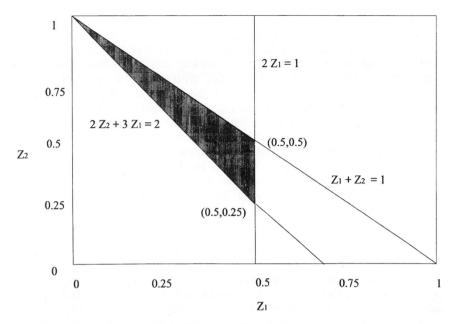

Figure 3.5   The possible triangle for IBD probabilities.

produce the same values of z_1 and z_2 will have equal likelihoods. The representation of the likelihood in terms of z_1 and z_2 therefore achieves parsimony without loss of information. SPLINK is thus ideal for data in the form of affected sib-pairs.

When the data contain larger pedigrees, however, the SPLINK approach is less attractive. For instance, if there are three affected members (or even two affected and one unaffected members) in a sibship, then it is unclear how the likelihood of the marker data in the entire sibship can be written in terms of z_1 and z_2, or whether additional parameters are required. At present, SPLINK attempts to overcome this problem by considering all affected sib-pairs separately and applying an adjustment to reduce the influence of families with multiple affected sib-pairs. As well as not having a firm theoretical basis, this procedure does not overcome the fundamental problem that the parameters p, f_0, f_1, f_2, θ can no longer be reduced to the parameters z_1 and z_2 with no loss of information, when the pedigree data contain members of known affection status other than an affected sib-pair. In practice, the method is likely to remain nearly optimal when the majority of families are in the form of affected sib-pairs, and only a small proportion of families contain additional affected members.

3.14.4   Non-parametric linkage analysis of affected relative-sets

Many attempts have been made to generalize the non-parametric ASP methods to other types of affected relative pairs and to larger sets of affected relatives. Since the likelihood of an affected relative-set cannot be written in terms of the

IBD probabilities of an affected sib-pair, the extension of likelihood methods requires the introduction of additional parameters. Any adequate statistical model for the data on an affected relative-set should take account of the correlated nature of the data. However, the most satisfactory way of doing this is probably to assume a 'Mendelian model' with 'genetic parameters' such as p, f_0, f_1, f_2, θ. It is perhaps because of this reason that the non-parametric likelihood approach is difficult to generalize to affected relative-sets.

There have been several popular extensions of the counting methods of non-parametric linkage analysis to affected relative-sets. The affected-pedigree-member (APM) method took a step backward by considering allele-sharing to be defined by IBS rather than IBD (Weeks and Lange, 1988). Suppose that the marker genotypes of an affected relative pair are A_iA_j and A_kA_l, the method defines, as a measure of allele-sharing, the weighted sum

$$Z = \frac{1}{4} [\delta(A_i, A_k)f(A_i) + \delta(A_i, A_l)f(A_i) + \delta(A_j, A_k)f(A_j) + \delta(A_j, A_l)f(A_j)]$$

(3.69)

where the function $\delta(X, Y)$ of two alleles X and Y is defined as 1 when the two alleles X and Y are IBS and 0 when the two alleles X and Y are not IBS, and the weight $f(X)$ of allele X is related to the rarity of X (e.g. $f(X) = p^{-1}$ or $f(X) = p^{-1/2}$ where p is the frequency of X), since the sharing of a rare allele is more 'significant' than the sharing of a common allele. Regardless of the precise choice of $f(X)$, the Z values of all affected relative pairs in a pedigree are added to give a total measure of allele-sharing among affected members of the pedigree. Next, the mean and variance of this total measure is derived, given a set of marker allele frequencies and assuming the absence of linkage between marker and disease (for details see Weeks and Lange, 1988). Let the number of affected relatives, the measure of allele-sharing, and its theoretical mean and variance, of pedigree m be r_m, Z_m, M_m and V_m, then an overall test statistic is

$$T = \frac{\sum_m W_m(Z_m - M_m)}{\left[\sum_m W_m^2 V_m\right]^{1/2}}$$

(3.70)

where the weight W_m is defined, quite arbitrarily, as

$$W_m = \frac{(r_m - 1)^{1/2}}{V_m^{1/2}}$$

(3.71)

The statistic T is asymptotically standard normal and provides a test for linkage based on excessive IBS allele-sharing.

This APM method suffers from some problems. First, the test statistic is greatly influenced by the choice of weighting function for allele frequency. Whether $f(X) = p^{-1}$ or $f(X) = p^{-1/2}$ is used may make a big difference in the P-value, and it may be tempting to report the smaller of the two P-values. Secondly, the test is prone to false positive results when marker allele frequencies are misspecified, particularly if the weight function $f(X) = p^{-1}$ is used. This is because the expected values of Z are calculated without regard to the genotypes of other family members, so that they are highly dependent on allele frequencies. Thirdly, the method may lose linkage information by ignoring the genotypes of all other pedigree members when considering the allele-sharing by an affected relative pair.

The problems of APM stem from the use of IBS rather than IBD, in situations where partial IBD information is available from the genotypes of family members other than the affected relative pair being considered. These problems motivated the development of an IBD-based method of non-parametric relative-pairs analysis, implemented in the program ERPA (Curtis and Sham, 1994). Using the risk calculation option of MLINK, ERPA calculates for each affected relative pair the prior IBD probabilities at a test position (based entirely on the degree of relationship between the two relatives without taking into account marker genotype data) and the posterior IBD probabilities at the same position (based on the degree of relationship between the two relatives as well as marker genotype data at neighbouring marker loci). From the prior and posterior IBD distributions of each affected relative-pair, ERPA calculates the prior and posterior expected numbers of alleles IBD. In the absence of linkage, disease and marker phenotypes are unrelated, so that the expected value of the posterior expected number of alleles IBD for an affected relative pair is equal to the prior expected number of alleles IBD. An excess of the posterior expected numbers of alleles IBD over the prior expected numbers of alleles IBD among affected relative pairs is therefore indicative of linkage. The interpretation of this excess is, however, hampered by the difficulties in determining the variance of the posterior expected number of alleles IBD for an affected relative pair, and the covariance of these expected numbers for two affected relative pairs in the same family. Although, in principle, these quantities can be obtained by repeated uses of MLINK, this would involve heavy computation. It was therefore decided to use an approach similar to that of ESPA, which is to regard the posterior expected number of alleles IBD (scaled down by a factor inversely related to the number of affected members in the family) as an actual number of alleles IBD, and to use these numbers to obtain a standard Pearson chi-squared statistic. This procedure appeared in simulations to give P-values that did not lead to an excess of false positive linkage results.

Although ERPA suffers from a test statistic with uncertain distributional properties, it draws attention to the advantages of using IBD rather than IBS information to measure allele-sharing by affected relative pairs. This has led to a modification of the APM method to redefine allele-sharing in terms of IBD rather than IBS (Davies *et al.*, 1996). In other words, the function $\delta(X,Y)$ in the measure of allele-sharing between two individuals

$$Z = \frac{1}{4} \left[\delta(A_i, A_k) f(A_i) + \delta(A_i, A_l) f(A_i) + \delta(A_j, A_k) f(A_j) + \delta(A_j, A_l) f(A_j) \right]$$

(3.72)

is now defined as 1 when the two alleles X and Y are IBD and 0 when the two alleles X and Y are not IBD. The statistical significance of the resulting test statistic, called SimIBD, is obtained by simulation of the marker genotypes of affected pedigree members conditional on the marker genotypes of the unaffected pedigree members. This statistic was shown by simulation studies to have greater power than the traditional, IBS-based APM statistic.

All of the non-parametric approaches to the analysis of affected relative-sets described so far are based on consideration of allele-sharing by pairs of affected relatives. This raises the problem of how the measures of allele-sharing by pairs of relatives of different types and in different families should be combined over the entire sample to give an overall test statistic. In principle, the weight assigned to a pair of relatives should reflect the amount of linkage information contained by the pair that is not already contained in other pairs of relatives in the sample. In practice, however, most existing methods use weighting schemes that are based on intuition rather than formal statistical analysis.

The problem of an optimal weighting scheme has been most thoroughly studied in the situation where all the affected relatives in a pedigree are contained in the same sibship. Let the number of affected and unaffected members in the sibship be a and u, respectively. The problem is to determine the weight that should be given to the measure of IBD allele-sharing of an affected sib-pair in the sibship. Since the affected sib-pairs within the same sibship are equivalent in information content, these sib-pairs can be weighted equally, so that the total measure of the allele-sharing for a sibship is simply the sum of the measures of allele-sharing for the $a(a-1)/2$ affected sib-pairs in the sibship. Let this sum be Y_i for family i, for $i = 1, \ldots, n$, then the overall test statistic for the entire sample is

$$T = \frac{\sum w_i Y_i - \sum w_i m_i}{(\sum w_i^2 s_i^2)^{1/2}} \qquad (3.73)$$

where m_i and s_i^2 are the mean and variance of Y_i under the null hypothesis (H_0) of no linkage, and w_i is the weight assigned to sibship i. This statistic is asymptotically standard normal under H_0 for any set of weights $w_1, w_2, w_3, \ldots$. Suarez and Hodge (1979) suggested that the total contribution from a sibship should be proportional to the number of independent affected sib-pairs, i.e. $a - 1$. Since the number of affected sib-pairs is $a(a-1)/2$, this requires the contribution of each pair to be scaled down by a factor of $w = 2/a$. This is commonly known as the Suarez weighting scheme. Another well-known weighting scheme is based on the suggestion by Hodge (1984) that the total contribution from a sibship should be proportional to its information content in the Shannon sense, which she showed to be $2a - 3 + 0.5^{a-1}$ bits. This can be achieved by scaling down the contribution from an affected sib-pair by a factor of $w = (4/3)(2a - 3 + 0.5^{a-1})/[a(a-1)]$. However, an alternative criterion for the choice of weights is maximum power (Sham et al., 1997). Let the mean and variance of Y_i be μ_i and σ_i^2 under the alternative hypothesis (H_1), then for a size α test, the power, $1 - \beta$, of the test is

$$1 - \beta = \Phi\left(\frac{z_\alpha (\sum w_i^2 s_i^2)^{1/2} + \sum w_i(\mu_i - m_i)}{(\sum w_i^2 \sigma_i^2)^{1/2}} \right) \qquad (3.74)$$

where Φ is the standard normal distribution function, and $z_\alpha = \Phi^{-1}(\alpha)$ is its 100αth percentile (e.g. when $\alpha = 0.0001$, $z_\alpha = -3.72$). Optimal weights are obtained by maximizing $1 - \beta$ with respect to $w_1, \ldots, w_n$. When $s_i^2 = \sigma_i^2$ for all values of i (i.e. when the variances are equal under the null and alternative hypotheses for all sibships), the optimal weights are given by

$$w_i = \frac{\left(\dfrac{\mu_i - m_i}{s_i^2}\right)}{\left(\dfrac{\mu_1 - m_1}{s_1^2}\right)} \tag{3.75}$$

for $i = 1, \ldots, n$. Otherwise the optimal weights can be found using a numerical optimization procedure. When Y_i is defined as the sum of the pairwise IBD values in sibship i, the mean and variance of Y_i for various values of a_i and u_i, under the null hypothesis H_0 and various single disease locus alternatives H_1 (defined by the parameters p, f_0, f_1, f_2, θ) have been evaluated. The optimal weights derived from these means and variances vary according to the disease model. However, the pattern of results suggests that, under most plausible single locus models, nearly optimal power is usually obtained by assigning equal weight to all affected sib-pairs, regardless of the number of affected or unaffected individuals in the sibship.

This method of obtaining optimal weighting schemes can be easily generalized to more complex situations involving a mixture of different types of relative pairs and more complex disease models. However, a more fundamental issue is whether the pairwise approach is appropriate for the analysis of pedigrees which may contain multiple affected members in several generations. A general class of non-parametric linkage tests can be constructed on the basis of the IBD configuration, u, and the 'IBD-sharing' functions $S_p(u)$ and $S_w(u)$, of the affected members in pedigrees (Whittemore and Halpern, 1994b). However, there may not be a unique IBD configuration that is compatible with the marker phenotype of the family. A summary statistic of the actual extent of IBD sharing among the affected members, as indicated by the marker phenotypes X of the entire pedigree, is then a weighted average of the values of the 'IBD-sharing' function of all possible IBD configurations, each configuration being weighted by its conditional probability given the marker phenotypes X

$$S(X) = \sum_u P(u|X)\, S(u) \tag{3.76}$$

The mean and variance of $S(X)$ can be obtained by considering the probabilities $P(X)$ and the associated IBD-sharing statistics $S(X)$ of all possible sets of marker phenotypes X, under the null hypothesis of no linkage, given the relative positions of the test locus and the marker loci and the allele frequencies of the marker loci. The set of possible marker phenotypes may be reduced by fixing the marker phenotypes of some family members. This is equivalent to conditioning the distribution of marker phenotypes X on the actual phenotypes Y of a subset of family members. The subset Y should contain no information on the IBD configuration of the affected members. This would include all unaffected founders and their unaffected offspring who have no affected descendants. In addition to reducing the set of possible marker phenotypes that must be considered, conditioning on irrelevant information also renders the test more robust to misspecification of marker allele frequencies. In practice, the mean of $S(X)$ is easy to obtain, as it is equal to the expected value of the $S(u)$ over all possible IBD configurations u ignoring the marker phenotype data, but the calculation of the variance of $S(X)$ may be computationally intensive since the number of possible marker phenotypes X may be enormous. The variance of $S(X)$ is easy to compute only in two extreme situations. The first situation is when there is only one allele per marker locus, so that the same set of marker phenotypes must always be observed. This implies that $S(X)$ is always equal to its mean, and that the variance of $S(X)$ is 0. The other situation is when the marker loci are fully informative so that every possible set of marker phenotypes X will completely determine the IBD configuration u. In this case, the variance of $S(X)$ is simply equal to the expected value of $[S(u)]^2$ over all possible IBD configurations u ignoring the marker phenotype data, minus the square of the expected value of $S(u)$. The true variance of $S(X)$ in a given situation is somewhere between these two extreme values.

Let the IBD-sharing statistic of pedigree i be S_i, and its mean and variance be M_i and V_i, then an overall test statistic for linkage based on excessive IBD-sharing among affected relatives is

$$T = \frac{\sum_i w_i S_i - \sum_i w_i M_i}{\left(\sum_i w_i^2 V_i\right)^{1/2}} \tag{3.77}$$

This statistic is asymptotically standard normal for any set of weights w_i, which may be chosen to optimize the power for detecting a particular alternative hypothesis (as defined typically by a particular set of values for the parameters p, f_0, f_1, f_2 and θ).

Non-parametric tests of linkage based on IBD allele-sharing among affected relative-sets, as measured by $S_p(X)$ or $S_w(X)$, have been implemented in the NPL procedure of the GENEHUNTER program (Kruglyak *et al.*, 1996). GENEHUNTER uses phenotype information at multiple marker loci to derive the probability distribution of the IBD configurations at a test position. Since the phenotypes at multiple marker loci are likely to be almost fully informative about the IBD configuration at the test location, the variance of the $S(X)$ statistic for a pedigree is approximated by the upper bound that assumes IBD configurations are always fully known conditional on the marker phenotypes. This simplification leads to a conservative test. Under dominant models, tests based on the $S_w(X)$ function are usually more powerful than tests based on the $S_p(X)$ function. Under a recessive model, the reverse is usually true especially if the data consist only of nuclear families (Whittemore and Halpern, 1994b). If the true model is extremely uncertain, then there may be no reason to prefer one test or the other. In this situation both tests can be performed and the more significant of the two P-values taken. However, this P-value should then be doubled in order to adjust for multiple testing.

3.14.5   General problems with non-parametric methods

The main justification for using non-parametric approaches to linkage analysis is that they do not require a genetic model of the disease to be specified. Linkage between markers and disease induces an increase in the sharing of marker alleles by related affected individuals. Non-parametric methods attempt to ignore the underlying mechanisms that caused the increase in the allele-sharing, and to concentrate on whether an increase is present or not. This approach has its strong advocates and is gaining popularity. Much of this popularity stems from the conceptual simplicity of the approach, and the sense of security that any positive results cannot have arisen because of questionable assumptions about the disease model. However, some of these advantages are to some extent illusory.

The major problem of non-parametric methods is that different genetic mechanisms will lead to different patterns of increased allele-sharing among affected relatives, and no single measure can be optimally sensitive to all these patterns. Even in the simplest case of affected sib-pairs, a whole family of non-parametric tests can be constructed by varying the relative weights to be attached to n_1 and n_2, the numbers of affected sib-pairs IBD for 1 and 2 marker alleles, respectively. When sibships with a variable number of affected and unaffected members are included in the sample, the optimal weights for combining statistics from different sibships vary depending on the underlying genetic model of the disease. With larger pedigrees, the choice of statistic for measuring increased allele-sharing is likely to be even more crucially dependent on the true model of the disease. Non-parametric tests are therefore not unlike parametric tests in making assumptions about the likely genetic model of the disease. However, while the presumed disease model is made explicit in parametric linkage analysis, the implicit assumptions underlying non-parametric methods are often obscure.

3.14.6   Parametric model-free methods

Although the classical lod score method was introduced for the linkage analysis of Mendelian diseases, it is possible to extend the method to make it more appropriate for complex disorders. We call such an approach parametric model-free.

The most simple-minded variant of this approach is to decide on a particular genetic model (i.e. a particular set of values for the disease allele frequency q and the penetrances f_0, f_1, f_2) from a visual inspection of the pedigrees, and then to use this model in a traditional lod score analysis. This method relies partially on the ability to infer values of the parameters q, f_0, f_1, f_2 that are nearly optimal, and partially on the robustness of lod score linkage analysis to misspecification of the disease model. Both of these assumptions are potentially hazardous. Pedigrees for linkage analysis tend to be selected for having multiple affected members, so that inferences drawn from such families about genetic parameters may be highly misleading. If the disease model is grossly misspecified, then the power to detect linkage may be drastically reduced. Thus, it is often recommended that, when the true disease model is unknown, lod score analysis should be conducted under several different models, so that at least one of these is likely to be close to the true model.

The use of multiple models for linkage analyses raises new questions. How many models should be considered? What combinations of parameter values should be set in these models? How should the results from the multiple analyses be interpreted? Even more fundamentally, is it appropriate to assume a model with one disease locus when the susceptibility to the disorder is influenced by alleles at multiple loci?

3.14.7   Linkage analysis of multiple disease loci

A multilocus disease model is characterized by many more genetic parameters than a single-locus disease model. In principle, it is possible to conduct a lod score analysis under a disease model with multiple loci. This is simply a generalization of multipoint linkage analysis with multiple disease as well as marker loci, forming two or more syntenic groups. For two disease loci, a procedure for lod score analysis has been implemented in the TLINKAGE program (Schork *et al.*, 1993). In practice, however, there are serious problems with this formal likelihood approach.

One problem is that many more parameters need to be specified for a multilocus disease model than for a single disease model. For each disease locus, it is necessary to specify the number of alleles and their frequencies. For the system as a whole, it is necessary to specify a penetrance parameter for each possible combination of genotypes at the contributing loci. Assuming that all the loci are biallelic and are in Hardy–Weinberg equilibrium, then a disease model with d loci will have d allele frequencies, and 3^d penetrances. As the number of disease loci increases from 1 to 2 to 3, the number of genetic parameters increases from 4 to 11 to 30. As the values of these parameters are usually unknown to the investigator, the problem of model specification is greatly magnified when a multilocus model is considered instead of a single-locus model (MacLean *et al.*, 1993b).

This problem is compounded by the large number of combinations of possible positions of the multiple disease loci. To simplify the argument, suppose that the genome can be divided, arbitrarily, into 300 chromosomal segments. A single disease locus can be situated in any one of these 300 segments, so that a genome scan will require 300 separate linkage analyses, one for each segment. If there are two disease loci which must be considered jointly, then the number of combinations of possible positions becomes 300^2. If there are three loci, then the number becomes 300^3. An exhaustive search for a multilocus system will therefore require an enormous amount of analysis.

Another difficulty of linkage analysis under a multilocus disease model is that the computation of the likelihood tends to become very time-consuming. In addition to being a multipoint calculation, the computational demand is increased because, unlike a marker locus, the genotype at a disease locus is not closely determined by the phenotype. As a result, it is usually necessary to include in the likelihood calculation all possible combinations of disease genotypes for every individual.

Given these serious difficulties, a formal multilocus model linkage analysis can be justified only if it is substantially more powerful than a single-locus analysis. Several simulation studies have attempted to quantify the gain in power associated with the correct, multilocus specification of the disease model, compared with a simplified, single-locus specification (Greenberg and Hodge, 1989; Greenberg, 1990; Goldin, 1992; Goldin and Weeks, 1993; MacLean *et al.*, 1993b; Schork *et al.*, 1993; Sham *et al.*, 1994). The general consensus from these studies is that the gain in power is usually rather modest, provided that the single-locus analysis is performed under an admixture model with nearly optimal parameter values. The precise magnitude of the gain depends on several factors. It is slightly greater for large than for small pedigrees. It is also slightly greater when the markers are tightly rather than loosely linked to the disease loci. Finally, the gain may be somewhat greater when there is a strong synergistic interaction between the high-risk alleles of two disease loci. Since the gain in power is usually modest, multilocus model linkage analysis should be reserved for situations where there is already some evidence for multiple disease loci, and some indication of their position, from single-locus linkage analyses.

If the high-risk mutations at a disease locus have been identified, then the linkage analysis for additional disease loci can benefit from taking appropriate account of the information at the known disease locus. If the identified locus contains alleles that are themselves sufficient to cause the disease, then families in which the disease is caused by these alleles should be excluded from further linkage analysis. On the other hand, if the alleles at the identified locus exert a minor influence on the risk of the disease, then their effects could be modelled by defining separate liability classes for individuals with different genotypes at the identified locus, and setting appropriate penetrance parameters for these classes.

3.14.8 Single-locus parametric model-free methods

A single-locus analysis for a multilocus trait is a simplification that is justified if it has nearly the same power as analysis under the correct multilocus model. This is often true provided the single-locus parameters are set at their optimal values. These optimal values are, however, not generally known to the investigator. Consequently, the same pedigree data are usually analysed under several different models, in order to ensure that at least one of these is nearly optimal. Some investigators consider two models, one dominant and one recessive, to be sufficient, while others prefer to include 'intermediate models' where the penetrance of the heterozygous genotype is somewhere between the penetrances of the two homozygous genotypes. It is usual to incorporate both reduced penetrance ($f_2 < 1$) and phenocopies ($f_0 > 0$) in all these models, whether dominant, recessive, or intermediate. However, there is often not enough knowledge about the disease to justify any precise set of values for f_0 and f_2 in a particular model. It is then customary to set f_0 at a value not far below the population risk of the disease, and f_2 at a value near the recurrence risk of the disease among monozygotic cotwins of affected individuals. The frequency of the disease allele (q) is then calculated to give the correct prevalence of the disease.

To illustrate the rationale and difficulties of setting the genetic parameters (q, f_0, f_1, f_2) in this way, consider a complex disorder under the influence of multiple alleles at different loci. The simplest of such situations is a two-locus biallelic model, which may be specified by the frequencies and penetrances of the $3 \times 3 = 9$ possible combinations of genotypes. Let the two loci be A and B with alleles A_1, A_2 and B_1, B_2, where A_1 and B_1 are the low risk and A_2 and B_2 the high risk alleles. Let the frequencies of A_1, A_2, B_1, B_2 be p_1, p_2, q_1, q_2, and the penetrance of the genotype $A_i A_j B_k B_l$ be f_{ijkl}, then the 'average penetrance' of the genotype $A_i A_j$ is

$$f_{ij..} = \sum_{k=1}^{2} \sum_{l=1}^{2} q_k q_l f_{ijkl} \tag{3.78}$$

If the 'average penetrances' $f_{11..}, f_{12..}, f_{22..}$ are known, then these values can be used in the linkage analysis. The 'average penetrances' $f_{11..}$ and $f_{22..}$ may, however, be quite different from the prevalence of the disease and the recurrence risk of the disease among monozygotic cotwins of affected individuals, which are given by

$$K = \sum_{i=1}^{2} \sum_{j=1}^{2} \sum_{k=1}^{2} \sum_{l=1}^{2} p_i p_j p_k p_l f_{ijkl} \tag{3.79}$$

$$K_M = \frac{\displaystyle\sum_{i=1}^{2} \sum_{j=1}^{2} \sum_{k=1}^{2} \sum_{l=1}^{2} p_i p_j p_k p_l f_{ijkl}^2}{\displaystyle\sum_{i=1}^{2} \sum_{j=1}^{2} \sum_{k=1}^{2} \sum_{l=1}^{2} p_i p_j p_k p_l f_{ijkl}} \tag{3.80}$$

Example 3.15
Consider a two-locus model where the frequencies of the two high risk alleles A_2 and B_2 are $p_2 = 0.1$ and $q_2 = 0.2$ respectively, and the penetrance matrix is

	B		
A	11	12	22
11	0.001	0.003	0.009
12	0.1	0.3	0.9
22	1	1	1

What are the 'average penetrances' of the genotypes at loci A and B? What is the population prevalence of the disease? And what is the recurrence risk of the disease among monozygotic cotwins of affected individuals?

Using the above formulae, the 'average penetrances' are

$$f_{11..} = 0.00196$$
$$f_{12..} = 0.196$$
$$f_{22..} = 1$$
$$f_{..11} = 0.02881$$
$$f_{..12} = 0.06643$$
$$f_{..22} = 0.17929$$

The population prevalence of the disease is

$$K = 0.046867$$

The recurrence risk of the disease among monozygotic cotwins of affected individuals is

$$K_M = 0.473108$$

Thus, $f_{11..}$ and $f_{.11}$ are less than K by different amounts. Moreover, while $f_{22..}$ is greater than K_M, $f_{.22}$ is less than K_M. Considering that the values of K and K_M are 0.047 and 0.47, it might seem reasonable to set the penetrance parameters at values such as $f_0 = 0.03$ and $f_2 = 0.5$, but such values would not be realistic for either locus.

This example illustrates that, under a multilocus model, no single set of parameter values can be appropriate for all underlying susceptibility loci. It follows that, when linkage analysis is being performed in a particular chromosomal location, there is no way of knowing what the appropriate values of the genetic parameters are, for the hypothetical susceptibility locus in that position.

There have been several responses to this problem. One response is to simplify matters by disregarding the unaffected individuals from the analysis. This can be done simply by setting all the penetrance parameters f_0, f_1 and f_2 close to 0, while keeping the ratio f_2/f_1 at an appropriately large value. If, for example, f_0, f_1 and f_2 are set at the values 0.0001, 0.0001 and 0.01, then the ratios of penetrances for affected individuals are $1 : 1 : 100$. In other words, although the probability of being affected is low even for individuals with two copies of the disease allele, this probability is nevertheless 100 times greater than the corresponding probabilities for individuals with 0 or 1 copy of the disease allele. For unaffected relatives, however, these penetrances translate into probabilities that are in the ratios $0.9999 : 0.9999 : 0.99$, so that individuals with the low risk genotypes are only slightly ($0.9999/0.99$, or 1.01 times) more likely to be unaffected than individuals with the high risk genotype. The genotypes of unaffected individuals will therefore have very little effect on the value of the likelihood function. This coding scheme is a popular way of implementing an 'affecteds-only' analysis.

Another response to this problem is to set the genetic parameters at some plausible values and then refrain from multipoint analysis, on the basis that two-point linkage analysis is relatively robust to model misspecification. As discussed in Section 3.13, two-point linkage analysis under an incorrect model often produces a maximum lod score that is nearly as large, but occurring at a higher recombination fraction, compared with the analysis under the true model. As far as linkage detection is concerned, minor misspecification of the disease model is therefore unproblematic, provided that the analysis is restricted to two-point lod scores.

Regardless of how the genetic parameters are set, the use of multiple models complicates the interpretation of lod scores. If the highest lod score obtained from the multiple analyses is chosen to represent the evidence for linkage, then some adjustment for multiple testing is necessary. If the number of models is m, then it is quite common to subtract $\log_{10}(m)$ from the highest lod score to obtain an adjusted lod score, or to multiply the P-value of the highest lod score by a factor of m to obtain an adjusted P-value. These two common methods of adjustment are related to each other by the result that the upper limit of a P-value associated with a lod score of Z is 10^{-Z}. Subtracting $\log(m)$ from Z therefore inflates the upper limit of the P-value to $10^{-[Z-\log(m)]}$, which is equal to $10^{-Z}m$.

Since the maximum lod scores obtained by applying different models to the same data set are positively correlated, these simple methods of adjustment will give a conservative test. When many models are tested, the size of this bias may become quite large. One attempt to overcome this problem is to use Monte Carlo simulations to find an empirical P-value for the largest lod score (Weeks *et al.*, 1990). This method can be very time-consuming as it may involve performing multiple linkage analyses on thousands of simulated replicates.

If linkage analysis is restricted to two loci (a marker and a disease), then the robustness of the lod score method to model misspecification means that it is necessary to use only two or three different models. Consequently, a simple Bonferroni type adjustment of the P-value for multiple testing is quite reasonable. However, it is undesirable to restrict the analysis to only two loci, as multipoint analysis is more powerful than two-point analysis for the detection of linkage. Since multipoint analysis is more sensitive to model misspecification, it is important to repeat the analysis over a greater number of different models, in order to ensure that at least one of these is an adequate approximation to the optimal model. A simple Bonferroni type adjustment is therefore likely to be over-conservative, but the alternative of using Monte Carlo simulations to obtain an empirical P-value may not be feasible because of the heavy computational demand of multipoint linkage analysis.

A different approach is therefore necessary for the multipoint analysis of complex disorders (Curtis and Sham, 1995). An obvious extension to the idea of analysing the data under several models and choosing the largest lod score is to maximize the lod score formally over all possible models. In other words, the quantities (q, f_0, f_1, f_2) are treated as nuisance parameters, and the lod score is maximized over all possible combinations of these parameters. The hypothesis is that, at a particular position in a chromosomal segment, denoted as x, there is a disease-predisposing locus characterized by a set of unknown parameters (q, f_0, f_1, f_2) and responsible for the disease in a proportion α of the families in the sample. Let the vector of parameters (q, f_0, f_1, f_2) be abbreviated as $\boldsymbol{u}$, then the likelihood of the disease data D and the marker data M, as a function of these parameters, can be written as $L(D, M; x, \alpha, \boldsymbol{u})$. The maximized lod score is the logarithm of the maximized likelihood ratio, which is

$$R_1 = \text{Max}_u \left(\frac{\text{Max}_\alpha L(D, M; \alpha, \boldsymbol{u})}{L(D, M; \alpha = 0, \boldsymbol{u})} \right) \tag{3.81}$$

This ratio is equivalent to

$$R_1 = \frac{\text{Max}_{u, \alpha} L(M | D; \alpha, \boldsymbol{u})}{L(M)} \tag{3.82}$$

The denominator of this ratio is simply the likelihood of the marker data, because under the null hypothesis the marker phenotypes are independent of the disease phenotypes. For this reason, twice the natural logarithm of this likelihood ratio does not have a standard chi-squared distribution. Instead, the null distribution of this statistic is influenced by the size and structure of the pedigrees in the sample. While it is possible to estimate the null distribution for a particular data set by Monte Carlo simulations, this is best avoided as multipoint likelihood calculations are computationally demanding.

In the presence of nuisance parameters, it is possible to obtain a likelihood ratio statistic that is asymptotically chi-squared by maximizing the likelihood over the main parameter and the nuisance parameters jointly in the numerator, and maximizing the likelihood over only the nuisance parameters in the denominator (with the main parameter being set at the value specified by the null hypothesis). Applied to the present situation, this leads to the likelihood ratio

$$R_1 = \frac{\text{Max}_{u,\alpha} L(M, D; \alpha, u)}{\text{Max}_u L(M, D; \alpha = 0, u)} \tag{3.83}$$

The problem of using this likelihood ratio for testing the hypothesis of linkage is that it will have little power under some circumstances if the method of ascertainment of the pedigrees is not taken into account. For instance, if the sample consists solely of affected sib-pairs, then both the numerator and the denominator will maximize at parameter values such as $q = 1$ or $f_0 = f_1 = f_2 = 1$, which will explain (erroneously) why all individuals in the sample are affected. These parameter values, however, imply that the disease locus is monomorphic, so that the data must be regarded as having no information about linkage. This problem can be avoided by taking appropriate account of the method of ascertainment into the likelihood function. However, as most pedigrees for linkage analysis are collected unsystematically, the precise method of ascertainment is often uncertain, so that appropriate adjustment is difficult. In order to improve the power of the test without having to make a formal adjustment for ascertainment, it has been suggested that the nuisance parameters should be constrained to exclude extreme values such as $q = 1$ or $f_0 = f_1 = f_2 = 1$. One reasonable constraint is to require the parameters to be consistent with the population risk of the disease, K. In other words the parameters (q, f_0, f_1, f_2) are constrained to values which satisfy the relationship $(1 - q)^2 f_0 + 2q(1 - q)f_1 + q^2 f_2 = K$. A three-dimensional graphical representation of the constraint $(1 - q)^2 f_0 + 2q(1 - q)f_1 + q^2 f_2 = K$, together with the requirement that $f_0 \le f_1 \le f_2$, is shown in Figure 3.6. In order to reduce computational burden, Curtis and Sham (1995) suggest restricting the parameter space further to the two dotted lines in Figure 3.6, which represents dominant models with penetrate parameters between $(f_0 = 0, f_1 = 1, f_2 = 1)$ and $(f_0 = K, f_1 = K, f_2 = K)$, and recessive models with penetrance parameters between $(f_0 = K, f_1 = K, f_2 = K)$ and $(f_0 = 0, f_1 = 0, f_2 = 1)$. The only nuisance parameter is then f_1, while f_0 and f_2 are functions of f_1 given by $f_0 = f_1$ and $f_2 = f_1(K - 1)/K + 1$ when $f_1 < K$, and by $f_0 = (1 - f_1)K/(1 - K)$ and $f_2 = f_1$ when $f_1 \ge K$.

If both the numerator and the denominator of the likelihood ratio are maximized subject to these constraints, then the resulting likelihood ratio statistic is asymptotically chi-squared with one degree of freedom, when only

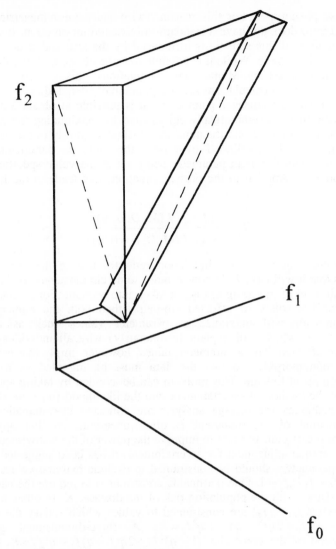

Figure 3.6   Parameter space for the MFLINK method.

one point of a genetic map is considered. This statistic has been shown in simulation studies to be usually only slightly less powerful than a lod score analysis under the correct model (Curtis and Sham, 1995). If multiple positions within a chromosomal segment are tested, then the Stationary Gaussian Markov Process Model (see Section 3.15.5) can be used to convert a point-wise significance to a segment-wise or genome-wise significance.

This approach to parametric model-free linkage analysis of complex disorders has been implemented in the MFLINK program, which uses the VITESSE program for multipoint likelihood calculations. The performance of this parametric model-free approach as compared with non-parametric methods for the detection of linkage is a topic that requires further investigation.

3.15 The interpretation of lod scores

In parametric linkage analysis, it is standard practice to summarize the results of a linkage analysis in the form of a lod score function, rather than as a P-value. The lod score at a certain value of θ is defined as the common logarithm (i.e. base 10) of the ratio of the likelihood value at that value of θ to the likelihood value at $\theta = 1/2$. Historically, the choice of base 10 rather than base e dates from Morton (1955), who considered that base 10 was simpler to interpret, as lod scores of 1, 2, 3, etc. would then represent simply likelihood ratios of 10, 100, 1000, etc. Moreover, the maximum lod score over the admissible range $0 \leqslant \theta \leqslant 1/2$ need only be multiplied by a factor of $2 \ln 10$ (≈ 4.6) for it to have the convenient property of being asymptotically distributed as a $50:50$ mixture of 0 and a chi-squared random variable with one degree of freedom.

3.15.1 Bayesian interpretation of lod scores

The simplest possible interpretation of a lod score occurring at a certain value of θ is to regard it as a direct measure of *support* for that value of θ provided by the data (Edwards, 1984). Thus, if a lod score of 3 is obtained at $\theta = 0.1$, then the hypothesis $\theta = 0.1$ is 1000 times better supported than the hypothesis $\theta = 0.5$, according to the data. This approach, however, ignores any prior knowledge about the likely values of θ. Since there are 22 autosomes in humans, it is reasonable to assume that there is a $1/22$ chance that any two loci are linked, and given that two loci are linked, the probability distribution of θ is uniform in the interval $0 \leqslant \theta \leqslant 1/2$. In other words, a reasonable prior distribution for θ is that it is $1/2$ with probability $21/22$, and between 0 and $1/2$ with probability density $1/11$ (Smith, 1959). The posterior probability of linkage, given the likelihood function $L(\theta)$, is then given by the *Bayes theorem* as

$$P(\theta < 0.5) = \frac{\int_0^{0.5} \dfrac{L(\theta)}{11}\, d\theta}{\int_0^{0.5} \dfrac{L(\theta)}{11}\, d\theta + \dfrac{21}{22} L\left(\theta = \dfrac{1}{2}\right)} \qquad (3.84)$$

Dividing the numerator and denominator of this expression by $L(\theta = 1/2)$ yields

$$P(\theta < 0.5) = \frac{\dfrac{1}{11} \int_0^{0.5} \dfrac{L(\theta)}{L(\theta = 0.5)}\, d\theta}{\dfrac{1}{11} \int_0^{0.5} \dfrac{L(\theta)}{L(\theta = 0.5)}\, d\theta + \dfrac{21}{22}} \qquad (3.85)$$

In order to evaluate this expression it is necessary to obtain the area under the likelihood ratio function $L(\theta)/L(\theta = 0.5)$ from $\theta = 0$ to $\theta = 0.5$. Since the shape of the likelihood ratio curve varies depending on the size and structure of the pedigrees and on the disease model, the area under this curve, and therefore the posterior probability of linkage, are also somewhat variable. However, for the simple situation of N fully informative gametes, all of which are non-recombinants, the area under the likelihood ratio curve can be obtained by integration to be $(2^N - 0.5)/(N + 1)$. In this simplified situation, the maximum lod score (lod_{max}) and the posterior probability of linkage $P(\theta < 0.5)$, for several values of N, are as follows:

N	lod_{max}	$P(\theta < 0.5)$
5	1.5	0.33
6	1.8	0.46
7	2.1	0.60
8	2.4	0.73
9	2.7	0.83
10	3.0	0.90
11	3.3	0.94
12	3.6	0.97
13	3.9	0.98
14	4.2	0.99

A maximum lod score of 3 therefore corresponds to a posterior probability of linkage of approximately 90%, but a maximum lod score of 3.3 is necessary to increase the posterior probability of linkage to about 95%. These results show that the conventional critical value of a maximum lod score of 3 should perhaps be increased to 3.3, in order to ensure that the declaration of linkage is correct in over 95% of occasions

3.15.2   The sequential test interpretation of lod scores

This Bayesian argument, however, was not the original reasoning used by Morton (1955) to derive the lod score of three criterion. Instead, the criterion was originally based on the theory of sequential tests developed by Wald (1947). For two simple hypotheses (say H_0: $\theta = 0.5$ and H_1: $\theta = 0.1$), the theory defines the likelihood ratio $R = L_1/L_0$ and two critical values A and B. Observations are made sequentially, one at a time. After each observation, the value of R based on all accumulated data is calculated. This value is checked against the critical values A and B, and a decision is made to continue the data collection as long as R is between A and B. However, if R exceeds the critical value A, then H_1 is accepted and the procedure terminated. Similarly, if R falls below the critical value B, then H_0 is accepted and the procedure terminated. The two possible errors in this procedure are the acceptance of H_1 when H_0 is true (defined as a type 1 error), and the acceptance of H_0 when H_1 is true (defined as type 2 error). The probabilities of these two types of errors (α and β) that arise from a particular choice of the critical values A and B are given approximately by the simultaneous equations

$$A = \frac{1 - \beta}{\alpha} \qquad B = \frac{\beta}{1 - \alpha} \qquad (3.86)$$

Morton suggested adopting the critical values $A = 1000$ and $B = 0.01$, so that the error probabilities can be set at the low levels $\alpha = 0.001$ and $\beta = 0.01$. This unusually low level of α was chosen to keep the 'posterior probability of a type 1 error' (i.e. the probability that a declared linkage is false) to less than 0.05. Morton argued that the prior probability of H_1 (linkage) should be set at $1/20$, so that the 'posterior probability of a type 1 error' could be derived by the Bayes theorem as

$$P = \frac{\alpha P(H_0)}{\alpha P(H_0) + (1 - \beta) P(H_1)} \qquad (3.87)$$

which is approximately 0.02 when $P(H_0) = 0.05$, $P(H_1) = 0.95$, $\alpha = 0.001$ and $\beta = 0.01$. This was the original justification for the criteria that linkage should be accepted when the lod score exceeds 3, and rejected when the lod score falls below -2. A review of human linkage studies confirmed that only 2% of linkages established at a lod score of 3 or more were subsequently shown to be false positive (Rao *et al.*, 1979).

Morton's sequential approach has, however, been criticized for various reasons (Chotai, 1984). Most importantly, the specification of a single value of θ in the range $0 \leqslant \theta \leqslant 1/2$ as the alternative hypothesis is unsatisfactory except in the case of a candidate gene of known location relative to the marker locus (in which case the prior probability of linkage, 0.05, may not be appropriate). In other situations, the test is nearly optimal only when the pre-specified value of θ happens to be near the true value. Moreover, when the lod score at the pre-specified value of θ is much less than the lod score at some other value of θ, it may be difficult (or indeed inappropriate) to refrain from considering the evidence for linkage at the value of θ at which the lod score is greatest, rather than at the pre-specified value of θ.

Because of the problems with setting a single pre-specified value of θ, the current standard criterion for declaring linkage is a lod score of 3 or more, at any value of θ between 0 and $1/2$ (rather than at a pre-specified value of θ). As far as linkage exclusion is concerned, a lod score of less than -2 at a certain value of θ is still regarded as sufficient evidence to exclude that value of θ.

3.15.3 The fixed sample test interpretation of lod scores

The question of whether lod scores should be assessed in a sequential framework or according to fixed sample theory remains a controversial, if somewhat academic, issue. The sequential approach proposed by Morton led to the desirable habit of summarizing linkage results as tables of lod scores at a standard set of values of θ (usually $0.05, 0.1, 0.2, 0.3$). This practice has enabled researchers readily to combine the evidence for linkage from several independent datasets. However, the collection and analysis of linkage data is seldom strictly sequential. Researchers may wait until sufficient data are collected before proceeding to analyse the entire sample. When a putative linkage is discovered by one group, several other groups may decide to attempt replication of the finding at the same time, rather than one after another. The situation is therefore such that neither sequential nor fixed sample theory is entirely justified. In practice, fixed sample theory is usually adopted as it is easier to implement.

In a fixed sample framework, the statistical significance of a maximum lod score of 3 is obtained from the sampling distribution of the likelihood ratio statistic. In large samples, the maximum lod score multiplied by 2 ln 10 ($\approx$4.6) is distributed approximately as a 50:50 mixture of 0 and a chi-squared random variable with one degree of freedom. The probability of a chi-squared random variable exceeding 13.8 approximately 0.0002, so that the significance level associates with a maximum lod score of 3 is 0.0001. In small samples, however, this asymptotic P-value may be substantially lower than the true P-value. It can be shown that the P-value associated with a maximum lod score of L is always less than or equal to 10^{-L} (Chotai, 1984; Collins and Morton, 1991). One situation where the true P-value approaches this upper bound is that of a phase-known sibship with 10 non-recombinant and 0 recombinant gametes. This sibship yields a maximum lod score of 3.01, which is associated with an asymptotic P-value of 0.0001. However, the true probability of all 10 meioses being non-recombinant by chance is only 2^{-10}, which is approximately 0.001.

3.15.4   Monte Carlo simulations

For most samples, the true significance level associated with a maximum lod score of L is much less than the 'upper bound' 10^{-L} but closer to the value based on asymptotic theory. However, as there are no simple rules for assessing the accuracy of asymptotic theory, Monte Carlo methods are sometimes used for obtaining an empirical P-value associated with the maximized lod score obtained from a particular dataset. In each simulation, the pedigree structures and the disease phenotypes in the sample are retained, but the marker phenotypes of the founders are generated according to population allele frequencies, and the marker phenotypes of the non-founders are generated according to Mendelian segregation, without regard to disease phenotypes. In other words, disease phenotypic data are retained, and marker phenotypic data generated under the null hypothesis of non-linkage between the disease and marker loci. For each set of simulated data, the maximum lod score is calculated and compared with the maximum lod score of the actual data. The proportion of simulated datasets for which the maximum lod score exceeds the maximum lod score of the actual data provides an empirical estimate of the significance level of the maximum lod score obtained from the actual data.

In addition to being computationally intensive (especially for a multipoint analysis), the Monte Carlo approach has one other problem when used to obtain the statistical significance of a maximum lod score. The problem arises when the informativeness of the actual data is much greater than expected, given the pedigree structures and marker allele frequencies. In this situation, the empirical P-value may be very small not so much because of a vast excess of non-recombinant gametes over recombinant gametes, but because of an improbably large number of informative gametes. In this situation, the declaration of linkage based on a small empirical *P*-value obtained by simulation can be misleading, as the following example shows.

Example 3.16
Suppose that the following three-generation family is used to test for linkage between two marker loci A and B

$$A_1A_1B_1B_1 \quad\underline{\quad\quad}\quad A_2A_2B_1B_2$$
$$A_1A_2B_1B_2 \quad\underline{\quad\quad}\quad A_1A_1B_1B_1$$
$$A_1A_1B_1B_1$$

The grandparental genotypes allow the phase of the doubly heterozygous parent to be determined as A_1B_1/A_2B_2. The offspring inherits the non-recombinant A_1B_1 haplotype from this parent. The family therefore contains just one fully informative gamete which is non-recombinant, so that the maximum lod score is $\log_{10}2$, i.e. approximately 0.3. The appropriate *P*-value is 0.5, as this is the probability of obtaining a lod score of 0.3 or more from one fully informative gamete. Now suppose that a Monte Carlo method is used to estimate the *P*-value, where the genotypes of locus A are held fixed and the genotypes of locus B are simulated. A simulation will produce a maximum lod score of 0 unless the potentially informative parent is heterozygous at locus B, in which case the maximum lod score has probability 1/2 of being 0.3 (when the transmitted gamete is non-recombinant) and probability 1/2 of being 0 (when the transmitted gamete is recombinant). If the frequency of B_2 is very rare, then the probability of heterozygosity is very low, so that in the vast majority of simulations a maximum lod score of 0 will be obtained. For instance, if the frequency of B_2 is 10^{-6}, then the probability of heterozygosity is approximately $2(10^{-6})$, so that the probability that a simulation will produce a lod score of 0.3 is just 10^{-6}. Thus according to the Monte Carlo method an empirical *P*-value of 10^{-6} is obtained, which is obviously very misleading.

The conventional Monte Carlo approach therefore assesses not only the extent of support for linkage, but also how informative the dataset happens to be. This problem does not arise in circumstances where it is possible to distinguish the observations which determine the informativeness of the dataset from those that relate directly to the hypothesis being tested. In this situation, the observations directly relevant to linkage should be generated by a simulation conditional on the observations that determine informativeness. However, some observations may serve both purposes (e.g. an individual who receives a potentially informative gamete from a parent may also transmit a potentially informative gamete to an offspring), and so it is not easy in many situations to make a clear distinction and conduct the Monte Carlo simulation in a way that is robust to the actual information content of the data. Consequently, in the context of linkage analysis, empirical significance levels derived from Monte Carlo simulations should not be regarded as necessarily reflecting the true extent of evidence in support of linkage. In most situations, the asymptotic sampling distribution will give a *P*-value that is sufficiently accurate.

3.15.5   The genome-wise significance of a lod score

At first sight, it may seem surprising that, as a criterion for declaring linkage, a maximum lod score of 3 is associated with a false positive rate of about 0.05 but an asymptotic *P*-value of only 0.0001. The reason for this large discrepancy is that, while the false positive rate takes proper account of the prior probability of linkage, the *P*-value is merely concerned with the 'local' evidence for linkage without regard to the size of the genome. However, since the search for a disease locus by linkage analysis is usually carried out using multiple markers throughout the genome, it may be argued that an adjustment of the 'point-wise' significance level is necessary to allow for multiple testing. In the extreme scenario, when the entire genome is saturated with marker information, the adjusted *P*-value is called the 'genome-wise' significance.

Saturating the entire genome with marker information means that all recombination events (i.e. crossover points) of every potentially informative gamete can be inferred. This enables the evidence for linkage to be assessed on a point-by-point basis, over the entire genome. At each point, the likelihood ratio chi-squared statistic (i.e. maximum lod score multiplied by a factor of 4.6) is calculated, together with the corresponding point-wise significance. Over the entire genome, a series of chi-squared statistics is obtained. The genome-wise significance is defined as the probability of exceeding the largest of these chi-squared statistics under the null hypothesis of non-linkage between marker and disease for the entire genome.

The square root of the likelihood ratio chi-squared statistic is a standard normal deviate under the null hypothesis. In the simple situation of a large sample consisting of n fully informative gametes, the standard normal deviate at locus i, denoted as Z_i, is approximately

$$Z_i = \frac{\left(\dfrac{n}{2} - R_i\right)}{\left(\dfrac{n}{4}\right)^{1/2}} \tag{3.88}$$

where R_i is the number of recombinant gametes at locus i. This statistic is standard normal, because, under the null hypothesis, the mean and variance of R_i are $n/2$ and $n/4$, respectively. The square of this normal deviate is a Pearson chi-squared statistic, which in large samples is approximately equal to a likelihood ratio chi-squared statistic.

The relationship between point-wise and genome-wise significance is determined crucially by the extent to which the standard normal deviates at different points are correlated with each other. The weaker the correlations, the larger is the adjustment necessary to convert a point-wise significance to a genome-wise significance. The standard normal deviates at non-syntenic loci are uncorrelated, but those at syntenic loci are correlated to a variable extent depending on the distances between the them.

Consider a single gamete, if a locus (locus 1) is non-recombinant with the disease, then a neighbouring locus (locus 2) is also non-recombinant with the disease, unless a crossover has occurred between the two loci. Let the recombination fraction between the loci be θ, and let R_{ij} denote a random variable which takes a value of 1 if locus i in gamete j is recombinant with the disease, and 0 otherwise, for $i = 1, 2$ and $j = 1, ..., n$. Under the null hypothesis that the disease locus is unlinked to either marker, the mean and variance of R_{ij} are $1/2$ and $1/4$, respectively, while the covariance between R_{1j} and R_{2j} is $(1 - 2\theta)/4$. The correlation between R_{1j} and R_{2j} is therefore $(1 - 2\theta)$. Since the number of recombinant gametes at locus i, R_i, is the sum of the variables R_{ij} over $j = 1, ..., n$, the correlation between R_1 and R_2 is also $(1 - 2\theta)$. Furthermore, since the standard normal deviate Z_i is proportional to R_i, the correlation between Z_1 and Z_2 is also $(1 - 2\theta)$. Assuming the Haldane map function, the correlation between Z_1 and Z_2 can be written as a function of map distance m as

$$r(m) = 1 - 2[(1 - e^{-2m})/2] = e^{-2m} \tag{3.89}$$

This expression conforms with intuition in that the correlation between the standard normal deviates is 1 for two loci at the same point, and decreases exponentially as the map distance between the loci increases. Considering the standard normal deviate as a variable that changes in value along a chromosome, then it is clear that this variable is characterized by a constant mean (0), uniform variance (1) and exponential decline in correlation, as a function of distance (e^{-2m}). A random variable with these properties is known as a Stationary Gaussian Markov Process (Grimmett and Stirzaker, 1992). As a result, the number of distinct regions in an interval of length t where Z^2 exceeds a certain critical value C can be shown to be distributed approximately as a Poisson random variable with mean

$$\mu = (1 + 2\,tC)(1 - \Phi\sqrt{C}) \tag{3.90}$$

where t is the length of the chromosomal segment in map units and Φ is the standard normal distribution function, so that $(1 - \Phi\sqrt{C})$ is the point-wise significance level associated with a chi-squared statistic of C. (For details see Feingold *et al.*, 1993; Kruglyak *et al.*, 1995; Lander and Kruglyak, 1995.) The probability that maximum lod score of the segment will exceed C, under the null hypothesis of no disease locus linked to any point in the segment, is

$$p = 1 - e^{-\mu} \tag{3.91}$$

This can be regarded as an approximate 'segment-wise' significance level for the maximum lod score. Treating each chromosome as a long chromosomal segment, the number of regions in the entire genome where the maximum lod score will attain a point-wise significance of α_1 is distributed approximately as a Poisson random variable with mean

$$\mu_G = (23 + 2TC)\alpha_1 \tag{3.92}$$

where T is total length of the genome. The genome-wise significance of the maximum lod score is therefore

$$\alpha = 1 - e^{-\mu_G} \tag{3.93}$$

With a maximum lod score of 3, $\alpha_1 = 0.0001$, $C = 13.8$, so that with $T = 33$, we have $\mu_G = 0.09$, and $\alpha = 0.09$. According to this formulation, a maximum lod score of 3 corresponds to a genome-wise significance of approximately 0.09. In order to reduce the genome-wise significance to 0.05, the critical maximum lod score needs to be set at the slightly higher value of 3.3.

Of the many ways that lod scores can be interpreted, a Bayesian approach is probably the most satisfactory for Mendelian disorders. In this situation, the posterior probability of linkage can be estimated, and this is arguably the ideal measure of the evidence for linkage. When the appropriate model for the disease is uncertain, however, the difficulty in framing the alternative hypothesis precisely renders the Bayesian approach problematic. By concentrating on the null hypothesis, fixed sample significance tests avoid the need to specify a precise alternative hypothesis. Both Bayesian and significance test arguments lead to a critical maximum lod score of about 3 for declaring linkage as 'significant'. This concordance is not coincidental, as one true positive result is expected in a single genome scan for a Mendelian disorder (provided that the sample is sufficiently large). A maximum lod score of 3.3, which corresponds to a false positive rate of 5% by Bayesian calculations, would therefore imply on average about one false positive result per 20 genome scans. This, however, is precisely the 'genome-wise' significance level associated with a maximum lod score of 3.3 derived from the theory of Stationary Gaussian Markov Processes. Similarly, a maximum lod score of about 2 is associated with a posterior probability of linkage of approximately 50% for a Mendelian disorder, and is expected to arise by chance about once per genome scan. However, the difference in interpretation between a Mendelian and a complex disorder is that, for a complex disorder, the posterior probability of linkage given a maximum lod score of 3.3 is uncertain, and may be much less than the value of 0.95 that is applicable to a Mendelian disorder.

3.15.6   Lod scores and non-parametric methods

The results from a non-parametric linkage analysis are usually summarized by a P-value, i.e. a 'point-wise' significance level. This 'point-wise' significance can be converted to a 'genome-wise' significance by Equations (3.92) and (3.93), or to a 'maximum lod equivalent.' Since the 'point-wise' significance associated with a maximum lod score of L is

$$\alpha_1 = 1 - \Phi(2 \ln(10)L)^{1/2} \tag{3.94}$$

The maximum lod score that is equivalent of a 'point-wise' significance of α_1 is

$$L = \frac{[\Phi^{-1}(1 - \alpha_1)]^2}{2\ln(10)} \tag{3.95}$$

These interrelationships enable the results from parametric and non-parametric linkage analyses to be compared with each other.

3.16   Assessing the information content for linkage analysis

Before embarking on a linkage study on a pedigree sample, it is often desirable to assess the amount of linkage information contained in the sample. For a

Mendelian disease, this assessment may help to decide whether the sample size is adequate for detecting linkage, or for the localization of the disease gene into a sufficiently small chromosomal segment. When the disease is complex and the genetic model uncertain, then the assessment may provide some insights into the magnitude of genetic effect (in terms of penetrance and admixture proportion) that the sample has sufficient power to detect. Another purpose of such an assessment in a multipoint setting is to evaluate whether there are gaps between adjacent markers where substantial information can be gained by typing additional markers. Finally, such an assessment may reveal individuals who convey insufficient linkage information to warrant genotyping. Several ways of measuring linkage information content for these purposes have been proposed.

3.16.1 Equivalent number of fully informative gametes

When the linkage data in a pedigree consist of fully informative gametes, the lod score function of the pedigree is given by

$$Z(\theta) = R \log_{10}\theta + (N - R) \log_{10}(1 - \theta) - N \log_{10}(0.5) \qquad (3.96)$$

for $0 \leqslant \theta \leqslant 0.5$, where N is the number of fully informative gametes and R the number of recombinants in the pedigree. Thus, given the observed pedigree lod score function, it is possible to deduce the value of N, provided that the pedigree data do indeed consist of fully informative gametes. This value can then be used as a measure of the linkage information content of the pedigree. If the pedigree data do not consist of fully informative gametes, then it is still possible to obtain a value of N (and a value of R) which will give a lod score function that is similar to that observed, and use the value of N, defined as the equivalent number of fully informative gametes, to measure the linkage information content of the pedigree. The amount of linkage information in a sample is then measured by the total equivalent number of fully informative gametes in its constituent pedigrees.

In order to obtain N from an observed pedigree lod score function, Edwards (1976) suggests equating the observed maximum lod score to its theoretical value. For fully informative gametes, the maximum lod score is

$$Z_{max} = N [\hat{\theta} \log_{10} \hat{\theta} + (1 - \hat{\theta})\log_{10}(1 - \hat{\theta}) - \log_{10} (0.5)] \qquad (3.97)$$

where $\hat{\theta}$ is the maximum likelihood estimate of θ. Given the observed values of θ and Z_{max}, this equation can be solved to give the value of the unknown quantity N

$$N = \frac{Z_{max}}{\hat{\theta} \log_{10}\hat{\theta} + (1 - \hat{\theta}) \log_{10}(1 - \hat{\theta}) - \log_{10}(0.5)} \qquad (3.98)$$

This procedure is not applicable when $\hat{\theta} = 0.5$ and $Z_{max} = 0$. In this situation, it is necessary to equate the observed lod score at any value of θ to its theoretical value. If the point $\theta = 0.25$ is chosen, then the equation is

$$Z\left(\theta = \frac{1}{4}\right) = N\left(\frac{1}{2} \log_{10} \frac{1}{4} + \frac{1}{2} \log_{10} \frac{3}{4} - \log_{10} \frac{1}{2}\right) \qquad (3.99)$$

This equation simplifies to give $N = 2Z(\theta = 0.25)/(\log_{10}(0.75))$, which can be used as an estimate of the equivalent number of fully informative gametes of the family, when the maximum lod score of the family is 0.

As it may seem somewhat arbitrary to use only a single point of the lod score function for deriving N, some investigators have extended the above procedure to take account of the entire lod score function, by defining some index of the goodness-of-fit between the an observed lod score function and an expected lod score function over the entire range $0 \leqslant \theta \leqslant 0.5$, and maximizing this index with respect to N and R (Curtis and Gurling, 1993; MacLean *et al.*, 1993b)

The equivalent number of fully informative gametes is intuitively appealing as it enables the information content of a pedigree (or a sample) to be assessed in relation to the simple and familiar situation where recombinants and non-recombinants can be counted. However, the method must be regarded as approximate when the data do not really consist of fully informative gametes.

3.16.2   Expected lod score and the power to detect linkage

Another commonly used measure of the linkage information content of a pedigree is the expected lod score of the pedigree under the true (or assumed) recombination fraction and genetic model. The expected lod score, often abbreviated as the ELOD, is the value of the expected lod score function at the true value of θ.

In order to obtain the expected lod score function, it is necessary to calculate the expected lod score for each value of θ in the range $0 \leqslant \theta \leqslant 0.5$. This in turn involves obtaining the probability distribution of the possible lod score values at each value of θ. For data consisting of fully informative gametes, finding the expected lod score function is straightforward. Suppose that the number of fully informative gametes is N, then there are $N + 1$ possible lod score functions, corresponding to $R = 0, 1, 2, \ldots, N$, where R is the number of recombinants. The expected lod score function is a weighted average of these $N + 1$ functions, where the weights are the probabilities of the $N + 1$ possible values of R, which follow a binomial distribution with parameters N and θ_t (the true recombination fraction).

A simpler way of obtaining the expected lod score function for any number of fully informative gametes is based on the recognition that the lod score function is additive over independent observations. The expected lod score function for N fully informative gametes is therefore N times the expected lod score function of one fully informative gamete. A fully informative gamete is either recombinant, with lod score function

$$Z(\theta) = \log_{10}(\theta) - \log_{10}(0.5) \qquad (3.100)$$

or it is non-recombinant, with lod score function

$$Z(\theta) = \log_{10}(1 - \theta) - \log_{10}(0.5) \qquad (3.101)$$

the probabilities of these outcomes are θ_t and $(1 - \theta_t)$, where θ_t is the true value of θ. The expected lod score function of a single fully informative gamete is therefore

$$E[Z(\theta)] = \theta_t \log_{10} \theta + (1 - \theta_t)\log_{10}(1 - \theta) - \log_{10} 0.5$$
$$= \theta_t \log_{10} (2\theta) + (1 - \theta_t)\log_{10} 2(1 - \theta) \qquad (3.102)$$

so that for N fully informative gametes the expected lod score function is

$$E[Z(\theta)] = N[\theta_t \log_{10} (2\theta) + (1 - \theta_t)\log_{10} 2(1 - \theta)] \qquad (3.103)$$

The ELOD is therefore

$$ELOD = N[\theta_t \log_{10} (2\theta_t) + (1 - \theta_t)\log_{10} 2(1 - \theta_t)] \qquad (3.104)$$

The expected lod score functions for $N = 10$ under various true values of θ (0, 0.1, 0.2, 0.3, 0.4, 0.5) are given in Figure 3.7. The maximum of each expected lod score function occurs at the true value of θ, as can be shown by setting the derivative of $E[Z(\theta)]$ to 0. The linkage information content of a dataset may therefore be conveniently summarized by the value of the expected lod score function at the true (or assumed) value of θ, which is defined as the ELOD.

The ELOD is closely related to two other quantities that are also often used to measure the linkage information content of a sample. One of these is the expected maximum lod score, abbreviated as EMLOD, which differs from the ELOD because the maximum lod score does not always occur at the true value of θ. The other measure is the power to detect linkage, at a preassigned critical lod score

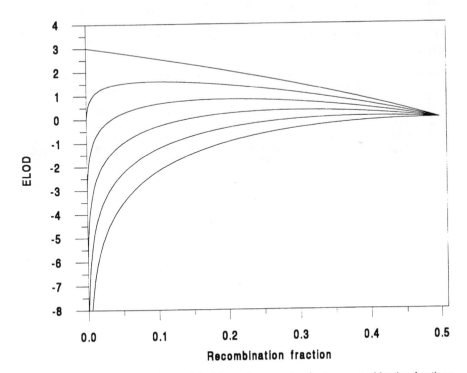

Figure 3.7   ELOD functions for ten fully informative gametes for true recombination fractions of 0, 0.1, 0.2, 0.3, 0.4 and 0.5.

value (or significance level). These two measure are related to the ELOD because the maximum lod score multiplied by a factor $2 \ln(10)$ is a standard likelihood ratio statistic which has asymptotically a non-central chi-squared distribution under an alternative hypothesis. This non-central chi-squared distribution is characterized by two quantities, the non-centrality parameter, which is determined by the true θ and genetic model as well as the size of the sample, and the number of degrees of freedom, which is one because the only unknown parameter is θ. The non-centrality parameter is equal to the ELOD multiplied by a factor of $2 \ln(10)$. Since the mean of a non-central chi-squared distribution is the sum of the non-centrality parameter and the degrees of freedom, it follows that, asymptotically

$$2 \ln(10)[\text{EMLOD} - \text{ELOD}] = 1 \qquad (3.105)$$

Moreover, the ELOD is related to the power to detect linkage because the probability that the maximum lod score will exceed a certain critical value C (e.g. 3) is equal to the probability that a non-central chi-squared random variable with non-centrality parameter $2 \ln(10)\text{ELOD}$ and one degree of freedom will exceed $2 \ln(10)C$.

Example 3.17
Calculate the ELOD, EMLOD and the power to detect linkage at a critical lod score of 3, for a sample consisting of 20 fully informative gametes, when the true θ is 0.1.

The possible numbers of recombinants, R, their probabilities, $P(R)$, their associated lod scores at the true value of θ, $\text{Lod}(\theta_t)$, their associated maximum lod scores $\text{Lod}(\hat{\theta})$, and the indicator variable for whether the maximum lod score is significant, I, are set out as follows.

R	$P(R)$	$\text{Lod}(\theta_t)$	$\hat{\theta}$	$\text{Lod}(\hat{\theta})$	I	$P(R)\text{Lod}(\theta_t)$	$P(R)\text{Lod}(\hat{\theta})$	$P(R)I$
0	0.12158	5.1055	0.00	6.02060	1	0.62070	0.73196	0.12158
1	0.27017	4.1512	0.05	4.29632	1	1.12153	1.16074	0.27017
2	0.28518	3.1970	0.10	3.19697	1	0.91171	0.91171	0.28518
3	0.19012	2.2427	0.15	2.34900	0	0.42639	0.44659	0.00000
4	0.08978	1.2885	0.20	1.67416	0	0.11568	0.15030	0.00000
5	0.03192	0.3342	0.25	1.13622	0	0.01067	0.03627	0.00000
6	0.00887	−0.6200	0.30	0.71470	0	−0.00550	0.00634	0.00000
7	0.00197	−1.5742	0.35	0.39695	0	−0.00310	0.00078	0.00000
8	0.00036	−2.5285	0.40	0.17489	0	−0.00090	0.00006	0.00000
9	0.00005	−3.4827	0.45	0.04350	0	−0.00018	0.00000	0.00000
10	0.00001	−4.4370	0.50	0.00000	0	−0.00003	0.00000	0.00000
11	0.00000	−5.3912	0.50	0.00000	0	−0.00000	0.00000	0.00000
12	0.00000	−6.3455	0.50	0.00000	0	−0.00000	0.00000	0.00000
13	0.00000	−7.2997	0.50	0.00000	0	−0.00000	0.00000	0.00000
14	0.00000	−8.2539	0.50	0.00000	0	−0.00000	0.00000	0.00000
15	0.00000	−9.2082	0.50	0.00000	0	−0.00000	0.00000	0.00000
16	0.00000	−10.1624	0.50	0.00000	0	−0.00000	0.00000	0.00000
17	0.00000	−11.1167	0.50	0.00000	0	−0.00000	0.00000	0.00000
18	0.00000	−12.0709	0.50	0.00000	0	−0.00000	0.00000	0.00000
19	0.00000	−13.0252	0.50	0.00000	0	−0.00000	0.00000	0.00000
20	0.00000	−13.9794	0.50	0.00000	0	−0.00000	0.00000	0.00000
	1.00000					3.19697	3.44476	0.67693

The exact results are therefore:

$$ELOD = 3.19697$$

$$EMLOD = 3.44476$$

$$power = 0.67693$$

Taking $2 \ln(10)ELOD$ as the non-centrality parameter, asymptotic theory predicts

$$EMLOD = [2 \ln(10)ELOD + 1]/[2 \ln(10)] = 3.41424$$

$$power = P(\chi^2_{14.722, 1} > 13.815) = 0.54778$$

These asymptotic results are fairly close to the exact values.

Most real pedigree samples do not consist of fully informative gametes so that the above simple approach is not applicable. Instead, Monte Carlo simulation is necessary to obtain the expected lod score function in these situations. Since the information content of the pedigree sample depends on the disease and marker phenotypes, it is desirable that these are fixed as much as possible without biasing the evidence in favour of or against linkage. In practice, this is often done by fixing the disease phenotypes of all pedigree members and the marker phenotypes of all founder members to the actual phenotypes, and simulating the marker phenotypes of non-founding members by random segregation under an assumed recombination fraction between the marker and the disease locus. A lod score function is calculated for each simulated replicate, and several parameters of this function are saved, including the value at the true (or assumed) value of θ, the maximum value, and a $(0, 1)$ indicator variable for whether the maximum value exceeds a certain critical value (e.g. 3). The average values of these parameters over a large number of replicates are then taken as empirical estimates of the ELOD, EMLOD and power to detect linkage.

For multipoint analysis, the same principles apply, except that the lod score is now a function of location rather than recombination fraction, and the data are simulated under an assumed location of the disease locus, rather than an assumed recombination fraction. In order to evaluate the linkage information content at a particular location, one can simulate replicates of the data, assuming that there is a disease locus at the hypothetical position, and calculate for each replicate the multipoint lod score at the same position. The average of these multipoint lod scores is then an empirical estimate of the multipoint ELOD at that position. The position can be shifted point-by-point from one end of a chromosomal segment to the other, to obtain a series of estimates across the region. These ELOD estimates can be used to assess the information content of the dataset for detecting linkage in the region.

To assess the effect of not genotyping a family member, two ELOD calculations can be performed, one including and the other excluding the genotype of the family member concerned. The amount of linkage information contributed by the family member is measured by the difference in ELOD of these two analyses. If the difference is very small, then the family member can be omitted with little loss in linkage information content.

The simulations for obtaining empirical estimates of ELOD, EMLOD and power can be performed using the the programs SIMLINK (Ploughman and Boehnke, 1989) and SLINK (Weeks *et al.*, 1990)

3.16.3   Fisher's information

Another common measure of linkage information content is Fisher's information. When only one unknown parameter is involved, Fisher's information is equal to the reciprocal of the sampling variance of the maximum likelihood estimate of the parameter. For several unknown parameters, Fisher's information matrix is the inverse of the variance–covariance matrix of the maximum likelihood estimates of the parameters. Given a maximum likelihood estimate, Fisher's observed information is minus the derivative of the score function with respect to the parameter, evaluated at the maximum likelihood estimate of the parameter. For a particular hypothesized value of the parameter, Fisher's expected information is the expected value of minus the derivative of the score function with respect to the parameter, evaluated at the hypothesized value of the parameter.

For data consisting of fully informative gametes, Fisher's information is easy to obtain. For N fully informative gametes with R recombinants, the log-likelihood function is

$$\ln L(\theta) = R \ln \theta + (N - R)\ln(1 - \theta) \tag{3.106}$$

The score function is the derivative of the log-likelihood function

$$S(\theta) = R \theta^{-1} - (N - R)(1 - \theta)^{-1} \tag{3.107}$$

The derivative of the score function is therefore

$$S'(\theta) = -R\theta^{-2} + (N - R)(1 - \theta)^{-2} \tag{3.108}$$

Minus one times the expectation of this function, evaluated at the true value θ_t, then gives Fisher's expected information as

$$I(\theta) = N\theta_t^{-1} - N(1 - \theta_t)^{-1} = N[\theta_t(1 - \theta_t)]^{-1} \tag{3.109}$$

Fisher's observed information is given by the same expression, with θ_t being replaced by the maximum likelihood estimate of θ. In order for these expressions to be applicable, it is necessary that the hypothesized value of θ, or the maximum likelihood estimate of θ, is not equal to 0. Fisher's information does not apply when the log-likelihood function at the maximum likelihood estimate of θ does not have a gradient of 0.

Fisher's information can be used to obtain an estimate of the non-centrality parameter of the likelihood ratio test for linkage, which is equal to $2 \ln(10)$ times the ELOD. For N fully informative gametes, an estimate of the non-centrality parameter is

$$2 \ln(10)\text{ELOD} \approx (\theta_t - 0.5)I(\theta_t - 0.5)$$
$$= N(\theta_t - 0.5)^2[\theta_t(1 - \theta_t)]^{-1} \tag{3.110}$$

This approximation, however, is reasonably accurate only for values of θ_t close to the null hypothesis value of $1/2$.

For general pedigree data Fisher's expected information at a given value of θ can be estimated empirically from the average curvature of the log-likelihood function at that value of θ, in a large number of simulated replicates of the data. For this purpose, it is convenient to use the result (stated in Section 2.4.2) that Fisher's expected information at a given value of θ is equal to the expectation of the square of the score function evaluated at that value of θ.

$$I(\theta_t) = E[S(\theta_t)]^2 \qquad (3.111)$$

Since $S(\theta_t)$ is the gradient of the log-likelihood function at θ_t, its value in a particular simulated replicate can be estimated empirically by evaluating the log-likelihood at θ_t and again at $\theta_t + \delta$ (where δ is a small positive increment) and dividing the difference in log-likelihood by δ. Fisher's expected information is then approximated by the average of the squares of these estimated gradients over all the simulated replicates.

The above result also leads to a simple way of estimating the standard error of a maximum likelihood estimate of θ. Fisher's expected information of a parameter is equal to the inverse of the sampling variance of the parameter estimate. The standard error of the maximum likelihood estimate of θ is therefore approximately

$$SD(\hat{\theta}) = \frac{\delta}{\ln L(\hat{\theta}) - \ln(\hat{\theta} + \delta)} \qquad (3.112)$$

A very rough estimate of the standard error of a maximum likelihood estimate is therefore the increment in parameter value that corresponds to a unit drop of the log-likelihood from its maximum. When dealing with lod scores it is important to remember that a unit drop in log-likelihood corresponds to a decrease in lod score of $1/\ln(10) = 0.434$. Thus, a quick approximation of the standard error of a maximum likelihood estimate of θ is the increase in the value of θ that corresponds to a drop in the lod score of 0.434 units from the maximum. An approximate 95% confidence interval of θ is then given by the range of values of θ within two standard errors of the maximum likelihood estimate.

Although Fisher's information for general pedigrees can be obtained by Monte Carlo simulations, investigators are usually more interested in the power to detect linkage than in the precision of the recombination fraction estimate. For these reasons, perhaps, Fisher's information is not routinely calculated by programs such as SIMLINK and SLINK.

3.16.4 Entropy-based information content mapping

The above methods of assessing linkage information content use both disease and marker phenotype information, and are dependent on the specification of a disease model. Another method, called entropy-based information content mapping and implemented in the GENEHUNTER program (Kruglyak *et al.*, 1996), is concerned with marker information alone. According to this method, the linkage information content of a pedigree at a certain chromosomal position is measured by how completely the inheritance vector of the pedigree at that position is determined by the marker phenotypes of the pedigree members.

At a given chromosomal position, a pedigree with n individuals of whom f are founders contains $2(n-f)$ transmissions events. The number of possible inheritance vectors is therefore $2^{2(n-f)}$. However, since the phases of the f founders are unknown, inheritance vectors that differ only by phase changes in the founders are completely equivalent and have equal probabilities. The $2^{2(n-f)}$ inheritance factors can therefore be grouped into 2^{2n-3f} equivalent classes each containing 2^f equivalent members. The probabilities of these 2^{2n-3f} equivalent classes of inheritance vectors constitute the inheritance distribution. The 'entropy' of an inheritance distribution is defined as

$$E = -\Sigma\, P_i \log_2 P_i \qquad (3.113)$$

where P_i is the probability of the ith inheritance vector, and the summation is taken over all 2^{2n-3f} inheritance vectors. In the absence of marker information, all possible inheritance vectors are equally likely, so that $E = 2n - 3f$ bits. When information is complete, the marker phenotypes are consistent with only one inheritance vector, so that $E = 0$. The entropy-based information content at position x is defined as

$$I_E(x) = 1 - \frac{E(x)}{E_0} \qquad (3.114)$$

where $E(x)$ is the entropy at position x given the observed marker phenotypes, and E_0 is the entropy in the absence of marker information, i.e. $2n - 3f$.

Entropy-based information content mapping places equal weight on all the transmission events in a pedigree. This may be undesirable under some circumstances. The gametes of unaffected individuals are never informative for a Mendelian dominant disease with complete penetrance. Conversely, the gametes of affected individuals are never informative for a Mendelian recessive disease with no phenocopies. In general, when the disease model is known, the entropy-based measure is inferior to the ELOD or related measures, which are able to weight transmission events according to the likelihood of heterozygosity at the disease locus. Entropy-based information content mapping is therefore most useful when the disease model is uncertain.

3.17 Strategic issues in linkage studies

There are many strategic issues in linkage studies. What should be the criteria for subjecting a disease to linkage analysis? What kind of pedigrees should be collected? How many markers should be used, and how should they be selected? Is it possible to increase efficiency of a genome scan by adopting sequential procedures? These are important issues that must be resolved by the investigator at the planning stages of a study.

3.17.1 Criteria for subjecting a disease to a linkage study

A disease should be subjected to a linkage study only if a positive result is both desirable and feasible. For many diseases with uncertain aetiology, the localization of a disease gene will constitute a major breakthrough in research that may lead to an improved understanding of the pathophysiology of the disease and consequently more effective methods of prevention and treatment. The main question is therefore whether the localization of a disease gene is feasible. The linkage approach is certainly feasible for Mendelian diseases, as witnessed by the hundreds of disease genes that have been successfully localized by this method.

For complex disorders, the feasibility of linkage analysis is less clear. In principle, segregation analysis can be performed in order to test whether a gene of major effect is present. Unfortunately, this approach is rarely helpful, as segregation analysis of complex disorders requires very large, systematically ascertained samples, and is very sensitive to numerous complicating factors such as assortative mating and differential fertility. The failure of segregation analysis to demonstrate a major gene effect therefore does not constitute a strong argument against using a linkage approach.

Another criterion which is sometimes used to assess the feasibility of linkage analysis is that the disease should have substantial heritability. Heritability is defined as the proportion of phenotypic variance in a population that is attributable to genetic variation. When heritability is 0, linkage analysis is clearly hopeless. However, because heritability is an aggregate measure of the magnitude of the total contribution of all genetic loci, it has no direct relationship with how easily a particular disease locus can be detected by linkage analysis. Nevertheless, heritability places an upper limit on the magnitude of the contribution of a single locus, so that a disease with a very low heritability is unlikely to be successfully tackled by linkage analysis. In practice, a low heritability is associated with a weak tendency of the disease to aggregate in families, and in this situation even the collection of an adequate family sample is problematic.

The frequency of a disorder is also sometimes used to assess the likelihood of success of a linkage approach. In general, the rarer the disease, the fewer aetiological factors are involved, and the greater the effect size of the susceptibility genes. A linkage approach is therefore more likely to be successful for rare diseases than for common conditions, for a given level of heritability. However, this greater feasibility of linkage analysis for rare diseases is partially balanced by the greater public health impact of common disorders. The extension of linkage analysis to common disorders is therefore an important scientific and methodological development.

3.17.2 The choice of pedigrees for linkage analysis

In principle, it should be possible to settle the issue of family selection by comparing the linkage information content of different pedigree structures under a range of underlying genetic models. It is therefore surprising that the issue has remained somewhat controversial. While linkage analysis is traditionally conducted using large pedigrees with multiple affected members, the recent trend is to focus on small family units such as affected sib-pairs and their parents.

The increasing popularity of small family units in linkage studies is due mainly to the gradual shift of research focus from Mendelian diseases to complex disorders. Many investigators prefer to use non-parametric rather than parametric methods for the linkage analysis of complex disorders, and most non-parametric methods are applicable only to small family units such as affected sib-pairs and their parents. Complex disorders are more likely to be associated with diagnostic uncertainties than Mendelian diseases, and diagnostic errors may have a greater detrimental effect on large pedigrees than on small family units. If the frequency of the disease allele is high, or if disease alleles at two or more loci are involved, then multiple disease alleles may be introduced into a large pedigree from several founders. This intrafamilial heterogeneity is expected to reduce the linkage information content of the family. Furthermore, if the frequency of the disease allele is so high that the probability of parental homozygosity becomes substantial, then selecting large pedigrees with multiple affected members may enrich the sample with homozygous parents, whose gametes are uninformative for linkage. Finally, for complex disorders, large pedigrees with multiple affected members are often difficult to find, whereas affected sib-pairs tend to be much more abundant.

In spite of these familiar arguments for the use of small family units, it is clear that large pedigrees with multiple affected members are much more powerful than small family units when the disease allele involved is rare and has a large effect. Further work is necessary to quantify systematically the linkage information content of different family structures under a range of different circumstances.

3.17.3 The choice of markers for linkage analysis

The choice of markers for a linkages study involves many factors, only some of which are statistical in nature. Such factors may include availability, cost, and reliability of measurement. From a statistical point of view, a marker should be highly polymorphic, as measured by the heterozygosity or the polymorphism information content (PIC). Furthermore, given two markers that are approximately equal in heterozygosity, the one with fewer alleles is preferable, because this decreases computational burden, and increases the robustness of the analysis to misspecification of allele frequencies. The ideal marker from a statistical point of view is therefore one with many (say about 10) equally frequent alleles.

In a multipoint analysis, it is intuitively obvious that the markers should be evenly spaced in the chromosomal segment, provided that they are equally polymorphic. The density of markers necessary to extract nearly all the linkage information in a region depends on the level of heterozygosity of the markers. In practice, markers always vary in heterozygosity, and are never absolutely evenly spaced. To assess whether a given marker set is sufficient, or whether additional markers are desirable, the maximum possible ELOD should be obtained by performing simulations with a single marker locus that is completely linked to the disease, and that has a heterozygosity of one (so that all the founder alleles in a pedigree are different from each other). Multipoint ELOD calculations based on the existing marker set can then be conducted to see if there are regions where the ELOD is far below the maximum ELOD. Further markers should be added to such regions. When the disease model is uncertain, entropy-based information mapping can be used instead of ELOD to identify gaps where further markers should be added.

3.17.4 Sequential procedures for genome scans

A complete genome scan involves the genotyping of a large number (usually about 300) of evenly spaced markers on a large number of pedigrees. Suppose that the number of markers and pedigrees are m and p, respectively, then there are mp combinations of markers and pedigrees. Here, a sequential procedure is defined as a set of rules for deciding which marker–pedigree combination to genotype next, or whether the genotyping effort should be terminated.

Numerous factors may enter into the choice of sequential procedure, only some of which are statistical in nature. Factors of a political or psychological nature include the amount of time and resources available, the aims of the investigator in relation to those of other groups, and the ease with which positive and negative results can be published. The optimal procedure also depends on how much is known about the disease, in particular, whether there are strong candidate genes on biological grounds. The feasibility of a procedure for the laboratory must also be considered. The technology may be such that it is particularly efficient to conduct genotyping on one large batch of DNA samples at a time.

A formal decision-theoretic approach to obtain an optimal sequential procedure needs to take account of these complicating factors, as well as statistical considerations. While such a formal analysis is difficult to conduct or justify, it is clear that investigators do make informal assessments of these factors in order to arrive at strategic decisions. Thus, it seems sensible to focus the genotyping efforts to regions with candidate genes that have not been examined previously. If these efforts are unsuccessful, then investigators may decide to conduct a whole genome scan.

If the sample size is small, then the investigator may simply choose to genotype the entire sample, one chromosome at a time, in an arbitrary order. A side benefit of this approach is that complete data will be available for the first few chromosomes long before the completion of the genome scan, so that the results on these chromosomes can be submitted for rapid publication. On the other hand, if the pedigree sample is large, then the investigator may choose to divide the sample into two or more subsets for a multi-stage genome scan. An entire genome scan is performed only for the first subset. For subsequent subsets, the search is limited to promising regions revealed by earlier stages. This multi-stage procedure directs the genotyping effort away from negative regions and towards promising areas. At the end of such a procedure, some of the mp marker–pedigree combinations will remain untyped, in regions where the evidence for linkage is negative. Another form of multi-stage strategy is to perform a genome scan using a set of coarsely-spaced markers (up to about 20 cM between adjacent markers), and follow up any suggestive positive findings using sets of progressively more finely-spaced markers. This is continued until the initial suggestive findings are either confirmed or rejected, or until all the linkage information in the region is exhausted. Again, this multi-stage procedure will result in some of the mp marker–pedigree combinations being left untyped in regions where the linkage evidence is entirely negative.

Taken globally, the genotyping efforts of several different groups on the same disorder can also be viewed in a similar sequential framework. When one group reports a positive finding, other groups often redirect their efforts to the same region, to see if the positive finding can be replicated. This approach can be regarded as an informal generalization of the sequential test of linkage proposed by Morton (1955). However, for complex disorders, the evidence for linkage often cannot be summarized simply as a single table of lod scores. In order to facilitate the accumulation of data and to encourage more powerful combined analyses, investigators should make their raw data openly available once their findings have been published.

3.18 Conclusions

The molecular process of recombination during meiosis enables the relative positions of genetic loci to be inferred from the patterns of allele-transmissions from parent to offspring. The enormous success of this linkage approach of gene mapping is partly due to the increased availability of easily measured genetic markers, but also to the development of powerful statistical methods. The lod score method, based on the theory of likelihood ratios, is the most established and popular of the many statistical techniques that have been developed for linkage analysis. This method has reliably detected linkages for hundreds of Mendelian disorders. For complex disorders, however, non-parametric methods based on allele-sharing have gained popularity in recent years. The application of linkage analysis to complex disorders is an active area of methodological research.

4

The Analysis of Allelic Associations

Genetic linkage is the tendency of short chromosomal segments to be inherited intact from parent to offspring. As a result, some combinations of alleles (i.e. haplotypes) on these short segments may be preserved over a large number of generations and become quite frequent in the population. The excessive co-occurrence of certain combinations of alleles in the same gamete (or in the same person) because of tight linkage, or for other reasons, is known as allelic association.

The study of allelic associations is an important tool for the mapping of genetic loci, which is complementary to linkage analysis. Historically, association studies between diseases and 'classical polymorphisms' such as ABO blood groups and HLA antigens have yielded many consistent findings. Such findings suggest that the associated genetic variant is either in close proximity to a disease-predisposing allele, or is the disease-predisposing allele itself. Association analysis is set to become an even more powerful tool in the near future, as the Human Genome Project is rapidly identifying all the functional loci in the human genome, together with numerous polymorphisms in and around these functional DNA sequences.

4.1 Definition of allelic association

Consider two loci A and B, with alleles $A_1, A_2, \ldots, A_m$ and $B_1, B_2, \ldots, B_n$ occurring at frequencies $p_1, p_2, \ldots, p_m$ and $q_1, q_2, \ldots, q_n$ in the population. The genotype of each individual consists of two haplotypes, one from the paternal gamete and the other from the maternal gamete. Each haplotype consists of two alleles, one at locus A and the other at locus B. With m possible alleles at locus A and n possible alleles at locus B, there are a total of mn possible haplotypes, which can be denoted as $A_1B_1, A_1B_2, \ldots, A_mB_n$, and whose frequencies can be denoted as $h_{11}, h_{12}, \ldots, h_{mn}$.

By definition, if the occurrence of allele A_i and the occurrence of allele B_j in a haplotype are independent events, then the frequency of the joint occurrence of alleles A_i and B_j in a gamete (i.e. the haplotype frequency of A_iB_j) is equal to the product of the allele frequencies of A_i and B_j

$$h_{ij} = p_iq_j \qquad (4.1)$$

If this equality does not hold, then the occurrences of A_i and B_j are not independent, and the two alleles are said to be associated. If $h_{ij} > p_iq_j$, then A_i and B_j are said to be positively associated. Conversely, if $h_{ij} < p_iq_j$, then the two alleles are said to be negatively associated.

Example 4.1
Consider two biallelic loci A and B with alleles A_1, A_2 and B_1, B_2. There are four haplotypes A_1B_1, A_1B_2, A_2B_1, A_2B_2. Suppose that the frequencies of these four haplotypes in a large population are 0.4, 0.1, 0.2 and 0.3, respectively. Are there any allelic associations between the two loci in the population?
   The allele frequencies are A_1: $0.4 + 0.1 = 0.5$, A_2: $0.2 + 0.3 = 0.5$, B_1: $0.4 + 0.2 = 0.6$, B_2: $0.1 + 0.3 = 0.4$. In the absence of allelic associations, the four haplotype frequencies should be A_1B_1: $(0.5)(0.6) = 0.3$, A_1B_2: $(0.5)(0.4) = 0.2$, A_2B_1: $(0.5)(0.6) = 0.3$, A_2B_2: $(0.5)(0.4) = 0.2$. The actual haplotype frequencies of 0.4, 0.1, 0.1 and 0.4 are different from these values, and by definition this implies the presence of allelic associations. Alleles A_1 and B_1 are positively associated, and so are alleles A_2 and B_2. In contrast, allele A_1 is negatively associated with allele B_2, and allele A_2 is negatively associated with allele B_1.

4.2   Maintenance of allelic associations: linkage disequilibrium

We now consider how allelic associations are maintained from generation to generation by tight linkage in a large, closed, randomly mating population. Again, let the alleles at locus A be $A_1, A_2, ..., A_m$ and their frequencies be $p_1, p_2, ..., p_m$ and the alleles at locus B be $B_1, B_2, ..., B_n$ and their frequencies be $q_1, q_2, ..., q_n$. In addition, let the recombination fraction between the two loci be θ. The question is, if the frequency of the haplotype A_iB_j in the current generation is h_{ij0}, what will be the frequency of the same haplotype in the next generation, assuming random mating within the population?
   To answer this question, we note that each haplotype in the next generation is either a recombinant (probability θ) or a non-recombinant (probability $1 - \theta$), with respect to loci A and B. When the haplotype is a non-recombinant, it has probability h_{ij0} of being A_iB_j. When it is a recombinant, the probability of it being A_iB_j is simply p_iq_j under the assumption of random mating. The total probability that a haplotype transmitted to the next generation is A_iB_j is therefore

$$h_{ij1} = (1 - \theta)h_{ij0} + \theta p_iq_j \qquad (4.2)$$

The change in haplotype frequency from generation 0 to generation 1 is

$$h_{ij1} - h_{ij0} = \theta(p_iq_j - h_{ij0}) \qquad (4.3)$$

From this we deduce that the haplotype frequency will not change if $h_{ij0} = p_iq_j$ (i.e. if there is no allelic association), and that for any discrepancy between p_iq_j and h_{ij0}, the change in haplotype frequency is proportional to θ. When $h_{ij0} = p_iq_j$ for all i, j at the two loci, there will be no change in haplotype frequencies from generation to generation, and we say that the two loci are in linkage equilibrium. Otherwise the two loci are said to be in linkage disequilibrium.

The rate that a randomly mating population approaches linkage equilibrium depends crucially on the recombination fraction θ. Rewriting (4.2) as

$$h_{ij1} - p_i q_i = (1 - \theta)(h_{ij0} - p_i q_j) \tag{4.4}$$

we see that the discrepancy between haplotype frequency and its equilibrium value is diminished by a factor of $(1 - \theta)$ per generation, so that after k generations we have

$$h_{ijk} - p_i q_j = (1 - \theta)^k (h_{ij0} - p_i q_j) \tag{4.5}$$

The difference between a haplotype frequency and its equilibrium value (i.e. $h_{ij} - p_i q_j$) is sometimes used as a measure of the magnitude of association between alleles. Figure 4.1 plots the decline of linkage disequilibrium in a large, stable randomly mating population, for several different values of recombination fraction.

The term linkage disequilibrium is perhaps somewhat unfortunate as it may be taken to imply that the loci involved are necessarily linked. According to the above definition and to common usage, linkage disequilibrium is synonymous with allelic associations. Another, perhaps less confusing, term for the phenomenon is *gametic phase disequilibrium.*

Example 4.2
Suppose that the recombination fraction between two loci is 0.01. How many generations would it take to halve the magnitude of allelic associations (as measured by the discrepancies of the haplotype frequencies from their equilibrium values) between the two loci, assuming a large population in random mating?

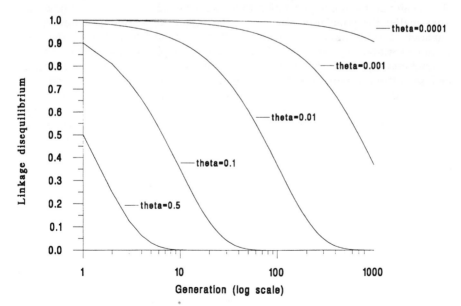

Figure 4.1   Decay of linkage disequilibrium by generation.

The magnitude of allelic associations is diminished by a factor of $(1 - \theta)$ per generation. It is therefore diminished by a factor of $(1 - \theta)^k$ after k generations. The number of generations for it to be halved is therefore obtained by equating $(1 - \theta)^k$ to $1/2$, giving

$$k = \log(0.5)/\log(1 - \theta)$$

Substituting $\theta = 0.01$ gives $k = 69.0$ generations.

4.3   Generation of allelic associations

The above model relates the rate of dissipation of allelic associations to the recombination fraction, but does not address how disequilibrium is generated in the first place. Linkage disequilibrium can be generated by random genetic drift, founder effect, mutation, selection, and population admixture and stratification. It is difficult to develop precise mathematical models for all these processes, except under some idealized and often unrealistic assumptions. It is especially difficult to work out precisely how these processes relate to and interact with each other in a real population. However, it is useful to have an intuitive understanding of these processes, in order to appreciate the strengths and limitations of allelic association studies for gene mapping.

An important mechanism for the generation of allelic associations is 'random genetic drift', which is a term used to describe the random changes in allele or haplotype frequencies from one generation to the next in a finite population. The gene pool of one generation can be regarded as a random sample of the gene pool of the previous generation. Allele and haplotype frequencies are therefore subject to sampling variation. Allele and haplotype frequencies can also be altered from one generation to the next by the occurrence of mutations. The smaller the population, the larger the effects of sampling variation and mutation, and the larger the random drift in allele and haplotype frequencies from generation to generation. The tendency for haplotype frequencies to drift at random is partially balanced by a tendency for recombination events in meioses to return haplotype frequencies to their equilibrium values and, to a smaller extent, by a tendency of randomly occurring mutations to reduce the frequencies of common haplotypes. The expected magnitude of linkage disequilibrium between two polymorphic loci in a stable population is therefore a function of population size, recombination fraction, and mutation rate.

A closely related phenomenon is the so-called 'founder effect'. This applies to a population which has grown rapidly, largely in isolation, from a small group of ancestors. In Finland, for example, most of the current population of about 5 000 000 people are descendants of a small population of about 1000 individuals some 2000 years ago (Hastbacka *et al.*, 1992). As noted above, a small population is prone to linkage disequilibrium due to random genetic drift. A small 'founder population' is therefore likely to be in appreciable linkage disequilibrium for many pairs of linked loci. As the population expands, the balance between random genetic drift, recombination and mutation is disturbed, and the extent of linkage disequilibrium between all pairs of loci will tend to diminish from generation to generation until a new balance is reached. However, if the expansion of the population is rapid, the reduction in linkage disequilibrium will tend to 'lag behind' the increase in population size. In other words, there will be a greater degree of allelic associations between loci of a given recombination fraction, than would be expected for the current size of the population. The degree of allelic associations present will therefore be appropriate for a population size intermediate between the founder and the current population. This value, sometimes known as an 'effective population size', is approximately equal to the harmonic mean of the sizes of all generations between the founder and the present population, and is often much closer to the size of the founder population than that of the present population.

The generation of linkage disequilibrium by genetic drift and mutation is crucially dependent on the effective population size. There are other mechanisms, however, that can generate linkage disequilibrium regardless of the size of the population. One such mechanism is selection, which occurs when an individual's genotype has an influence on reproductive fitness (defined as the average number of offspring who survive to reproductive age). If the effect of an allele on reproductive fitness is potentiated by the presence of another allele at a different locus, then there will be a disproportionate increase in the frequency of individuals with both these alleles, relative to the increase in the number of individuals with only one of the two alleles. The frequency of the haplotype consisting of the two synergistic alleles will therefore be increased to above its equilibrium value.

Another important mechanism that can lead to linkage disequilibrium is population admixture and stratification. When a population consists of two or more subgroups which, for geographical or cultural reasons, have evolved more or less separately for many generations, two loci that are in linkage equilibrium in every subgroup may be in linkage disequilibrium for the population as a whole. This phenomenon can be regarded as a special case of Simpson's paradox, which is defined as the observation that a measure of association between two variables (e.g. the degree of linkage disequilibrium between two loci) may be identical within the levels of a third variable (e.g. population subgroup), but can take on an entirely different value when the third variable is disregarded, and the association measure calculated from the pooled data (Everitt, 1995). For this phenomenon to arise the population subgroups must show some variability in the allele frequencies of the two loci. If there is a positive correlation in the frequencies of two alleles in the population subgroups, then the two alleles will appear to be positively associated in the population as a whole.

Example 4.3
Consider three populations that have reached linkage equilibrium with respect to the alleles A and B. Suppose that the population size (N), the frequency of allele A, the frequency of allele B, and the frequency of the haplotype AB are as follows.

N	A	B	AB
1 000	0.3	0.5	0.15
2 000	0.2	0.4	0.08
10 000	0.05	0.1	0.005

If these three populations are merged to form one single population, what will be the allele and haplotype frequencies in this new population, before any interbreeding takes place? Do these frequencies represent linkage equilibrium?

The frequencies in the new population are weighted averages of the frequencies in the original populations. Thus

$$P(A) = [0.3(1000) + 0.2(2000) + 0.05(10\ 000)]/13\ 000 = 0.0923$$

$$P(B) = [0.5(1000) + 0.4(2000) + 0.1(10\ 000)]/13\ 000 = 0.1770$$

$$P(AB) = [0.15(1000) + 0.08(2000) + 0.005(10\ 000)]/13\ 000 = 0.0277$$

The equilibrium frequency of AB is $(0.0923)(0.1770) = 0.0163$. Alleles A and B are therefore positively associated in the new population.

The state of allelic associations in a population at a given time is therefore the result of the complex interplay between many aspects of the evolutionary history of the population. Unless the evolutionary history of a population is known in great detail, it is impossible to construct an adequate statistical model for the linkage disequilibrium between pairs of loci in the population. It is therefore seldom possible to use data on the present state of linkage disequilibrium in the population for making precise inferences about parameters such as recombination fraction, effective population size and mutation rate, except for some unusually well characterized populations. However, it is generally accepted that, for most human populations and for most regions of the genome, substantial linkage disequilibrium is only likely to occur between loci with a recombination fraction of less than 1%. This is the rationale behind the use of association analysis as a tool for the fine mapping of disease genes.

4.4   Association analysis as a tool for fine mapping

Linkage analysis is a powerful tool for detecting the presence of a disease locus in a chromosomal region. However, it is not very efficient for fine mapping, since the discrimination between small differences in recombination frequency requires data on a large number of informative gametes. For instance, observing no recombinant in 50 fully informative gametes suggests a recombination fraction of 0, but it is also not incompatible with a recombination fraction of up to 5%. This problem is compounded for complex disorders, where individual recombinant gametes cannot be identified with certainty. Fortunately, linkage analysis can be followed up by association analysis for the fine mapping of disease loci. This approach was described by Bodmer (1986) succinctly as follows.

Then, knowing where this (a marker locus linked to the disease) is in the genome, it should be possible to saturate the relevant region with further polymorphic markers and look for the one that has a population association with the trait, rather than increasing the number of families analysed to search for close linkage. This is the most efficient way of finding closely linked markers, since family data are very inefficient at distinguishing between small recombination fractions such as 0.5% versus 5%.

The basis of this approach is that, for most human populations, appreciable allelic associations are only likely to exist between loci with recombination fractions of less than 1%. The detection of allelic associations between two loci therefore constitutes evidence that they are in tight linkage. However, as we have shown earlier, allelic associations can occur between loosely linked or even unlinked loci in the presence of a founder effect or population admixture and stratification. These causes of allelic associations other than tight linkage must be taken into consideration in the design, analysis and interpretation of allelic association studies.

4.5   Association analysis using a random population sample

There are several popular study designs for allelic association studies. The appropriate design for a particular situation depends on the nature of the loci under investigation. The simplest design is to take a random sample of the population. This is appropriate when the alleles of interest are common in the population. Since many disease-predisposing alleles are rare, this approach is most applicable to the investigation of allelic associations between two marker loci.

4.5.1   Association between two codominant markers

The testing of linkage disequilibrium between two codominant autosomal loci is a simple situation where the numerical procedure can be described in some detail. Moreover, the test is useful for confirming the physical proximity of two marker loci (although nowadays this is often better achieved by physical mapping methods), and for obtaining some idea of the range of genetic distances over which linkage disequilibrium is likely to be appreciable in a population.

Suppose that the autosomal marker loci A and B, with alleles $A_1, A_2, ..., A_m$ and $B_1, B_2, ..., B_n$, have been typed in a random sample of the population. Each individual will have a genotype of the form $A_iA_jB_kB_l$. There are $m(m+1)/2$ possible genotypes at locus A, and $n(n+1)/2$ possible genotypes at locus B, so that the total number of joint genotypes is $[m(m+1)/2][n(n+1)/2]$. The genotypic data from the sample consist of the counts of these $[m(m+1)/2]$ $[n(n+1)/2]$ joint genotypes, which can be arranged in a two-dimensional contingency table. Let the count of genotype $A_iA_jB_kB_l$ be denoted as n_{ijkl}, then for two biallelic loci the data can be represented as follows

Locus A	Locus B			
	B_1B_1	B_1B_2	B_2B_2	Total
A_1A_1	n_{1111}	n_{1112}	n_{1122}	$n_{11..}$
A_1A_2	n_{1211}	n_{1212}	n_{1222}	$n_{12..}$
A_2A_2	n_{2211}	n_{2212}	n_{2222}	$n_{22..}$
Total	$n_{..11}$	$n_{..12}$	$n_{..22}$	$n_{....}$

Let the population frequency of the haplotype $A_i B_k$ be h_{ik}. The aim of the analysis is to estimate the m allele frequencies of A (denoted as $p_1, p_2, ..., p_m$) the n allele frequencies of B (denoted as $q_1, q_2, ..., q_n$), the mn haplotype frequencies of A and B (denoted as $h_{11}, h_{12}, ..., h_m$), and the genotype frequencies of A and B (denoted as $g_{1111}, g_{1112}, ..., g_{mmnn}$), as well as to test the null hypothesis of linkage equilibrium between A and B.

The genotypic counts $n_{1111}, n_{1112}, ..., n_{mmnn}$ follow a multinominal distribution with parameters $n_{...}$ (the sample size) and the genotypic frequencies $g_{1111}, g_{1112}, ..., g_{mmnn}$. The log-likelihood of the data is therefore

$$\ln L = \sum n_{ijkl} \ln(g_{ijkl}) \tag{4.6}$$

where the summation is taken over all $[m(m+1)/2][n(n+1)/2]$ possible genotypes. The maximum likelihood estimate of a population genotype frequency is simply the sample genotype frequency, i.e.

$$\hat{g}_{ijkl} = n_{ijkl}/n_{...} \tag{4.7}$$

for all $[m(m+1)/2][n(n+1)/2]$ genotypes. Substituting these maximum likelihood estimates of the genotype frequencies into the log-likelihood function gives the log-likelihood of the full or saturated model, which we denote as $\ln L_2$. The simplest submodel of this full model is one where the genotypes are assumed to be produced by the random union of alleles. In this case, the two loci will be in Hardy–Weinberg equilibrium as well as in linkage equilibrium. The frequency of a joint genotype is then equal to the product of the genotype frequencies of the two loci under Hardy–Weinberg equilibrium, i.e.

$$\left. \begin{aligned}
g_{iikk} &= p_i p_i q_k q_k = p_i^2 q_k^2 \\
g_{iikl} &= p_i p_i q_k q_l + p_i p_i q_l q_k = 2p_i^2 q_k q_l \\
g_{ijkk} &= p_i p_j q_k q_k + p_j p_i q_k q_k = 2p_i p_j q_k^2 \\
g_{ijkl} &= p_i p_j q_k q_l + p_i p_j q_l q_k + p_j p_i q_k q_l + p_j p_i q_l q_k = 4p_i p_j q_k q_l
\end{aligned} \right\} \tag{4.8}$$

for $i \neq j$ and $k \neq l$. The maximum likelihood estimate of a population allele frequency is simply the sample allele frequency, i.e. the proportion of individuals homozygous for the allele plus half the proportion of individuals heterozygous for the allele. Substitution of the maximum likelihood estimates of allele frequencies into the above formulae gives estimates of genotype frequencies that are constrained by the hypothesis of random union of alleles (i.e. the joint hypothesis of linkage equilibrium and random mating). When these constrained genotype frequency estimates are substituted into the log-likelihood function, a value of the log-likelihood is obtained which we denote as $\ln L_0$. Since the saturated model log-likelihood $\ln L_2$ is associated with $[m(m+1)/2][n(n+1)/2] - 1$ estimated parameters, and the submodel log-likelihood $\ln L_0$ is associated with $(m-1)+(n-1)$ parameters, the test statistic $2(\ln L_2 - \ln L_0)$ has asymptotically a chi-squared distribution with $[m(m+1)/2][n(n+1)/2] - (m+n) + 1$ degrees of freedom. This provides a test for the joint hypothesis of linkage equilibrium and random mating.

In order to test the hypothesis of linkage equilibrium under the assumption of random mating, it is necessary to consider a model intermediate between the saturated model and the simplest model. This model places no restriction on haplotype frequencies, but assumes that genotypes are produced by the random union of haplotypes. The expressions for the genotype frequencies therefore become

$$
\left.
\begin{aligned}
g_{iikk} &= h_{ik}h_{ik}h_{ik}^2 \\
g_{ijkl} &= h_{ik}h_{il} + h_{il}h_{ik} = 2h_{il}h_{ik} \\
g_{ijkk} &= h_{ik}h_{jk} + h_{jk}h_{ik} = 2h_{ik}h_{jk} \\
g_{ijkl} &= h_{ik}h_{jl} + h_{jl}h_{ik} + h_{il}h_{jk} + h_{jk}h_{il} = 2(h_{ik}h_{jl} + h_{il}h_{jk})
\end{aligned}
\right\}
\tag{4.9}
$$

for $i \neq j$ and $k \neq l$. If the maximum likelihood estimates of the haplotype frequencies are available, then these values can be substituted into the above expressions to obtain estimates of genotype frequencies constrained only by random mating. Substitution of these estimated genotype frequencies into the log-likelihood function gives a value which we denote as $\ln L_1$, associated with $mn - 1$ estimated parameters (since there are mn haplotype frequencies which sum to 1). The test statistic $2(\ln L_1 - \ln L_0)$ has asymptotically a chi-squared distribution with $(mn - 1) - [(m - 1) + (n - 1)] = (m - 1)(n - 1)$ degrees of freedom. This provides a test of linkage equilibrium under the assumption of random mating.

Unlike the genotype and the allele frequencies, however, the population haplotype frequencies cannot be estimated by simple counting. This is because the haplotypes present in an individual heterozygous for both loci cannot be deduced from the individual's genotype. Thus, the genotype $A_iA_jB_kB_l$ can be made up of the haplotypes A_iB_k and A_jB_l, or the haplotypes A_iB_l and A_jB_k. It is therefore not possible simply to count the number of heterozygous haplotypes present in a sample. Instead, it is necessary to use an iterative method of counting based on the EM algorithm.

The only problematic genotypes for haplotype counting are those where both loci are heterozygous. The count of the genotype $A_iA_jB_kB_l$ (denoted as n_{ijkl}) can be considered as the sum of two unobserved counts, i.e. the number of individuals with the haplotype combination of A_iB_k and A_jB_l (denoted as $n_{ik,jl}$), and the number of individuals with the haplotype combination A_iB_l and A_jB_k (denoted as $n_{il,jk}$). The EM algorithm begins by setting starting values for the haplotype frequencies, including $h_{ik,0}, h_{il,0}, h_{jk,0}, h_{jl,0}$. It is reasonable to set the initial haplotype frequencies as the products of the relevant allele frequencies. These initial haplotype frequencies are used to find the initial expected values of the unobserved counts. For example

$$
\left.
\begin{aligned}
n_{i,k,jl,0} &= \frac{n_{ijkl}(h_{ik,0}h_{jl,0})}{h_{ik,0}h_{jl,0} + h_{il,0}h_{jk,0}} \\[2ex]
n_{il,jk,0} &= \frac{n_{ijkl}(h_{il,0}h_{jk,0})}{h_{ik,0}h_{jl,0} + h_{il,0}h_{jk,0}}
\end{aligned}
\right\}
\tag{4.10}
$$

The initial expected values are then regarded as real data that allow the number of heterozygous haplotypes in the entire sample to be counted, including those in non-problematic genotypes with at least one homozygous locus. The sample frequencies of the haplotypes calculated from these counts are then used as a set of revised haplotype frequencies, which are denoted as $h_{ik,1}$, $h_{il,1}$, $h_{jk,1}$, $h_{jl,1}$, etc. These revised haplotype frequencies are used to obtain a set of revised expected values of the unobserved counts, which are denoted as $n_{ik,jl,1}$ and $n_{il,jk,1}$, etc. The cycle of revising the haplotype frequencies, revising the expected values of the unobserved counts, and counting the haplotypes is repeated until the changes in haplotype frequencies from one iteration to the next become negligible. These are then the maximum likelihood estimates of the haplotype frequencies.

This method of testing for allelic associations between two codominant loci has been implemented in a computer program called EH (Terwilliger and Ott, 1994). This program produces an output that displays $\ln L_0$ and $\ln L_1$, as well as the chi-squared statistic $2(\ln L_1 - \ln L_0)$ and its associated degrees of freedom. The method can be generalized to deal with three or more markers. The EH program computes a likelihood ratio test that compares a model where all marker loci are in linkage disequilibrium (i.e. when the frequencies of the haplotypes containing alleles are unconstrained) with one where all marker loci are in linkage equilibrium (i.e. when the frequencies of the haplotypes are constrained to be equal to the products of the frequencies of the constituent alleles). The method can also be generalized for two X-linked loci, which is in some sense simpler because haplotypes can be counted directly in males.

Since $\ln L_1$ and $\ln L_0$ are both calculated under the assumption of random mating, the above test based on $2(\ln L_1 - \ln L_0)$ is, strictly speaking, only appropriate for populations under random mating. One might wonder whether it would be possible to construct an alternative test for linkage disequilibrium allowing for non-random mating. This would involve calculating the likelihood of a model assuming linkage equilibrium under non-random mating, and comparing this with the likelihood of the saturated model. Unfortunately, because of the indeterminacy of haplotypes in doubly heterozygous individuals, a model allowing for non-random mating (whether in linkage equilibrium or not) is always able to produce a perfect fit to the observed genotype counts. This leaves no degree of freedom to test for linkage disequilibrium. There is therefore no alternative to testing for linkage disequilibrium under the assumption of random mating, when the only data available are derived from a random sample of unrelated individuals in the population. The results from such an analysis must therefore be interpreted with caution, especially if there is evidence of deviation from Hardy–Weinberg equilibrium at either locus, or if the likelihood ratio test for non-random union between haplotypes, i.e. $2(\ln L_2 - \ln L_1)$, is significant.

Example 4.4

To illustrate the application of the EM algorithm to the estimation of haplotype frequencies, consider the following contingency table of genotype data on two biallelic loci

Locus A	Locus B			
	BB	Bb	bb	Total
AA	10	15	5	30
Aa	10	50	13	73
aa	3	13	10	26
Total	23	78	28	129

The allele frequencies are

$$p(A) = (30 + 73/2)/129 = 0.5155$$
$$p(a) = (26 + 73/2)/129 = 0.4845$$
$$p(B) = (23 + 78/2)/129 = 0.4806$$
$$p(b) = (28 + 78/2)/129 = 0.5194$$

The haplotype frequencies are

$$p(AB) = [2(10) + 15 + 10 + 50x]/[129(2)]$$
$$p(Ab) = [15 + 2(5) + 50(1 - x) + 13]/[129(2)]$$
$$p(aB) = [50x + 3 + 13 + 28(2)]/[129(2)]$$
$$p(ab) = [50(1 - x) + 13 + 13 + 10(2)]/[129(2)]$$

where x is the unknown proportion of genotypes AaBb that are AB/ab rather than Ab/aB. The problem is to estimate the four haplotype frequencies despite not knowing the value x. Using the EM algorithm, the first step is to obtain some initial values for the haplotype frequencies. It seems sensible to choose the products of the allele frequencies.

$$p_0(AB) = (0.5155)(0.4806) = 0.24776$$
$$p_0(Ab) = (0.5155)(0.5194) = 0.26774$$
$$p_0(aB) = (0.4845)(0.4806) = 0.23285$$
$$p_0(ab) = (0.4845)(0.5194) = 0.25163$$

The 'expected' value of x, given these haplotype frequencies, is

$$x_0 = (0.24776)(0.25163)/[(0.24776)(0.25163) + (0.26774)(0.23285)] = 0.50000$$

Substituting this x_0 into the haplotype frequencies yields

$$p_1(AB) = [2(10) + 15 + 10 + 50x]/[129(2)] = 0.27131$$
$$p_1(Ab) = [15 + 2(5) + 50(1 - x) + 13]/[129(2)] = 0.24418$$
$$p_1(aB) = [50x + 3 + 13 + 28(2)]/[129(2)] = 0.20930$$
$$p_1(ab) = [50(1 - x) + 13 + 13 + 10(2)]/[129(2)] = 0.27519$$

The 'expected' value of x, given these revised haplotype frequencies, is then

$$x_1 = (0.27131)(0.27519)/[(0.27131)(0.27519) + (0.24418)(0.20930)]$$
$$= 0.406354$$

This process of revising the haplotype frequencies and x in turn is repeated until haplotype frequencies do not change appreciably from one cycle to another.

Iteration	P(AB)	P(Ab)	P(aB)	P(ab)	x
0	0.24776	0.26774	0.23285	0.25163	0.500002
1	0.27131	0.24418	0.20930	0.27519	0.406354
2	0.28946	0.22603	0.19115	0.29334	0.337244
3	0.30285	0.21264	0.17776	0.30673	0.289214
4	0.31216	0.20333	0.16845	0.31604	0.257710
5	0.31827	0.19723	0.16234	0.32214	0.237974
6	0.32209	0.19340	0.15852	0.32597	0.226008
7	0.32441	0.19108	0.15620	0.32829	0.218906
8	0.32579	0.18971	0.15482	0.32966	0.214746
9	0.32659	0.18890	0.15402	0.33047	0.212328
10	0.32706	0.18843	0.15355	0.33094	0.210932
11	0.32733	0.18816	0.15328	0.33121	0.210124
12	0.32749	0.18800	0.15312	0.33137	0.209660
13	0.32758	0.18791	0.15303	0.33146	0.209394
14	0.32763	0.18786	0.15298	0.33151	0.209240
15	0.32766	0.18783	0.15295	0.33154	0.209152
16	0.32768	0.18782	0.15293	0.33155	0.209100
17	0.32769	0.18781	0.15292	0.33156	0.209072
18	0.32769	0.18780	0.15292	0.33157	0.209056
19	0.32770	0.18780	0.15291	0.33157	0.209046
20	0.32770	0.18779	0.15291	0.33158	0.209040
21	0.32770	0.18779	0.15291	0.33158	0.209036
22	0.32770	0.18779	0.15291	0.33158	0.209034
23	0.32770	0.18779	0.15291	0.33158	0.209034

The EM algorithm has therefore converged to the haplotype frequencies of

$$P(AB) = 0.32770$$

$$P(Ab) = 0.18779$$

$$P(aB) = 0.15291$$

$$P(ab) = 0.33158$$

Incidentally, for the saturated model with eight estimated parameters (nine genotype frequencies which sum to 1), the log-likelihood is

$$\ln L_2 = -243.58$$

For the random mating, linkage disequilibrium model with three estimated parameters (three haplotype frequencies which sum to 1), the log-likelihood is

$$\ln L_1 = -248.23$$

For the random mating, linkage equilibrium model with two estimated parameters (two allele frequencies which sum to 1, per locus), the log-likelihood is

$$\ln L_0 = -252.68$$

Thus

$$2(\ln L_2 - \ln L_1) = 9.40, \text{df} = 5, p = 0.09$$

$$2(\ln L_1 - \ln L_0) = 8.89, \text{df} = 1, p = 0.003$$

There is thus suggestive evidence for linkage disequilibrium between the two loci but no evidence for non-random mating.

4.6 Association analysis using a case-control design

The most popular design for studying allelic associations between a disease and a marker is to compare a set of cases with a set of controls collected from the same population. Marker alleles that are positively associated with the disease are analogous to risk factors in epidemiology. However, the methods of analysis do differ slightly from standard epidemiological methods, depending on the nature of the disorder and marker.

4.6.1 Association between a simple disorder and a marker

The use of association analysis for the fine mapping of a disease locus depends on the fact that the genotype (and allele) frequencies at the disease locus are different between affected and unaffected individuals in the population. If a marker locus is in linkage disequilibrium with the disease locus, then the marker locus will also differ in genotype (and allele) frequencies between affected and unaffected individuals in the population.

In order to demonstrate these effects quantitatively, let the low and high risk alleles at a disease locus D be denoted as D_1 and D_2, with population frequencies p_1 and p_2. Let the conditional probabilities of disease given the three genotypes D_1D_1, D_1D_2 and D_2D_2 (i.e. the penetrances) be f_{11}, f_{12} and f_{22}. The population prevalence of the disease, assuming Hardy–Weinberg equilibrium, is

$$K = p_1^2 f_{11} + 2p_1 p_2 f_{12} + p_2^2 f_{22} \tag{4.11}$$

The genotype frequencies at the disease locus among affected individuals (A) in the population are then

$$\left. \begin{aligned} P(D_1 D_1 | A) &= \frac{p_1^2 f_{11}}{K} \\[2mm] P(D_1 D_2 | A) &= \frac{2p_1 p_2 f_{12}}{K} \\[2mm] P(D_2 D_2 | A) &= \frac{p_2^2 f_{22}}{K} \end{aligned} \right\} \tag{4.12}$$

Similarly, defining $s_{11} = 1 - f_{11}$, $s_{12} = 1 - f_{12}$, $s_{22} = 1 - f_{22}$, and $Q = 1 - K$ the genotype frequencies at the disease locus among unaffected individuals (U) in the population are

$$
\left.
\begin{aligned}
P(D_1 D_1 | U) &= \frac{p_1^2 \, s_{11}}{Q} \\[2mm]
P(D_1 D_2 | U) &= \frac{2 p_1 p_2 \, s_{12}}{Q} \\[2mm]
P(D_2 D_2 | U) &= \frac{p_2^2 \, s_{22}}{Q}
\end{aligned}
\right\}
\tag{4.13}
$$

These expressions quantify the differences in genotype frequencies at the disease locus between affected and unaffected individuals in the population. From the genotype frequencies, the allele frequencies at the disease locus among affected and unaffected individuals in the population can be calculated as

$$
\left.
\begin{aligned}
P(D_1 | A) &= \frac{p_1^2 f_{11} + p_1 p_2 f_{12}}{K} \\[2mm]
P(D_2 | A) &= \frac{p_2^2 f_{22} + p_1 p_2 f_{12}}{K} \\[2mm]
P(D_1 | U) &= \frac{p_1^2 s_{11} + p_1 p_2 s_{12}}{Q} \\[2mm]
P(D_2 | U) &= \frac{p_2^2 s_{22} + p_1 p_2 s_{12}}{Q}
\end{aligned}
\right\}
\tag{4.14}
$$

These expressions quantify the differences between the allele frequencies at the disease locus between affected and unaffected individuals in the population.

Now consider a marker locus B with alleles $B_1, B_2, \ldots, B_n$, with allele frequencies $q_1, q_2, \ldots, q_n$. Let the haplotype frequencies of loci D and B be $h_{11}, h_{12}, \ldots, h_{1n}, h_{21}, h_{22}, \ldots, h_{2n}$. The conditional probabilities of affection, given a marker genotype, assuming random mating, are

$$
\left.
\begin{aligned}
P(A | B_i B_i) &= \frac{f_{11} h_{1i}^2 + f_{12}(2 h_{1i} h_{2i}) + f_{22} h_{2i}^2}{q_i^2} \\[3mm]
P(A | B_i B_j) &= \frac{f_{11}(2 h_{1i} h_{1j}) + f_{12}(2 h_{1i} h_{2j} + 2 h_{1j} h_{2i}) + f_{22}(2 h_{2i} h_{2j})}{2 q_i q_j}
\end{aligned}
\right\}
\tag{4.15}
$$

for $i \neq j$. These conditional probabilities can be thought of as the 'apparent penetrances' of the marker genotypes. The genotype frequencies at locus B among affected and unaffected individuals in the population, assuming random mating, are

$$P(B_i B_i | A) = \frac{f_{11} h_{1i}^2 + f_{12} (2 h_{1i} h_{2i}) + f_{22} h_{2i}^2}{K}$$

$$P(B_i B_j | A) = \frac{f_{11} (2 h_{1i} h_{1j}) + f_{12} (2 h_{1i} h_{2j} + 2 h_{1j} h_{2i}) + f_{22} (2 h_{2i} h_{2j})}{K}$$

$$P(B_i B_i | U) = \frac{s_{11} h_{1i}^2 + s_{12} (2 h_{1i} h_{2i}) + s_{22} h_{2i}^2}{Q}$$

$$P(B_i B_j | U) = \frac{s_{11} (2 h_{1i} h_{1j}) + s_{12} (2 h_{1i} h_{2j} + 2 h_{1j} h_{2i}) + s_{22} (2 h_{2i} h_{2j})}{Q}$$

$$(4.16)$$

for $i \neq j$. These expressions quantify the differences in genotype frequencies at the marker locus between affected and unaffected individuals in the population. These differences can be shown to be 0 if the disease and marker loci are in linkage equilibrium, i.e. $h_{1i} = p_1 q_i$, for $i = 1, \ldots, n$.

The allele frequencies $P(B_1 | A), P(B_2 | A), \ldots, P(B_n | A)$ among affected individuals are weighted sums of the genotype frequencies $P(B_1 B_1 | A)$, $P(B_1 B_2 | A), \ldots, P(B_n B_n | A)$, where the weight is 1 if the genotype is homozygous for the allele being considered, $1/2$ if the genotype contains one copy of the allele being considered and one copy of some other allele, and 0 if the genotype does not contain the allele being considered. The allele frequencies among unaffected individuals can be calculated from the genotype frequencies $P(B_1 B_1 | U), P(B_1 B_2 | U), \ldots, P(B_n B_n | U)$ in a similar fashion. These allele frequencies will be different from those in affected individuals unless the marker locus is in linkage equilibrium with the disease locus.

These results show that differences between genotype or allele frequencies between affected and unaffected individuals in a population can arise from linkage disequilibrium between disease and marker loci. Since most diseases affect a small proportion of the population, a simple random sample of the population will contain far more unaffected than affected individuals, and it is more efficient to study a random sample of affected individuals (the cases) and a random sample of unaffected individuals (the controls). The data from such a case-control study will consist of the counts of the various possible marker genotypes in the cases and in the controls. How the data should be analysed depends on how much is known about the mode of inheritance of the disease.

For Mendelian diseases, the parameters p_1, p_2, f_{11}, f_{12} and f_{22} are usually known to a high degree of precision. It is therefore possible to express the likelihood of the data (i.e. the two sets of $n(n + 1)/2$ genotype counts) in terms of these fixed parameters and the $2n$ haplotype frequencies, under the assumption of random mating. This likelihood function can be maximized with respect to these $2n$ haplotype frequencies, with and without the constraints imposed by linkage equilibrium. Without the constraints of linkage equilibrium, the $2n$ haplotype frequencies represent $2n - 2$ free parameters (because the frequencies of the haplotypes containing D_1 must sum to p_1, and the frequencies of the haplotypes containing D_2 must sum to p_2). Linkage equilibrium implies that the $2n$ haplotype frequencies are the products of the two fixed disease allele frequencies and the n unknown marker allele frequencies, so that the number of free parameters is $n - 1$. If the unconstrained and constrained log-likelihoods are denoted as $\ln L_1$ and $\ln L_0$, then the likelihood ratio statistic $2(\ln L_1 - \ln L_0)$ has a chi-squared distribution with $(2n - 2) - (n - 1) = n - 1$ degrees of freedom, and can be used as a test for linkage disequilibrium. The maximization of the likelihood function can be achieved by a modification of the iterative counting algorithm for two codominant loci that take account of the specified parameters $p_1, p_2, f_{11}, f_{12}, f_{22}$ and the case-control sampling scheme (Terwilliger and Ott, 1994). This method can be generalized to deal with two or more marker loci simultaneously. In the EH program, linkage disequilibrium between a disease and a set of marker loci is assessed by a likelihood ratio test comparing a model that assumes linkage disequilibrium between all loci (disease and markers) with a model that assumes disequilibrium between the marker loci but equilibrium between the marker loci and the disease locus (Terwilliger and Ott, 1994).

Example 4.5
A case-control study with two biallelic markers was conducted on a rare autosomal recessive disorder population risk of 0.00001. The results are as follows.

| | Marker 1 | | | | | |
| | Case | | | Control | | |
Marker 2	1/1	1/2	2/2	1/1	1/2	2/2
1/1	0	3	25	0	1	28
1/2	2	45	1	0	16	1
2/2	16	3	0	7	1	0

Using EH, we specify the case-control option, with disease gene frequency 0.001 (the square root of the population risk) and penetrances $0, 0, 1$ (recessive). The output is as follows.

Estimates of gene frequencies (assuming independence)
(Disease gene frequencies are user specified)

| Locus | Allele | |
	1	2
Disease	0.9990	0.0010
1	0.6007	0.3993
2	0.3993	0.6007

# of typed Individuals: 149

There are eight possible haplotypes of these three loci. They are listed below, with their estimated frequencies (H_0, no association; H_1, markers associated, independent of disease; H_2, markers and disease associated).

Allele at disease	Allele at marker 1	Allele at marker 2	Haplotype frequency		
			H_0	H_1	H_2
+	1	1	0.239625	0.020505	0.009391
+	1	2	0.360445	0.579565	0.684507
+	2	1	0.159304	0.378424	0.286453
+	2	2	0.239625	0.020505	0.018649
D	1	1	0.000240	0.000021	0.000027
D	1	2	0.000361	0.000580	0.000520
D	2	1	0.000159	0.000379	0.000431
D	2	2	0.000240	0.000021	0.000022

# of iterations = 2

	df	Ln(L)	Chi-square
H_0	2	−308.07	0.00
H_1	3	−199.80	216.53
H_2	6	−195.68	224.79

The likelihood ratio chi-squared for H_1 versus H_0 of 216.53 on one degree of freedom is highly significant, meaning that the two marker loci are in disequilibrium with each other. Inspection of the first and second columns of estimated haplotype frequencies reveals that allele 1 at locus 1 is positively associated with allele 2 at locus 2.

The likelihood ratio chi-squared for H_2 versus H_1 of 8.26 on three degrees of freedom is only marginally significant $(P = 0.04)$. Thus there is only weak evidence for linkage disequilibrium between the disease and the marker system.

4.6.2   Association between a complex disorder and a marker

When the mode of inheritance of the disease is unknown, the values of p_1, p_2, f_{11}, f_{12} and f_{22} cannot be specified with certainty. There are several possible approaches for dealing with this problem. The most popular approach is to ignore the complexities of the underlying genetic model, and treat the data as an ordinary contingency table. The counts of the n alleles in the cases and controls can be represented in an $n \times 2$ contingency table; the statistical significance of the differences between allele frequencies can be assessed by a Pearson (or likelihood ratio) chi-squared test of homogeneity of proportions, with $n - 1$ degrees of freedom. Note that the overall total in such a contingency table of alleles is twice the number of individuals in the sample, as each individual contributes two alleles to the table.

In addition to comparing allele frequencies, investigators sometimes also compare genotype frequencies. Since there are $n(n + 1)/2$ possible genotypes, the data can be represented in a table with $n(n + 1)/2$ rows and 2 columns. A standard chi-squared test of homogeneity of proportions, with $[n(n + 1)/2] - 1$ degrees of freedom, can then be performed. Since the number of degrees of freedom increases more rapidly than the number of alleles, the test is only attractive for small values of n (i.e. 2 or 3). The overall total of the contingency table is equal to the sample size, as each individual contributes one genotype.

When two or more tightly linked loci are considered simultaneously for linkage disequilibrium with a complex disease, then the testing for unequal allele frequencies can be replaced by the testing for unequal haplotype frequencies, between cases and controls. This is a direct generalization, since a single allele can be thought of as a haplotype of a single locus. The relevant likelihood ratio test compares a model where two separate sets of haplotype frequencies apply to the cases and controls, to one where the entire sample is characterized by a single common set of haplotype frequencies. The procedure is, however, complicated by the indeterminacy of the haplotypes in individuals heterozygous for two or more loci. Fortunately, the problem can be conveniently overcome by repeated uses of the EH program. First, the program is used on the cases to obtain a set of haplotype frequency estimates, and the corresponding log-likelihood ($\ln L_{case}$). Then it is repeated on the controls to obtain a separate set of haplotype frequency estimates, and a corresponding log-likelihood ($\ln L_{control}$). Finally it is performed on the entire sample to obtain a set of overall haplotype frequency estimates, and the corresponding log-likelihood ($\ln L_{combined}$). The test statistic $2(\ln L_{case} + \ln L_{control} - \ln L_{combined})$ is then a chi-squared with $n-1$ degrees of freedom (where n is the number of haplotypes), and provides a test of heterogeneity in haplotype frequencies.

Example 4.6
Using EH to implement a chi-squared test of homogeneity of haplotype frequencies on the data in Example 4.5, we obtained log-likelihoods of -129.53, -66.15 and -199.80 for cases, controls and cases and controls combined. The chi-squared test statistic is therefore $2(-129.53 - 66.15 + 199.80) = 8.24$ with degree of freedom $= 3$, giving $P = 0.04$. These results are comparable to those obtained in Example 4.5.

There are advantages and disadvantages to the popular approach of testing for unequal allele or genotype frequencies between cases and controls. It is easy to implement, and requires no assumption about the mode of inheritance of the disease. Moreover, it can be generalized to take account of potential confounders, using standard epidemiological methods for case-control studies. Treating alleles or genotypes as risk factors, measures of associations such as odds ratios, relative risks and attributable fractions can be estimated. Samples from different countries or ethnicities can be subjected to stratified analysis (Woolf, 1955). When other potential confounders or effect-modifiers are present, logistic regression analysis can be used, with case-control status as the outcome variable, and genotypes and covariates (plus possible interactions) as predictor variables. However, in formulating the effect of genotype, it is necessary to make certain assumptions regarding the interactions between alleles. For example, a separate parameter can be assigned to each genotype or, more parsimoniously, to each allele (with the assumption that the effect of a genotype is determined additively by the alleles present). Assigning a separate parameter to each genotype will certainly increase the likelihood, but it also uses up more degrees of freedom.

It is possible to evaluate a series of models with different patterns of interactions between alleles (e.g. dominant, recessive, additive, etc) and choose one that optimizes goodness-of-fit and parsimony, but this introduces multiple testing which should be allowed for in assessing the statistical significance of the results. For a biallelic marker, dominant, recessive and additive models are easy to specify (e.g. an additive model is specified by assigning to the heterozygous genotype a value that is halfway between the values of the two homozygous genotypes), but the situation is more complex for markers with more than two alleles, since the number of possible dominance relations increases rapidly with the number of alleles. In this situation, it is usual to assign a main effect to each marker allele and to assume the absence of interactions.

Example 4.7
The following data are taken from a meta-analysis of 11 association studies on schizophrenia and a biallelic polymorphism in the dopamine D3 receptor gene (Shaikh *et al.*, 1996).

	Genotype counts					
	Cases			Controls		
Study	AA	Aa	aa	AA	Aa	aa
1	74	44	23	51	75	13
2	26	23	4	23	30	8
3	59	42	10	49	42	9
4	34	36	6	27	22	4
5	37	41	7	28	35	15
6	35	33	8	37	40	9
7	33	23	10	38	46	13
8	48	35	8	48	35	7
9	54	45	8	50	40	8
10	62	66	9	59	57	9
11	57	69	7	33	56	20

The first study suggested that homozygosity at the locus (i.e. genotypes AA and aa) increased susceptibility to schizophrenia. Subsequent studies suggested a recessive or an additive effect. The meta-analysis was performed by logistic regression, with case-control status as a dependent variable. The effect of genotype was coded in three ways to test for a homozygosity, recessive or gene-dosage effect, as follows.

Genotype	Homozygosity	Recessive	Additive
AA	1	1	1
Aa	0	0	0.5
aa	1	0	0

A number of models, each involving at most one of these genotype effects, was examined by logistic regression analysis using the GLIM program. The goodness-of-fit of each model was assessed by the scaled deviance (defined as twice the difference in log-likelihoods between the saturated model and the current model), and by the Akaike information criterion (AIC, defined as the scaled deviance minus twice the degrees of freedoms). The models examined, and their fit indices, were as follows.

K = Constant
C = Centre
H = Homozygosity
R = Recessive
A = Additive
CH = Centre homozygosity interaction
CR = Centre recessive interaction
CA = Centre additive interaction

Model	Scaled deviance	df	AIC
K	52.209	32	−11.791
K + H	49.332	31	−12.668
K + R	45.829	31	−16.171
K + A	45.731	31	−16.269
K + C	37.510	22	−6.490
K + C + H	34.298	21	−7.702
K + C + R	31.060	21	−10.940
K + C + A	31.296	21	−10.704
K + C + H + CH	18.224	11	−3.446
K + C + R + CR	20.860	11	−1.140
K + C + A + CA	20.431	11	−1.569

The best fitting model, according to AIC, was the additive model, followed closely by the recessive model. There is no evidence of heterogeneity between centres or interaction between genotype and centre. The significance of the additive model by the likelihood ratio test (chi-squared: $52.209 - 45.731 = 6.478$, one degree of freedom) is 0.01. At this level of significance, the evidence for an association between schizophrenia and this dopamine D3 polymorphism cannot be regarded as conclusive. Since the additive and the recessive models fit the data almost equally well, we present the odds ratio estimates for genotypes Aa and aa relative to genotype AA. These odds ratio estimates are 1.10 (95% confidence interval $0.82 - 1.48$) and 1.35 (95% confidence interval $1.00 - 1.81$), respectively.

If the study population is considered sufficiently homogeneous that the absence of potential confounding variables can be assumed, then it is reasonable to adopt a likelihood approach to tackle the problem of markers with more than two alleles. The probabilities of the case-control genotype data, under the disease locus parameters $(p_1, p_2, f_{11}, f_{12}, f_{22})$ and the haplotype frequencies $(h_{11}, h_{12}, ..., h_{1n}, h_{21}, h_{22}, ..., h_{2n})$, as stated in Equation

(4.16), are

$$
\left.
\begin{aligned}
P(B_i B_i | A) &= \frac{f_{11} h_{1i}^2 + f_{12}(2h_{1i} h_{2i}) + f_{22} h_{2i}^2}{K} \\[2mm]
P(B_i B_j | A) &= \frac{f_{11}(2h_{1i} h_{1j}) + f_{12}(2h_{1i} h_{2j} + 2h_{1j} h_{2i}) + f_{22}(2h_{2i} h_{2j})}{K} \\[2mm]
P(B_i B_i | U) &= \frac{s_{11} h_{1i}^2 + s_{12}(2h_{1i} h_{2i}) + s_{22} h_{2i}^2}{Q} \\[2mm]
P(B_i B_j | U) &= \frac{s_{11}(2h_{1i} h_{1j}) + s_{12}(2h_{1i} h_{2j} + 2h_{1j} h_{2i}) + s_{22}(2h_{2i} h_{2j})}{Q}
\end{aligned}
\right\}
\qquad (4.17)
$$

The overall likelihood function is the product of such probabilities, one for each observed genotype. In principle, the log-likelihood function can be maximized with respect to the disease locus parameters ($p_1, p_2, f_{11}, f_{12}, f_{22}, s_{11}, s_{12}, s_{22}$) and the haplotype frequencies ($h_{11}, h_{12}, \ldots, h_{1n}, h_{21}, h_{22}, \ldots, h_{2n}$), with and without the constraints implied by linkage equilibrium, to obtain the log-likelihoods $\ln L_0$ (assuming linkage equilibrium) and $\ln L_1$ (not assuming linkage equilibrium). The likelihood ratio statistic $2(\ln L_1 - \ln L_0)$ provides a test for linkage disequilibrium, although its asymptotic distribution is unclear since under linkage equilibrium the marker genotype provides no information about the disease locus model (and so the likelihood is independent of the nuisance parameters $p_1, p_2, f_{11}, f_{12}, f_{22}$). As well as this theoretical difficulty, there is no currently available computer program to implement the method. A similar approach was suggested by Risch (1983), but the emphasis was on inferring the mode of inheritance of the disease rather than on testing for linkage disequilibrium.

To our knowledge, no current method is able to model explicitly both potential confounding variables (i.e. population stratification, etc) and the unknown mode of inheritance (i.e. penetrances), when testing for allelic associations between disease and markers in a case-control design. It is possible that the additional power to be gained by such an approach over the more simplistic logistic regression method (which allows for potential confounding variables but simplifies the treatment of interactions between marker alleles) is not sufficiently large in most situations to warrant the additional complexities involved.

4.6.3 Association analysis between a disease and highly polymorphic marker loci

Modern DNA markers may have 20 or more alleles, and so it is not uncommon for the contingency table of allele counts produced from an exploratory case-control study to have many rows, some of which may contain very few observations. The problem is even more severe for contingency tables with genotype counts, as n alleles lead to $n(n+1)/2$ possible genotypes. It is commonly accepted that the chi-squared statistic produced from such a sparse table may not conform well to the asymptotic distribution. It may also happen that while there is no overall significant deviation from random distribution of alleles, one particular allele does appear to exhibit a marked deviation which, if taken on its own, would be considered statistically significant. These problems have led to a variety of different methods of analysis being applied to case-control data.

One common approach is to group rare alleles together. For example one might systematically merge rows containing small numbers of observations until the expected count for each cell is at least 5. This will ensure the validity of the chi-squared test, but may result in a substantial reduction in power, since positively and negatively associated alleles may be grouped together, cancelling out the effects of each other.

Another common approach is to consider each common allele individually against the rest, yielding up to n comparisons each based on a 2×2 table. This should result in chi-squared tests that are individually valid, but taking the most significant of these tests is a form of multiple testing and requires an adjustment to be made, or else there will be an increase in the false positive rate. If, for example, r comparisons are made and the smallest P-value obtained is p, then an adjusted P-value is given by

$$p^* = 1 - (1 - p)^r \tag{4.18}$$

For small values of p this is approximately equal to rp, the Bonferroni adjusted significance level. Although this procedure is commonly used, it concentrates on just one comparison and ignores information from the other, less significant comparisons. This may reduce the power to detect an overall difference in allele frequencies if two or more marker alleles are positively associated with the disease.

Another way of evaluating the significance of a sparse contingency table is to calculate a standard Pearson chi-squared statistic and then to use Monte Carlo or exact methods to see how frequently such a statistic would be exceeded by chance, under the null hypothesis of homogeneity of allele frequencies. It is usual to conduct the simulations or exact probability calculations conditional on the marginal totals of the table. In simulation studies based on data for fragile x, this method was found to be more powerful than using a table with rare alleles grouped together or comparing each allele against the rest (Sham and Curtis, 1995). We also evaluated the power of a novel test statistic, obtained by considering the different ways in which the $n \times 2$ table can be collapsed into a 2×2 table, and choosing the one with the largest Pearson chi-squared statistic. However, this statistic was found to have very similar power to the simple Pearson chi-squared statistic of the original $n \times 2$ table, when the P-values of both tests were obtained by simulation. In retrospect, this result is unsurprising, as the two tests are similar in making no prior assumption about the nature of the deviation from the null hypothesis. Our recommendation was that either the Pearson chi-squared of the raw table, or the largest Pearson chi-squared of all collapsed tables, with P-value obtained by simulation, should be used. These tests have been implemented in the CLUMP program (Sham and Curtis, 1995).

Another interesting test statistic for case-control allelic association studies with highly polymorphic markers was recently proposed by Terwilliger (1995). The proposed likelihood ratio test is based on a particular probabilistic model of the case-control data. The basic form of this model assumes that one of the n marker alleles is positively associated with the disease. The overall likelihood function is defined as a weighted sum of n conditional likelihoods (for the n marker alleles), in terms of the parameter λ (a measure of the magnitude of allelic association)

$$L(\lambda) = \sum_i p_i L_i(\lambda) \qquad (4.19)$$

where the weight attached to allele i is the prior probability that allele i is the one that is positively associated with the disease, which is assumed to be equal to the population frequency of the allele i, denoted as p_i. The conditional likelihood for allele i is equal to the probability of observing the actual data if allele i is the allele that is positively associated with the disease

$$\ln [L_i(\lambda)] = \sum_j [X_j \ln (q_i) + Y_j \ln (r_j)] \qquad (4.20)$$

where X_j and Y_j are the observed counts of marker allele j on disease and control chromosomes, and $q_j = p_j + \lambda(1 - p_j)$ and $r_j = p_j - \lambda(1 - p_j)p_D/(1 - p_D)$ when $j = i$ (i.e. the associated allele) and $q_j = p_j - \lambda p_j$ and $r_j = p_j + \lambda p_j p_D/(1 - p_D)$ when $j \neq i$ (i.e. the non-associated alleles) are the expected frequencies of allele j on disease and chromosomes, and p_D is the frequency of the disease allele. The likelihood ratio test statistic is defined as $2(\ln L_1 - \ln L_0)$, where $\ln L_1$ is the log-likelihood function maximized with respect to λ (subject to $\lambda > 0$), and $\ln L_0$ is the log-likelihood function at $\lambda = 0$ (i.e. no allelic association). This statistic was assumed to provide a one-tailed chi-squared test with one degree of freedom, for $\lambda > 0$ versus $\lambda = 0$. However, simulations showed that this gave a conservative test, especially when n (the number of marker alleles) is large.

Interestingly, if we assume the marker to be biallelic and set $p_1 = p_2 = p_D = 0.5$, the likelihood ratio statistic becomes identical in form to the likelihood ratio statistic for linkage in a single phase-unknown family. The asymptotic distribution of this statistic is not a $50:50$ mixture of 0 and chi-squared with one degree of freedom, but approximately a $68:32$ mixture of 0 and a random variable that is not chi-squared (see Section 3.6). This phenomenon may be one of the reasons for the apparent conservativeness of the significance level derived from interpreting the statistic as a one-tailed chi-squared test (Sham *et al.*, 1996).

Nevertheless, despite using a conservative null distribution, the proposed test may have more power to detect allelic associations than a standard Pearson chi-squared test, when the assumptions of the model are approximately correct. It is unclear whether these assumptions are likely to hold for most common diseases in large populations. Although the test allows these assumptions to be relaxed, for example, by defining two (or more) alleles to be positively associated with the disease, repeating the procedure under these alternative assumptions is equivalent to doing multiple tests of significance. The need for an adjustment for multiple testing may therefore offset any apparent increased power of the test. The test, which has been implemented in the computer program DISLAMB, is therefore most useful when there are good reasons to believe that the underlying assumptions are approximately true. Even in this situation, however, it may be more straightforward to compare, using the standard Pearson chi-squared test for 2×2 tables, the frequencies of the most common marker alleles in cases and controls, and then to adjust the resulting allele-wise significance levels for multiple testing to obtain an overall locus-wise significance level.

Example 4.8

In a case-control association study of a disease and a highly polymorphic locus the following allele counts are obtained.

Allele	1	2	3	4	5	6	7	8	9	10	11	12
Case	1	1	4	5	3	16	12	16	0	0	0	0
Control	2	2	9	6	1	16	46	8	7	2	2	2

This dataset was analysed using CLUMP and DISLAMB. The output of CLUMP, with 10 000 simulated replicates, is as follows.

Normal chi-square (T_1) was 28.963388
This was reached six times in 10 000 simulations

Chi-square from table after collapsing columns with small expected values together (T_2) was 19.201609
This was reached five times in 10 000 simulations based on the collapsed table.

Chi-square from comparing each column against the rest (T_3) was 11.490322
This was reached 38 times in 10 000 simulations (number of columns with expected values of 5 or more = 3)

Chi-square from 2×2 table clumped to produce maximum (T_4) was 22.739672
This was reached five times in 10 000 simulations

The recommended test statistics T_1 and T_4 give empirical *P*-values of 0.0006 and 0.0005 respectively.

DISLAMB requires a disease allele frequency to be specified. Two analyses were therefore performed, using the values 0.001 and 0.1 for disease allele frequency. The outputs are as follows.

Disease allele frequency = 0.00100000

Estimated parameters for likelihood ratio test: allele frequencies

Allele	H_0	H_1
1	0.01863354	0.01999872
2	0.01863354	0.02004044
3	0.08074534	0.08663514
4	0.06832298	0.07331055
5	0.02484472	0.02666253
6	0.19875776	0.21332031

Continued

Continued

Allele	H_0	H_1
7	0.36024845	0.38664991
8	0.14906832	0.08672829
9	0.04347826	0.04665857
10	0.01242236	0.01333733
11	0.01242236	0.01332676
12	0.01242236	0.01333143
Lambda	0.00000000	0.207132

LRT chi-square = 6.02464; P-value = 0.007064122343592; lambda = 0.207132
No significant evidence of linkage disequilibrium by LRT test
$2 \times n$ table chi-square = 28.96339; P-value = 0.002299838130846
No significant evidence of linkage disequilibrium by $2 \times n$ table chi-square test

Disease allele frequency = 0.10000000

Estimated parameters for likelihood ratio test: allele frequencies

Allele	H_0	H_1
1	0.01863354	0.01944754
2	0.01863354	0.01969685
3	0.08074534	0.08509672
4	0.06832298	0.07194969
5	0.02484472	0.02615364
6	0.19875776	0.20923768
7	0.36024845	0.37953349
8	0.14906832	0.10377026
9	0.04347826	0.04580620
10	0.01242236	0.01310835
11	0.01242236	0.01309273
12	0.01242236	0.01310685
Lambda	0.00000000	0.195629

LRT chi-square = 6.42989; P-value = 0.005620525703907; lambda = 0.195629
No significant evidence of linkage disequilibrium by LRT test
$2 \times n$ table chi-square = 28.96339; P-value = 0.002299838130846
No significant evidence of linkage disequilibrium by $2 \times n$ table chi-square test

Under either disease allele frequency, the results from DISLAMB ($P = 0.0071$ and $P = 0.0056$) were considered non-significant, as the critical value is considered to be 0.0001. (The results from CLUMP are also non-significant by this criterion.) DISLAMB also calculates the ordinary Pearson chi-squared statistic, but the asymptotic P-value is conservative, in comparison with the results from CLUMP.

4.6.4 The problem of 'spurious associations'

The issue of false positive findings is a thorny problem for association studies based on the case-control design. If there are stratifications within the population, then case-control studies may reveal evidence for association to the marker even if it is unlinked to the disease locus (see Section 4.3). Although technically speaking, alleles at the disease and marker loci are associated in the population, the purpose of association studies is generally to detect markers which are tightly linked to disease loci. Thus, associations that arise through population stratification and not tight linkage are often referred to as 'spurious'.

In order to avoid the problem of spurious associations, it is essential that the confounding effect of population stratification be allowed for in the design and analysis of the study. In a case-control framework, this requires the identification of sub-populations, conceptually defined as a subgroup of individuals within which matings tend to occur at random with respect to parental genotypes. In practice, sub-populations are usually defined in terms of factors which might influence disease and marker allele frequencies, such as ethnicity, geographical origin and possibly religion, social class and age. These factors may be relevant when there has been in-migration at certain times in the history of the population. Once these sub-populations are identified, they can be allowed for in the study design by matching or by focusing on one well-defined sub-population. The latter option may be preferable because it is possible that different marker alleles are associated with the disease in different sub-populations, so that no overall association may be apparent among cases and controls sampled from a mixture of sub-populations.

Even when strict inclusion criteria are applied in order to ensure the genetic homogeneity of the study sample, it is always possible to overlook some relevant factors that may lead to spurious associations. Such factors are often referred to as 'hidden population stratifications', and are impossible to rule out entirely. However, certain checks can be performed in order to assess whether they are likely to be present in a sample. Thus, individual markers can be tested for Hardy–Weinberg equilibrium, and pairs of markers known to be on different chromosomes can be tested for linkage equilibrium. In addition, if a disease shows allelic associations with many marker loci in different chromosomal regions, then it is likely that these associations are due to hidden population stratification rather than to tight linkage with several disease loci.

4.7 Association analysis using cases and parental controls

One way of overcoming the problem of hidden population stratification is to compare cases with their relatives rather than with unrelated controls. The cases and controls are then matched for genetic background. Although many types of relatives can be used for comparison with the cases, it is currently most popular to use parents for this purpose, as originally suggested by Rubinstein *et al.* (1981) and Falk and Rubinstein (1987) in their method called *haplotype relative risk* (HRR).

4.7.1   The haplotype relative risk method

The sampling unit of the HRR is a family with two parents and a single affected offspring (the case). A sample of such units is ascertained through a random sample of affected cases in the population. Each unit contributes a case genotype (the genotype of the affected offspring) and an artificially constructed 'control genotype' made up of two remaining alleles of the two parents not transmitted to the affected offspring. The original HRR considers the case genotypes and the control genotypes as two independent samples, and uses the standard methodology for unmatched case-control studies, with the 'exposure' being the presence or absence of a particular pre-specified genotype. This yields an unbiased estimate of the population relative risk for that exposure (hence the name HRR), when the recombination fraction between the marker and disease loci is 0. A popular variation of the HRR, called *haplotype-based HRR* (HHRR), considers allele rather than genotype as the unit of observation (Terwilliger and Ott, 1992). Thus, each trio of two parents and an affected offspring contributes two transmitted and two non-transmitted alleles, and the total collections of transmitted and non-transmitted alleles are considered as two independent case-control samples.

For a biallelic marker locus, allele transmission data can be presented in the form of a 2×2 square contingency table. In Table 4.1, the count of parents transmitting allele i and not transmitting allele j to an affected offspring (the case) is denoted as t_{ij}, so that the data are summarized as the four counts t_{11}, t_{12}, t_{21} and t_{22}. If the marginal totals are defined as $t_{i.} = t_{i1} + t_{i2}$ and $t_{.j} = t_{1j} + t_{2j}$, then the HHRR statistic is defined as

$$\text{HHRR} = \frac{(t_{1.} - t_{.1})^2}{t_{1.} + t_{.1}} + \frac{(t_{2.} - t_{.2})^2}{t_{2.} + t_{.2}} \tag{4.21}$$

which is asymptotically chi-squared with one degree of freedom under linkage equilibrium. This provides a powerful test for linkage disequilibrium when the recombination fraction (θ) is near 0.

Table 4.1 Transmission data for a biallelic marker. The cell count t_{ij} is the number of parents who transmitted allele i and not allele j

	Not transmitted		
Transmitted	Allele 1	Allele 2	Total
Allele 1	t_{11}	t_{12}	$t_{1.}$
Allele 2	t_{21}	t_{22}	$t_{2.}$
Total	$t_{.1}$	$t_{.2}$	$t_{..}$

4.7.2   The transmission distortion test

The HHRR method of analysis may seem somewhat inappropriate because it ignores the fact that the transmitted and non-transmitted alleles contributed by a parent can be regarded as paired observations. Ignoring individual matching may be misleading under non-random mating. The McNemar test for matched-pair data considers only parents whose transmitted and non-transmitted alleles are different (i.e. heterozygous parents), and assesses the evidence for preferential transmission of one allele over the other. Since this test assesses deviations from equal transmission, and is sensitive to linkage disequilibrium, it was renamed by Spielman *et al.* (1993) as the *transmission/disequilibrium test* (TDT), although the name *transmission distortion test* may be more appropriate, because there are circumstances (to be discussed below) when the test is not sensitive to linkage disequilibrium. The TDT statistic is defined as

$$\text{TDT} = \frac{(t_{21} - t_{12})^2}{t_{21} + t_{12}} \tag{4.22}$$

which is asymptotically chi-squared with one degree of freedom when the marker and disease loci are unlinked. The attractive feature of the TDT is that it is a test of linkage, and not merely of linkage disequilibrium. This is because linkage disequilibrium alone can only distort the distribution of marker genotypes among the parents of affected individuals (from the distribution of genotypes in the general population). The TDT considers the probabilities of marker allele transmission from heterozygous parents to affected individuals, and the distortion of these probabilities from 0.5 can only occur if the marker and disease loci are linked (assuming that there is no overall distortion from Mendelian segregation at the marker locus in the population).

Whether the TDT is a test of linkage, or linkage disequilibrium, or both has been a matter of some controversy (Hodge, 1993, 1994; Suarez and Hampe, 1994; Spielman *et al.*, 1994). The answer to this question depends on the nature of the sample. If the sample consists of a set of unrelated cases and their parents, then the TDT is a test of both linkage and linkage disequilibrium (Sham and Curtis, 1995). On the other hand, if the data are derived from a single large pedigree in which all affected individuals share a single ancestral disease allele descended from a single founder, then allelic associations between disease and marker alleles in the population are irrelevant, and the TDT is a test of just linkage. The situation is intermediate for other sampling schemes. Overall, the TDT is a valid test of linkage in all situations, but the extent to which it is sensitive to linkage disequilibrium depends on the number of separate ancestral disease alleles in the sample. Since most samples subjected to TDT analyses will contain many separate families, the TDT can be thought of as a test of linkage that has increasing power with increasing linkage disequilibrium.

Although the TDT may be an improvement on HHRR for the detection of linkage or linkage disequilibrium, it still has the potential shortcoming of ignoring the paired nature of the transmission data from the two parents of the same affected individual. The TDT effectively considers the allele transmissions from the father and mother of affected individuals to be independent events. In circumstances where this is untrue, the TDT may lose some of the information available in the sample. A more general method of analysis that is closely related to the TDT has been proposed (Schaid and Sommer, 1993; Knapp *et al.*, 1995b). In order to motivate this more general method, we first reframe the TDT as a likelihood ratio test. Letting the conditional probabilities of transmitting alleles B_1 and B_2 given parental genotype B_1B_2 be p_{12} and p_{21}, then the log-likelihood function of the transmission data from heterozygous parents to affected offspring is $t_{12}\ln(p_{12})+t_{21}\ln(p_{21})$. The maximum likelihood estimate of p_{12} is simply $t_{12}/(t_{12}+t_{21})$. The maximum log-likelihood is therefore

$$\ln L_1 = t_{12} \ln \frac{t_{12}}{t_{12}+t_{21}} + t_{21} \ln \frac{t_{21}}{t_{12}+t_{21}} \tag{4.23}$$

while the log-likelihood at the null hypothesis is

$$\ln L_0 = (t_{12}+t_{21})\ln \frac{1}{2} \tag{4.24}$$

The likelihood ratio statistic for the TDT is then $2(\ln L_1 - \ln L_0)$. This however, still ignores the paired nature of the parental data. Taking this into account, the transmission data can be summarized as the counts of offspring with the three possible genotypes B_1B_1, B_1B_2, B_2B_2 from the six possible parental mating types $B_1B_1 \times B_1B_1$, $B_1B_1 \times B_1B_2$, $B_1B_1 \times B_2B_2$, $B_1B_2 \times B_1B_2$, $B_1B_2 \times B_2B_2$, $B_2B_2 \times B_2B_2$. Assuming that the recombination fraction between the marker and disease loci is 0, then the 'apparent penetrances' (i.e. the probabilities of being affected by the disease) of the three genotypes B_1B_1, B_1B_2, B_2B_2 can be written as f_{11}, f_{12} and f_{22} (as in Equation (4.15)). The conditional probability of an offspring genotype (G_O) given that the offspring is affected (A) and that the parental mating type is G_P, is

$$P(G_O|A, G_P) = \frac{P(A|G_O)P(G_O|G_P)}{P(A|G_P)} \tag{4.25}$$

where $P(A|G_O)$ is the 'apparent penetrance' of genotype G_O, $P(G_O|G_P)$ is the probability of the observed offspring genotype given the parental mating type, while the denominator $P(A|G_P)$ is the probability of the observed offspring phenotype (affection status) given the parental mating. This latter probability can be decomposed as

$$P(A|G_P) = \sum P(A|G_O)P(G_O|G_P) \tag{4.26}$$

where the summation is taken over all possible offspring genotypes for the observed parental mating types. Of the six possible parental mating types, three $(B_1B_1 \times B_1B_1, B_1B_1 \times B_2B_2, B_2B_2 \times B_2B_2)$ will always produce offspring with the same genotype, and are therefore uninformative for transmission distortion. The mating type $B_1B_1 \times B_1B_2$ has two possible offspring genotypes, and the probabilities of these, according to Equations (4.25) and (4.26), are

$$\left. \begin{aligned} P(G_O = B_1B_1 | A, G_P = B_1B_1 \times B_1B_2) &= \frac{f_{11}}{f_{11}+f_{12}} \\[2mm] P(G_O = B_1B_2 | A, G_P = B_1B_1 \times B_1B_2) &= \frac{f_{12}}{f_{11}+f_{12}} \end{aligned} \right\} \tag{4.27}$$

Similarly, the mating type $B_1B_2 \times B_2B_2$ has two possible offspring genotypes, and the probabilities of these are

$$
\begin{aligned}
P(G_O = B_1B_2 \mid A, G_P = B_1B_2 \times B_2B_2) &= \frac{f_{12}}{f_{12} + f_{22}} \\[2mm]
P(G_O = B_2B_2 \mid A, G_P = B_1B_2 \times B_2B_2) &= \frac{f_{22}}{f_{12} + f_{22}}
\end{aligned}
\left.\rule{0pt}{14mm}\right\}
\qquad (4.28)
$$

Finally, the mating type $B_1B_2 \times B_1B_2$ has three possible offspring genotypes, and the probabilities of these are

$$
\begin{aligned}
P(G_O = B_1B_1 \mid A, G_P = B_1B_2 \times B_1B_2) &= \frac{f_{11}}{f_{11} + 2f_{12} + f_{22}} \\[2mm]
P(G_O = B_1B_2 \mid A, G_P = B_1B_2 \times B_1B_2) &= \frac{2f_{12}}{f_{11} + 2f_{12} + f_{22}} \\[2mm]
P(G_O = B_2B_2 \mid A, G_P = B_1B_2 \times B_1B_2) &= \frac{f_{22}}{f_{11} + 2f_{12} + f_{22}}
\end{aligned}
\left.\rule{0pt}{22mm}\right\}
\qquad (4.29)
$$

These seven probabilities can be divided through by f_{11}, so that they are functions of two relative risk parameters $r_{12} = f_{12}/f_{11}$ and $r_{22} = f_{22}/f_{11}$

$$
\begin{aligned}
P(G_O = B_1B_1 \mid A, G_P = B_1B_1 \times B_1B_2) &= \frac{1}{1 + r_{12}} \\[2mm]
P(G_O = B_1B_2 \mid A, G_P = B_1B_1 \times B_1B_2) &= \frac{r_{12}}{1 + r_{12}} \\[2mm]
P(G_O = B_1B_2 \mid A, G_P = B_1B_2 \times B_2B_2) &= \frac{r_{12}}{r_{12} + r_{22}} \\[2mm]
P(G_O = B_2B_2 \mid A, G_P = B_1B_2 \times B_2B_2) &= \frac{r_{22}}{r_{12} + r_{22}} \\[2mm]
P(G_O = B_1B_1 \mid A, G_P = B_1B_2 \times B_1B_2) &= \frac{1}{1 + 2r_{12} + r_{22}} \\[2mm]
P(G_O = B_1B_2 \mid A, G_P = B_1B_2 \times B_1B_2) &= \frac{2r_{12}}{1 + 2r_{12} + r_{22}} \\[2mm]
P(G_O = B_2B_2 \mid A, G_P = B_1B_2 \times B_1B_2) &= \frac{r_{22}}{1 + 2r_{12} + r_{22}}
\end{aligned}
\left.\rule{0pt}{52mm}\right\}
\qquad (4.30)
$$

From a sample of parents and affected offspring, the counts of these seven mutually exclusive events can be obtained. The log-likelihood function is then simply the sum of seven terms, each being the count of one of these events multiplied by the logarithm of the corresponding probability. The two parameters r_{12} and r_{22} can be estimated by maximizing this log-likelihood function. Denoting this maximum log-likelihood by $\ln L_1$ and the null log-likelihood (when $r_{12} = r_{22} = 1$) by $\ln L_0$, the statistic $2(\ln L_1 - \ln L_0)$ has a chi-squared distribution with two degrees of freedom, and provides a test for transmission distortion. This latter method is sometimes known as *genotype relative risk*, GRR (Schaid and Sommer, 1993; Knapp *et al.*, 1995b), but this term does not reflect the nature of the sampling unit. We would prefer to regard this test as a more general form of the usual TDT, which can be derived from this test by imposing the constraint $r_{22} = r_{12}^2$, so that the only parameter is r_{12}. With this substitution, the seven probabilities of Equation (4.29) become

$$
\left.
\begin{aligned}
P(G_O = B_1 B_1 \mid A, G_P = B_1 B_1 \times B_1 B_2) &= \frac{1}{1 + r_{12}} \\[2ex]
P(G_O = B_1 B_2 \mid A, G_P = B_1 B_1 \times B_1 B_2) &= \frac{r_{12}}{1 + r_{12}} \\[2ex]
P(G_O = B_1 B_2 \mid A, G_P = B_1 B_2 \times B_2 B_2) &= \frac{1}{1 + r_{12}} \\[2ex]
P(G_O = B_2 B_2 \mid A, G_P = B_1 B_2 \times B_2 B_2) &= \frac{r_{12}}{1 + r_{12}} \\[2ex]
P(G_O = B_1 B_1 \mid A, G_P = B_1 B_2 \times B_1 B_2) &= \frac{1}{(1 + r_{12})^2} \\[2ex]
P(G_O = B_1 B_2 \mid A, G_P = B_1 B_2 \times B_1 B_2) &= \frac{2 r_{12}}{(1 + r_{12})^2} \\[2ex]
P(G_O = B_2 B_2 \mid A, G_P = B_1 B_2 \times B_1 B_2) &= \frac{r_{12}^2}{(1 + r_{12})^2}
\end{aligned}
\right\}
\qquad (4.31)
$$

which are equivalent to the transmission probabilities assumed in the usual likelihood ratio TDT. This more general test therefore reduces to the usual TDT. This can be interpreted intuitively as meaning that when $r_{22} = r_{12}^2$ (i.e. $f_{11} f_{22} = f_{12}^2$), marker allele transmissions from the two parents of an affected offspring are independent of each other. If this condition holds or nearly holds, then the usual TDT will be more powerful than the more general test because it has only one degree of freedom. However, the general test is likely to be more powerful when there is substantial deviation from the condition $r_{22} = r_{12}^2$.

Example 4.9
A sample of 100 individuals affected by a disease, and their parents, is studied for association with a candidate biallelic locus. The counts of parental and offspring genotypes are as follows.

	Offspring		
Parents	1/1	1/2	2/2
11 × 11	22	0	0
11 × 12	17	25	0
11 × 22	0	7	0
12 × 12	1	11	13
12 × 22	0	1	1
22 × 22	0	0	2

Using a simple non-linear optimization function in SAS to maximize the log-likelihood function for the general transmission distortion test (genotype relative risk), the following results were obtained

Maximum-likelihood estimates (MLE):
$\hat{r}_{12} = 1.73$
$\hat{r}_{22} = 5.04$

Log-likelihoods
H_0 ($r_{12} = r_{22} = 1$): -58.00
H_1 (MLE): -64.46

Likelihood ratio test
$2(\ln L_1 - \ln L_0) = 2(-58.00 + 64.46) = 12.92$
df = 2
$P = 0.0016$

For HHRR and TDT the counts are collapsed into a table of allele transmissions.

	Non-transmitted		
Transmitted	1	2	
1	93	31	124
2	63	13	76
	156	44	200

The HHRR chi-squared statistic is
$(156 - 124)^2/(156 + 124) + (44 - 76)^2/(44 + 76) = 12.19$
df = 1
$P = 0.0005$

The TDT Pearson chi-squared statistic is
$(63 - 31)^2/(63 + 31) = 10.89$
df = 1
$P = 0.001$

The TDT likelihood ratio chi-squared statistic is
$2\{31[\ln(31/94)] + 63[\ln(63/94)] - 94[\ln(1/2)]\} = 11.11$
df = 1
$P = 0.0008$

The evidence for transmission distortion, being significant at the 0.001 level, suggests an association between the marker locus and the disease. The TDT likelihood ratio test has the advantage that, in conjunction with the general transmission distortion test, it offers a likelihood ratio test for the independence of marker allele transmission from the two parents to an affected offspring. The relevant likelihood chi-squared ratio statistic is $12.92 - 11.11 = 1.81$ with one degree of freedom. There is therefore no significant evidence for non-independent allele transmissions from parents to affected offspring (so that there is insufficient evidence for rejecting the assumption $r_{22} = r_{12}^2$ on which the TDT is based).

4.7.3   The transmission distortion test for multi-allelic marker loci

For polymorphic markers with n alleles ($n > 2$), it is convenient to use the restricted form of the TDT which assumes that marker allele transmissions from the two parents to an affected offspring are independent. This assumption is valid if the recombination fraction is very small and if the penetrances f_{11}, f_{12} and f_{22} are such that $f_{12}^2 = f_{11}f_{22}$. However, the method is expected to be nearly optimal if the true model is unknown and if the assumption of independence holds even approximately. The transmission data for an n-allele marker can then be summarized in a square $n \times n$ table.

In Table 4.2, the count of parents transmitting allele i and not transmitting allele j to an affected offspring (the case) is denoted as t_{ij}. The direct generalization of the HHRR statistic to Table 4.2 gives a test of 'marginal homogeneity'

$$\text{HHRR} = \sum_i \frac{(t_{i.} - t_{.i})^2}{t_{i.} + t_{.i}} \tag{4.32}$$

which is asymptotically chi-squared with $n - 1$ degrees of freedom under linkage equilibrium. Similarly, the direct generalization of the TDT to Table 4.2 gives a test of 'symmetry'

$$\text{TDT} = \sum_{i<j} \frac{(t_{ij} - t_{ji})^2}{t_{ij} + t_{ji}} \tag{4.33}$$

Table 4.2 Transmission data for a multi-allelic marker. The cell count t_{ij} is the number of parents who transmitted allele i and not allele j

| Transmitted | Not transmitted | | | | |
	Allele 1	Allele 2	...	Allele m	Total
Allele 1	t_{11}	t_{12}	...	t_{1m}	$t_{1.}$
Allele 2	t_{21}	t_{22}	...	t_{2m}	$t_{2.}$
...	...	...	...	...	...
Allele m	t_{m1}	t_{m2}	...	t_{mm}	$t_{m.}$
Total	$t_{.1}$	$t_{.2}$	...	$t_{.m}$	$t_{..}$

the summation being over all possible $n(n-1)/2$ heterozygous parental marker genotypes. This statistic has asymptotically a chi-squared distribution with $n(n-1)/2$ degrees of freedom when $\theta = 1/2$.

It is, however, undesirable that the generalized TDT has $n(n-1)/2$ degrees of freedom, since there are only $2n$ haplotype frequencies that may deviate from their equilibrium values. In fact, because of certain constraints (which are that the deviations involving any particular allele must sum to 0), these deviations can be characterized by just $n-1$ independent parameters. Because of this, alternative ways of extending the TDT to highly polymorphic markers have been proposed.

The most satisfactory way of achieving this is probably to adopt a logistic regression model, which is appealing since there are two possible outcomes for each parental genotype (i.e. either allele B_i or B_j is transmitted to an offspring when the parental genotype is B_iB_j). The logarithm of the odds (log-odds) of transmitting allele B_i, given that the parent has genotype B_iB_j, is assumed to be determined by a linear function of some parameters. Denoting the probabilities of transmitting alleles B_i and B_j conditional on parental genotype B_iB_j to be p_{ij} and p_{ji} respectively, and the log-odds $\ln(p_{ij}/p_{ji})$ as g_{ij}, the log-likelihood function of this logistic regression model is

$$\ln L = \sum [t_{ij} \ln(p_{ij}) + t_{ji} \ln(p_{ji})] \tag{4.34}$$

where the summation is taken over all $n(n-1)/2$ combinations of different alleles, and the transmission probabilities (p_{ij}) are functions of some specified parameters. In a saturated model, a separate parameter is specified for each parental genotype. This can be written as

$$g_{ij} = \ln \left(\frac{p_{ij}}{p_{ji}} \right) = \beta_{ij} \tag{4.35}$$

for all $n(n-1)/2$ combinations of different values of i and j. The parameters β_{ij} can be estimated as $\ln(t_{ij}/t_{ji})$. Substituting these estimates into the log-likelihood function yields the log-likelihood of the saturated model, which we denote as $\ln L_2$.

In this logistic regression model, the null hypothesis of equal transmission probabilities is specified by setting $\beta_{ij} = 0$, for all $n(n-1)/2$ heterozygous parental genotypes. Substituting these values into the log-likelihood function gives the log-likelihood of the null model, which we denote as $\ln L_0$. The likelihood ratio statistic $2(\ln L_2 - \ln L_0)$ has asymptotically $n(n-1)/2$ degrees of freedom and provides a test of equal transmission probabilities.

The main purpose of introducing this logistic regression model is, however, to construct an alternative test that has only $n-1$ degrees of freedom. This can be achieved by defining one parameter for each allele, with the parameter value of the last allele being fixed at 0. Denoting these parameters as $\beta_1, \beta_2, ..., \beta_n$, the log-odds of transmitting one rather than the other allele in a heterozygous parental genotype is defined as

$$g_{ij} = \ln \left(\frac{p_{ij}}{p_{ji}} \right) = \beta_i - \beta_j \tag{4.36}$$

for all $n(n-1)/2$ combinations of different values of i and j. The free parameters $\beta_1, \beta_2, \ldots, \beta_{n-1}$ can be estimated by a standard software for logistic regression, or by the computer program ETDT (Sham and Curtis, 1995). Substitution of these estimates into the log-likelihood function yields a log-likelihood which we denote as $\ln L_1$. The likelihood ratio statistic $2(\ln L_1 - \ln L_0)$ has asymptotically $n-1$ degrees of freedom and provides an appealing test for transmission distortion.

This test is expected to have greater power than the test based on $2(\ln L_2 - \ln L_0)$, when the assumptions underlying Equation (4.36) are approximately true (Sham and Curtis, 1995). These assumptions are that the disease locus and the marker loci are tightly linked (recombination fraction $\theta \approx 0$), and that the data are collected from a random sample of affected individuals in a randomly mating population. If the disease locus is characterized as usual by the parameters $p_1, p_2, f_{11}, f_{12}, f_{22}$, then a quantity that determines the degree to which selection through affected offspring has diminished the transmission of the normal allele can be shown to be

$$B = \frac{p_2[p_2(f_{22}-f_{12}) + p_1(f_{12}-f_{11})]}{p_1^2 f_{11} + 2p_1 p_2 f_{12} + p_2^2 f_{22}} \qquad (4.37)$$

If we also define a parameter e_{2i}, which describes the magnitude of the linkage disequilibrium between the disease allele (D_2) and a marker allele (B_i), as follows

$$e_{2i} = \frac{h_{2i}}{p_2 q_i} \qquad (4.38)$$

then the probability of transmitting allele B_i to an affected offspring from a parent genotype $B_i B_j$ can be shown to be

$$p_{ij} = \frac{d_{ij}}{d_{ij} + d_{ji}} \qquad (4.39)$$

where

$$d_{ij} = 1 + B[(e_{2i} - 1) + \theta(e_{2j} - e_{2i})] \qquad (4.40)$$

When $\theta = 0$, d_{ij} becomes identical to d_{ii}, so that

$$p_{ij} = \frac{d_{ii}}{d_{ii} + d_{jj}} \qquad (4.41)$$

This is equivalent to Equation (4.36) if we let $\ln(d_{ii}) - \ln(d_{jj}) = \beta_i - \beta_j$. The extended TDT based on the logistic regression model is therefore justified under these assumptions, if the alleles contributed from the two parents can be considered independent (i.e. if $f_{12}^2 = f_{11} f_{22}$).

Example 4.10
Suggestive linkage findings were reported between the mental illness schizophrenia and markers on chromosome 22. At the Institute of Psychiatry, these findings were followed up by an association analysis using the ETDT program. One of the loci examined was D22S278, which has seven alleles. The

frequencies of the genotypes among the parents of affected individuals in the sample are as follows.

1	2	3	4	5	6	7	
0	1	6	2	0	0	0	1
	3	10	7	7	2	0	2
		0	11	13	2	1	3
			2	5	0	0	4
				0	1	1	5
					0	0	6
						0	7

For each pairing of heterozygous parent and affected offspring, ETDT works out the transmitted and the non-transmitted allele. The frequencies of these transmission events are as follows (the count of row i and column j being the number of occurrence of the event: allele i transmitted and allele j not transmitted).

0	1	3	0	0	0	0	4
0	3	3	3	4	0	0	10
3	7	0	10	7	0	0	27
2	4	1	2	2	0	0	9
0	3	6	3	0	0	0	12
0	2	2	0	1	0	0	5
0	0	1	0	1	0	0	2
5	17	16	16	15	0	0	

Note that the row and column totals do not include the diagonal (i.e. homozygous) elements.

The results of the logistic regression analysis are as follows.

Fitted allele parameters with SEs:

	Value	SE
Allele 1	−7.500093	15.617084
Allele 2	−7.821035	15.607231
Allele 3	−6.956522	15.601933
Allele 4	−7.940615	15.607536
Allele 5	−7.478802	15.603623
Allele 6	−0.161049	18.421198

Correlation matrix of parameters:

1.000000	0.998716	0.998990	0.998776	0.998671	0.846082
0.998717	1.000000	0.999532	0.999445	0.999451	0.846731
0.998990	0.999532	1.000000	0.999530	0.999574	0.846882
0.998776	0.999444	0.999530	1.000000	0.999402	0.846607
0.998672	0.999451	0.999574	0.999402	1.000000	0.846718
0.846083	0.846731	0.846882	0.846607	0.846718	1.000000

Log-likelihood under null hypothesis: $\ln L_0 = -47.827$
Log-likelihood under parsimonious (allele-wise) hypothesis: $\ln L_1 = -40.004$
Log-likelihood using saturated (genotype-wise) model: $\ln L_2 = -35.517$

Chi-squared for allele-wise TDT $= 2(\ln L_1 - \ln L_0) = 15.647, 6$ df, $P = 0.016$
Chi-squared for genotype-wise TDT $= 2(\ln L_2 - \ln L_0) = 24.621, 14$ df, $P = 0.039$
Chi-squared for goodness-of-fit of allele-wise model $= 2(\ln L_2 - \ln L_1) = 8.974, 8$ df, $P = 0.345$

These results are suggestive of an association between alleles at the D22S278 locus and schizophrenia, with the strongest evidence coming from the allele-wise TDT test. However, the level of significance is not impressive for an allelic association analysis, and the results must be considered tentative until they are replicated in other samples.

4.8 Association analysis of pedigree data

The HHRR and TDT demonstrate one of the advantages of carrying out association analysis on sets of related individuals rather than on entirely unrelated subjects, that of avoiding the spurious associations arising through population stratification. There is a second potential advantage of using family data for association analysis, which is that it may allow the haplotypes present in some doubly heterozygous subjects to be determined. However, since the haplotypes in the non-founder members of a pedigree are determined by the haplotypes in the founders through Mendelian transmission, it is clear that, provided all the founders are genotyped, the non-founders cannot contribute any additional information about allelic associations other than possibly determining the haplotypes present in doubly heterozygous founders. Optimal data for association analysis therefore consist of families with a high ratio of founders to non-founders, for example, sets of two parents and a child, which can be analysed using TDT.

In some instances, however, one may wish to perform an association analysis on data consisting of larger pedigrees collected for some other purpose such as linkage analysis. Provided that the sample was ascertained without knowledge of the genotypes at either locus, analysis can proceed without the need to consider the possibility of bias in allele and haplotype frequencies. This is usually true for two marker loci. The simplest method of analysis is to reconstruct, as far as possible, the haplotypes present in all the founders, and organize the resulting haplotype counts in a contingency table and perform a standard Pearson chi-squared test. The disadvantage of this approach is that the haplotypes present in a founder cannot always be unambiguously reconstructed. A likelihood approach to the analysis is therefore more satisfactory. The likelihood function can be maximized over haplotype frequencies and recombination fraction, with and without the constraints implied by linkage equilibrium. Under linkage equilibrium, haplotype frequencies are equal to the products of the constituent allele frequencies, so that the likelihood can be written as a function of the allele frequencies and the recombination fraction. Let the log-likelihood maximized over unconstrained haplotype frequencies and recombination fraction be $\ln L_1$, and the log-likelihood maximized over allele frequencies and recombination fraction be $\ln L_0$. The statistic $2(\ln L_1 - \ln L_0)$ has asymptotically a chi-squared distribution with $(mn - 1) - (m - 1) - (n - 1) = (m - 1)(n - 1)$ degrees of freedom, where m and n are the numbers of alleles at the two loci, and provides a test for linkage disequilibrium between the two loci. The maximization of the likelihood function over haplotype or allele frequencies and the recombination fraction can be performed using the program ILINK in the LINKAGE package (Terwilliger and Ott, 1994).

It should be appreciated that correct modelling of linkage disequilibrium is important in the testing and estimation of the recombination fraction. It is common practice when performing parametric linkage analysis to assume that the loci concerned are in linkage equilibrium. This is a reasonable assumption in most situations, but may be inappropriate when the loci are very tightly linked. The correct procedure is then to compare the log-likelihoods of two models, one estimating haplotype frequencies and the recombination fraction jointly $(\ln L_1)$, and the other estimating only the haplotype frequencies with the assumption that recombination fraction is $1/2$ $(\ln L_0)$. The statistic $2(\ln L_1 - \ln L_0)$ then provides a one degree of freedom chi-squared test which takes proper account of possible linkage disequilibrium as nuisance parameters. Taking appropriate account of linkage disequilibrium enables the haplotypes present in doubly heterozygous founders to be determined more accurately, and therefore increases the power to detect linkage.

When the analysis involves a disease locus, the situation is complicated by the fact that most pedigrees, samples are not representative of the population but have been enriched for the disease to provide more power for linkage analysis. In linkage analysis it is usual to specify the disease locus parameters (i.e. $p_1, p_2, f_{11}, f_{12}, f_{22}$) that lead to the correct population risk. The disease allele frequencies are therefore not estimated from the data, but fixed to specific values that have biological plausibility. In order to carry out a likelihood-based linkage disequilibrium analysis treating the recombination fraction as a nuisance parameter, or a likelihood-based linkage analysis treating the haplotype frequencies as nuisance parameters (as in the case of two markers' loci described above), it is desirable to impose constraints on the haplotype frequencies that maintain the specified allele frequencies at the disease locus. Further work is necessary to establish the properties (e.g. robustness and power) of such analyses.

4.9 Using linkage disequilibrium to estimate recombination fraction

The use of linkage disequilibrium for the fine mapping of disease loci is based on theoretical considerations and empirical observations that appreciable allelic associations (detectable using realistic sample sizes of hundreds of individuals) are only likely to be present between two loci that are tightly linked, typically with a recombination fraction of less than 1 cM. The detection of linkage disequilibrium between disease and marker loci can therefore be used to infer the position of the disease to within about 1 cM either side of the marker. A distance of 2 cM corresponds to approximately 2 000 000 base pairs, which remains a large distance for the identification of the disease gene. For this reason, some attempts have been made to use the magnitude of the linkage disequilibrium between two loci to obtain a more precise estimate of recombination fraction.

For a large population that has been stable in size over a very large number of generations, the level of linkage disequilibrium between two loci is determined by the balance of random drift and mutation with recombination events. Consider two biallelic loci with allele frequencies p_1, p_2, q_1, q_1 and haplotype frequencies $h_{11}, h_{12}, h_{21}, h_{22}$, a convenient measure of the magnitude of linkage disequilibrium is the squared correlation coefficient

$$R^2 = \frac{(h_{11}h_{22} - h_{12}h_{21})^2}{(p_1 p_2 q_1 q_2)} \tag{4.42}$$

The expectation of this quantity was shown by Ohta and Kimura (1969) to be approximately

$$E(R^2) \approx \frac{E[(h_{11}h_{22} - h_{12}h_{21})^2]}{E(p_1 p_2 q_1 q_2)} \approx (4Nc)^{-1} \tag{4.43}$$

where N is the effective size of the population, and $c = \theta + \mu$ is the sum of the recombination fraction (θ) and the total mutation rate (μ) of the two loci, provided that Nc is much greater than 1 (see also Crow and Kimura, 1971). This can be used to obtain a method of moments estimator of θ, given that R^2, N and μ are known. However, this method is problematic because the true values of N and μ are seldom known. Furthermore, the sampling variance of R^2 tends to be very large due to stochastic events in past generations (called evolutionary sampling), which results in a very large standard error in the estimate of θ. Using a likelihood approach, Hill and Weir (1994) have come to the similar conclusion that 'precise information on map position will not be obtained from estimates of linkage disequilibrium'. Nevertheless, based on the observed magnitudes of linkage disequilibrium between loci whose positions are precisely known, it may be possible infer the likely recombination fraction between two loci in the same chromosomal region, from the magnitude of linkage disequilibrium between the two loci.

The situation is more favourable in an isolated population such as Finland, for which there is a simple and popular approach of estimating the recombination θ from the magnitude of linkage disequilibrium (de La Chapelle, 1993). The method assumes that the current population represents the gth generation from a founder population. Copies of the disease allele in the current population are assumed to be derived either from a single ancestral disease allele in the founder population, or from subsequent mutations. The proportion of the disease alleles in the current population (i.e. generation g) derived from the single ancestral allele in the founder population is denoted as α_g.

Suppose that the single ancestral chromosome containing the founder disease allele also contains a marker allele (denoted A) at a neighbouring locus, and that the recombination fraction between the disease and marker loci is θ. In the founder population, the only chromosome containing the founder disease allele also contains allele A, so that if the population frequency of A in the founder population is p, then the excess of allele A associated with the founder disease allele is $1 - p$. In the current population g generations later, the excess of allele A associated with the disease allele is $(1 - \theta)^g$ times the original excess $(1 - p)$ in a proportion α_g of disease alleles that are descended from the founder disease allele, and 0 in the rest of the disease alleles. Let the allele frequency of A among chromosomes containing the disease allele in generation g be p_g, then the excess of allele A associated with the disease allele in generation g is

$$p_g - p = \alpha_g (1 - \theta)^g (1 - p) \tag{4.44}$$

which can be rewritten as

$$(1 - \theta)^g = \frac{1}{\alpha_g} \frac{p_g - p}{1 - p} \tag{4.45}$$

The quantity $(p_g - p)/(1 - p)$ is called p-excess, and is denoted as p_e. This simplifies the above expression to

$$(1 - \theta)^g = \frac{p_e}{\alpha_g} \tag{4.46}$$

In order to use this expression to obtain an estimate of θ, it is necessary to have a value for α_g. It may be reasonable assume that the overall frequency of the disease allele is fairly constant from generation to generation, so that the reduction in the number of alleles descended from the founder disease allele from one generation to the next is compensated by fresh mutations. Let the disease allele frequency be q, the mutation rate be μ, and the proportions of disease alleles descended from the founder disease allele in generations k and $k + 1$ be α_k and α_{k+1}. The reduction in the number of alleles descended from the founder disease allele is compensated approximately by fresh mutations if

$$q\alpha_k - q\alpha_{k+1} = \mu \tag{4.47}$$

This simplifies to

$$\alpha_{k+1} = \alpha_k - \mu q^{-1} \tag{4.48}$$

Assuming that $\alpha_0 = 1$ (i.e. that the founder population has only one surviving disease allele in the current population), this recursive equation gives the approximate proportion of disease alleles derived from the founder disease allele in generation g as

$$\alpha_g = 1 - g\mu q^{-1} \tag{4.49}$$

This enables an observed value of p_e to be translated to an estimate of θ, provided that the model is reasonable for the study population, and that approximate values of the parameters g, μ and q are available. This simple approach worked well for the mapping of the genes for several rare Mendelian diseases in Finland (Hastbacka *et al.*, 1992, 1994; de La Chapelle, 1993). However, more sophisticated statistical methods for the fine mapping of disease genes using allelic associations in isolated populations are also emerging (Kaplan *et al.*, 1995; Kaplan and Weir, 1995, Devlin *et al.*, 1996).

4.10 Relationship between association and linkage analysis

Linkage analysis depends on studying sets of related individuals (except for inbred individuals who are informative for linkage even in the absence of any relatives), because the phenomenon that one is trying to detect is non-random co-inheritance of alleles at two loci. Although association analysis appears to utilize unrelated subjects, it also depends on the fact that the subjects are, in reality, distantly related. Closely related individuals are descended from common ancestors through a small number of meioses, and tend to have large segments of chromosomes in common. Distantly related individuals, on the other hand, are separated by a large number of meioses, and the numerous random recombination events ensure that the chromosomal segments that they share will be relatively small. This is the basis for the finer resolving power of association analysis compared with linkage analysis. It also explains why association analysis is not as sensitive as linkage analysis to loose linkage. In some sense, linkage and association analysis can be thought to represent the two ends of the same continuous phenomenon, with association analysis being considered as some form of identity-by-state analysis between very distant relatives. However, because the exact relationships between individuals are not known in an association analysis, the results are dependent on numerous random events that cannot be individually identified. In contrast, linkage analysis deals only with families where the genetic relationships between individuals are known, and so the relevant random events can be clearly identified. Linkage analysis is therefore more amenable to a formal likelihood-based approach with better defined statistical properties (in terms of the power to detect linkage and the precision of the recombination fraction estimate, as a function of disease model and sample size) than association analysis.

Because of the imperfect relationship between genetic distance and the magnitude of linkage disequilibrium, the absence of allelic associations between two loci cannot be taken as strong evidence for non-linkage. It is therefore important to examine several nearby polymorphic markers in an association analysis, since a disease locus may be in disequilibrium with some but not all the markers in its vicinity. Multiple markers are also desirable in linkage analysis, but once a small region is 'saturated' so that every meiosis is 'tagged' by at least one heterozygous marker at both ends, it is unnecessary to add further markers.

4.11 Conclusions

Associations between alleles at different loci can be generated by a number of mechanisms including random drift, mutation, and population admixture. Once generated, the association between two alleles may be maintained in the population for many generations if the recombination fraction between the two loci is small. The presence of allelic associations between two loci in a large, stable population is therefore suggestive of tight linkage. The detection of allelic associations using cohort, case-control, or family designs is becoming a popular approach for mapping disease loci when the effect of size of the susceptibility allele is too small for linkage analysis.

5

The Analysis of Continuous and Quasi-continuous Characters

Human characters that are determined by the action of the genes at a single locus are necessarily discrete in nature. Such traits include the ABO blood groups, HLA antigens, and rare dominant and recessive diseases. Because of the intimate relationship between genotype and phenotype for these characters, events occurring at the genetic level, such as segregation and recombination, can often be inferred directly from observations at the phenotypic level. The genetic basis of such characters can therefore be determined using the methods of segregation, linkage and association analysis described in the previous chapters.

The situation with *continuous characters* (e.g. height and weight) is less clear. While many such characters demonstrate familial resemblance (e.g. tall parents are more likely than short parents to have tall children), they cannot be solely determined by the action of genes at a single locus, for the simple reason that the genotype at a single locus is not continuous but discrete in nature. Indeed, the unimodal, bell-shaped frequency distribution characteristic of many such traits would suggest that their variations in populations are determined by multiple factors, genetic and/or environmental. The investigation of the genetic contribution is therefore complicated by the fact that the underlying genetic events at any single locus are masked by the operation of other genetic and environmental factors, if observations can be made only at the phenotypic level.

Because of the difficulties of discerning single gene action for continuous traits, traditional quantitative genetics in humans is concerned primarily with estimating the components of phenotypic variance due to the aggregate effects of genes. In recent years, however, linkage and association approaches incorporating DNA markers are increasingly being integrated into quantitative genetics. The success of this exciting new development promises to improve our understanding of the causes of serious common disorders such as hypertension, diabetes and depression.

5.1 Early history of the genetics of continuous characters

The statistical study of the familial likeness in continuous characters began with Francis Galton, who saw the inheritance of continuous characters in statistical terms.

> the problems of family likeness fell entirely within the scope of the higher laws of chance; that we were thereby rendered capable of defining the average amount of family likeness between kinsmen in each and every degree, and of expressing the frequency with which the family likeness will depart from its average amount to any specified extent.
>
> (Galton, 1890)

Galton thought that normally distributed continuous characters were determined by 'the collective actions of a host of independent petty influences' (Galton, 1877). In order to study how these influences are passed from parent to offspring, he considered the adult heights of children in relation to the heights of their parents. He noticed that when the parent exceeded the average parental height by one unit, the child exceeded the average children's height on average by only 1/3 unit. In other words, the average height of children who had a parent of a certain height fell somewhere between the parental height and the population average. Galton (1889) called this phenomenon reversion, and later regression, toward the mean. By plotting offspring height against parental height, Galton recognized that there were two regression lines: the regression of offspring height on parental height, and the regression of parental height on offspring height. Later, Galton realized that the two regression coefficients of any pair of variables would be equal whenever the two variables had the same 'resultant variability'. This led Galton to propose the use of a single quantity, the 'correlation' to describe the relationship between the two variables (Galton, 1890; Stigler, 1989). The concepts of multiple regression and multiple correlation were later introduced to describe the relationship between the value of a trait of an individual to those of his or her 'ancestry', i.e. parents, grandparents, etc (Galton, 1897; Pearson, 1903a). In the words of the statistician G. Udny Yule, the law of ancestral inheritance states that

> The mean character of the offspring can be calculated with the more exactness, the more extensive our knowledge of the corresponding characters of the ancestry.
>
> (Yule, 1902)

Although the work by Galton on regression and correlation was important from a statistical point of view, it suffered from the lack of consideration of the underlying mechanisms of heredity. Indeed, Galton was so taken by the elegance of the statistical relationships that he thought the 'laws of Heredity were solely concerned with deviations expressed in statistical units' (Galton, 1908). The basic misconception that traits were transmitted directly from parent to offspring hindered further progress, until the importance of the work by Gregor Mendel was recognized. After a fierce debate between the 'Galtonians' and the 'Mendelians', it was Ronald Fisher who in 1918 wrote a classic paper entitled 'The correlation between relatives on the supposition of

Mendelian inheritance' which reconciled the two schools and led to the development of biometrical genetics as a separate discipline.

5.2 The twin method

It may seem at first sight that the magnitude of the genetic contribution to the variation of a continuous character can be easily assessed through the degree of resemblance between relatives. However, members of the same family may be more likely than unrelated individuals to come under the same environmental influences, and this tendency would also contribute to familial resemblance. Galton (1875), in an essay entitled 'The history of twin, as a criterion of the relative powers of nature and nurture', pointed out this problem of confounding between genetic and environmental factors:

> The objection to statistical evidence in proof of its inheritance has always been: 'The persons whom you compare may have lived under the same social conditions and have had similar advantages of education, but such prominent conditions are only a small part of those that determine the future of each man's life. It is to trifling accidental circumstances that the bent of his disposition and his success are mainly due, and these you leave wholly out of account – in fact, they do not admit to being tabulated, and therefore your statistics, however plausible at first sight, are really of very little use'

Twins, Galton argued, could provide

> a means of distinguishing between the effects of tendencies received at birth, and those that were imposed by the circumstances of their after lives; in other words, between nature and nurture.

5.2.1 Basic principles of the twin method

Identical twins, technically called monozygotic (MZ), are derived by division of a single fertilized ovum (zygote) at an early stage of development. Two individuals of identical genetic structure are therefore produced. Fraternal twins are termed dizygotic (DZ), because they are derived from two distinct fertilized ova. Like full siblings, DZ twins have, on average, half their genes in common. The rate of twinning is relatively constant for MZ twins but more variable for DZ twins, so that the ratio of MZ to DZ twins are different in different populations; it is about 1 : 2 among Europeans but the opposite, about 2 : 1, among Orientals.

The argument that MZ and DZ twins can be used to separate out genetic from environmental influences is based on the assumption that MZ and DZ twins experience the same degree of similarity in their environments, with respect to factors having an effect on the trait being considered. Under this *equal environment assumption*, any excess similarity between MZ twins over that between DZ twins must be due to the greater proportion of genes shared by MZ twins than by DZ twins.

However, the validity of this crucial equal environment assumption, in relation to both prenatal and postnatal factors, is often debated. Penrose (1959), in his book *Outline of Human Genetics*, wrote:

> the study of twins, from being regarded as one of the easiest and most reliable kinds of researches in human genetics, must now be considered as one of the most treacherous.

He gave the following imaginary example to illustrate the potential danger with the twin method.

> Suppose that a student of human heredity should hail from another planet and that he should be required to use the twin method to find out whether or not people's clothes were a direct consequence of heredity. He would find that identical twins were often dressed alike, often down to quite small details, and that this was uncommon with fraternal twins. He would confidently conclude that the choice of clothes was almost an exclusively hereditary trait

This example illustrates how the environment can exaggerate the genetic component. However, there may be factors that operate to a greater extent on MZ than on DZ twins which tend to increased variability within twin-pairs (e.g. the phenomenon of lateral inversion, where some aspect of normal anatomical asymmetry is reversed in one member of a twin-pair), and such factors are expected to have the opposite effect of underestimating the role of genetic factors (Price, 1950). Nevertheless, when used with care, the twin method remains a useful tool in human genetics.

5.2.2   One-way analysis of variance for twin data

Early methods for the statistical analysis of twin data were based on the analysis of variance for MZ and DZ twins into between-pairs and within-pairs components. If a genetic component is present, there should be less within-pair variation among MZ twins than among DZ twins.

Consider a sample of MZ (or DZ) twin-pairs (ascertained, for example, from a population twin register) in which the variable X has been measured on each individual. Let the value of the variable for twin j ($j = 1, 2$) in pair i ($i = 1, ..., n$) be x_{ij}, then the *total sum of squares* (SST), *within-pairs sum of squares* (SSW) and *between-pairs sum of squares* (SSB) are defined as

$$\left. \begin{aligned} \text{SST} &= \sum_i \sum_j (x_{ij} - x_{..})^2 \\ \text{SSW} &= \sum_i \sum_j (x_{ij} - x_{i.})^2 \\ \text{SSB} &= \sum_i \sum_j (x_{i.} - x_{..})^2 \end{aligned} \right\} \tag{5.1}$$

where $x_{..} = (\sum_i \sum_j x_{ij})/(2n)$ is the overall mean of the sample, and $x_{i.} = \sum_j x_{ij}/2$ is the mean of pair i. One-way *analysis of variance* (ANOVA) partitions the total sum of squares into the within-pairs and between-pairs sum of squares, i.e.

$$\text{SST} = \text{SSW} + \text{SSB} \tag{5.2}$$

These sums of squares can be interpreted in terms of a statistical model for the data. In a *random effects model*, it is assumed that the variable X is determined by two underlying variables, say B and W, where B is perfectly correlated between members of the same twin-pair but uncorrelated between members of different twin-pairs, while W is uncorrelated between any two individuals. The variable B therefore contributes to the variation between but not within twin-pairs, whereas the variable W contributes to the variation between all individuals, both between and within twin-pairs. Under this model, the expected values of the sums of squares are

$$\left.\begin{array}{l} E(\text{SST}) = (2n - 1)\text{Var}(X) \\[4pt] E(\text{SSW}) = n\,\text{Var}(W) \\[4pt] E(\text{SSB}) = (n - 1)[\text{Var}(W) + 2\,\text{Var}(B)] \end{array}\right\} \qquad (5.3)$$

When X, B and W are normally distributed, it can be shown that SST, SSW and SSB are proportional to chi-squared random variables with *degrees of freedom* equal to $2n - 1$, n and $n - 1$, respectively, and that SSW and SSB are independent (Searle *et al.*, 1992). These sums of squares are divided by their respective degrees of freedom to yield the corresponding *mean squares*

$$\left.\begin{array}{l} \text{MST} = \dfrac{\text{SST}}{2n - 1} \\[10pt] \text{MSW} = \dfrac{\text{SSW}}{n} \\[10pt] \text{MSB} = \dfrac{\text{SSB}}{n - 1} \end{array}\right\} \qquad (5.4)$$

The ratio

$$F = \frac{\text{MSB}}{\text{MSW}} \qquad (5.5)$$

is an F-statistic with $(n - 1, n)$ degrees of freedom, and can be used to test the hypothesis that there is no correlation between twin-pairs, i.e. $\text{Var}(B) = 0$.

When data on n_{MZ} MZ twin-pairs and n_{DZ} DZ twin-pairs are available, two separate one-way ANOVAs can be performed, yielding the mean squares, MSB_{MZ}, MSW_{MZ} for MZ twins, and MSB_{DZ}, MSW_{DZ} for DZ twins. The hypothesis of a genetic contribution to X predicts that there is less within-pair variation among MZ than among DZ twins, i.e. that MSW_{MZ} is less than MSW_{DZ}. The ratio

$$F = \frac{\text{MSW}_{\text{DZ}}}{\text{MSW}_{\text{MZ}}} \qquad (5.6)$$

is an F-statistic with $(n_{\text{DZ}}, n_{\text{MZ}})$ degrees of freedom, and can be used to test the hypothesis that there is no genetic contribution to X.

Example 5.1

Dr Alison Macdonald has collected data on the personality dimension neuroticism (as measured by the Eysenck Personality Questionnaire, EPQ) on 522 female MZ twin-pairs and 272 female DZ twin-pairs from the Institute of Psychiatry Volunteer Twin Register (Macdonald, 1996). The neuroticism scale consists of 23 present–absent equally-weighted items, and is related to the vulnerability to develop anxiety and depression (Eysenck and Eysenck, 1975). The data are summarized in Table 5.1 by cross-tabulating the neuroticism scores of MZ and DZ twin-pairs, with twin 1 being arbitrarily defined as the twin with the lower neuroticism score.

One-way ANOVA of neuroticism scores was performed using SPSS-WIN, separately for the MZ and the DZ samples. The results are as follows:

MZ sample

Source	DF	Sum of squares	Mean square	*F* value	Pr > *F*
Between-pairs	521	13445.22605364	25.80657592	2.72	0.0001
Within-pairs	522	4953.00000000	9.48850575		
Total	1043	18398.22605364			

DZ sample

Source	DF	Sum of squares	Mean square	*F* value	Pr > *F*
Between-pairs	271	5970.45404412	22.03119573	1.48	0.0007
Within-pairs	272	4053.50000000	14.90257353		
Total	543	10023.95404412			

The *F*-test for a genetic contribution is therefore

$$F_{272, 522} = \frac{\mathrm{MSW}_{DZ}}{\mathrm{MSW}_{MZ}} = 1.5700737619$$

$$P = 0.000006513$$

These results indicate the presence of a genetic contribution to the variability of neuroticism scores in the population.

5.2.3   Testing for unequal variances and heteroscedasticity

The results of a one-way ANOVA can be considered valid only if certain assumptions are not violated. One such assumption in the analysis of twin data is that the trait variance is equal for MZ and DZ twins. Unequal variances may arise for many reasons. It is possible, for example, that DZ twins with extreme values of the traits are less likely to be sampled and that this is not so for MZ twins. Alternatively, there may be factors that operate on MZ but not DZ twins

Table 5.1 Cross-tabulation of neuroticism scores for MZ and DZ twin-pairs

MZ

T_1 \ T_2	1	2	3	4	5	6	7	8	9	10	11	12	13	14	15	16	17	18	19	All
3		1	1																	2
4	1	3	4	2																10
5		1	1	12	4															18
6		1	2	6	11	6														26
7			5	5	8	7	6													31
8		1	1	1	4	8	6	3												24
9		1	2	1	5	12	9	8	7											45
10			5	3	2	3	8	5	5	4										35
11		1	1	4	3	3	9	8	3	5										37
12		2	3	3	4	4	6	8	9	4	3									46
13	1		2	4	5	4	7	7	6	6	6	3								51
14	1		1	3	2	3	1	4	4	9	4	13	5							50
15			2	1	2	1	4	4	1	2	5	7	7	3						39
16			1			1	2	1	2	4	4	5	6	4	4	1				35
17					1			1	2	3	2	1	4	6	6	9	1			36
18			1				1	1	2		1	2	2		5	1	4	1		21
19		1				1		1	2	1	1	1					2	3	1	14
20									1											1
21													1							1
All	1	11	24	41	49	55	47	47	52	35	34	28	35	22	18	11	7	4	1	522

DZ

T_1 \ T_2	2	3	4	5	6	7	8	9	10	11	12	13	14	15	16	17	19	All
4		1	1															2
5		1	3	1														5
6		1		2	3													6
7		4	1	4	6	1												16
8	3		3	1	6	4	4											21
9		3	4	2	6	2	5	3										25
10	1		3	4	2	1	2	2	3									18
11		2	1	2	4	4	4	4	2									23
12	2	2	1	2	2	4		2	4	1	1							21
13	2	2	1	2	1	1	3	1	3	7	1							22
14		1		2	2	5	2	1	2	4	2	1	1					23
15				1	2	1	1	2	4	5	2		4	2				24
16	1	3	2	1		1		4	1	2	1		4	3	2			25
17		1	2		1	1	2	1	1	2	2		3	1	1			18
18			1		1		3	1	3		1	2	1			1		14
19										1	1	1	1		2	1	1	7
20											1					1		2
All	7	21	23	24	36	25	23	23	22	15	18	7	11	8	3	5	1	272

(or vice versa); such factors will contribute variability to one type of twins but not the other. Yet another possibility is *reciprocal twin-interaction*, where the trait value of one twin has a direct effect on the trait value of the other twin. The twin-interaction is said to be *cooperative* if a high value in one twin increases the value of the other twin, and *competitive* if the reverse is true (i.e. a high value in one twin decreases the value of the other twin). Cooperative interaction tends to increase the deviations (from the overall population mean) of twin-pairs where both twins are deviated in the same direction from the mean, but to decrease the deviations of twin-pairs who deviate in opposite directions. Since deviation of both twins in the same direction is more frequent for MZ than for DZ twins (assuming that genetic factors are operating), cooperative twin-interaction leads to a greater trait variance in MZ than in DZ twins. Competitive interaction has the opposite effect, i.e. a smaller trait variance in MZ than in DZ twins.

Following one-way ANOVA yielding the total mean squares for MZ and DZ twins (MST_{MZ}, MST_{DZ}), equality of variances can be tested by the F-statistic

$$F = \frac{\text{MST}_{MZ}}{\text{MST}_{DZ}} \tag{5.7}$$

which has an F-distribution with $(2n_{MZ} - 1, 2n_{DZ} - 1)$ degrees of freedom under the hypothesis of equal variances.

Another assumption of a one-way ANOVA is homoscedasticity, that is, the variation within a twin-pair is not related to the average of the pair. Heteroscedasticity arises when the effect sizes of unshared factors (i.e. factors that cause variation within pairs) in a twin-pair depend on the level of the shared factors present in the pair. Such effect modification is suggestive of gene–environment interaction, although it may also reflect interactions between shared and non-shared genes (for DZ twins), and between shared and non-shared environments (Jinks and Fulker, 1970).

The variation within a twin-pair can be measured by the absolute pair-difference, defined as

$$x_{i-} = |x_{i1} - x_{i2}| \tag{5.8}$$

Denoting the average absolute pair-difference of the sample as $x_{.-}$, the product-moment correlation between pair-means and absolute pair-difference is

$$r = \frac{\sum (x_{i.} - x_{..})(x_{i-} - x_{.-})}{\left(\sum (x_{i.} - x_{..})^2 \sum (x_{i-} - x_{.-})^2\right)^{1/2}} \tag{5.9}$$

The significance of this correlation can be tested using Fisher's z transformation

$$z = \frac{1}{2} \ln \left[\frac{1+r}{1-r}\right] \tag{5.10}$$

which is normally distributed with a mean of 0 and a variance of $1/(n-3)$ in large samples under the null hypothesis of zero correlation. If there appears to be a curvilinear relationship between x_{i-} and $x_{i.}$ on the scatterplot, then one or both of these variables can be transformed (e.g. to x_{i-}^2 and $x_{i.}^2$ to achieve linearity before the product-moment correlation and the z-transform are calculated.

Example 5.2
Returning to the neuroticism data of Example 5.1, the F-test for equal variances is

$$F_{543,\,1043} = \frac{\text{MSW}_{\text{DZ}}}{\text{MSW}_{\text{MZ}}} = 1.0465195042$$

$$p = 0.268726137$$

The Z-tests for heteroscedasticity are performed using SPSS-WIN. The means and absolute differences of the twin-pairs are computed. The product moment correlation coefficient between the means and absolute differences is 0.04682 for MZ twin-pairs and 0.00381 for DZ twins. The Z-tests for heteroscedasticity are then

$$Z_{\text{MZ}} = 0.0468542566$$

$$p = 0.142892555$$

$$Z_{\text{DZ}} = 0.0038100184$$

$$p = 0.475086731$$

There is no evidence for unequal variances or heteroscedasticity in the neuroticism scores of the sample.

5.2.4   Intraclass correlations

If the assumptions of a one-way ANOVA on twin data are justified, then the results obtained can be used to yield an *intraclass correlation*, which is defined as the correlation between two individuals in the same class (i.e. the same twin-pair). Since the covariance of two individuals in the same twin-pair is $\text{Var}(B)$, and the variance of each individual is $\text{Var}(B) + \text{Var}(W)$, the intraclass correlation is

$$\rho = \frac{\text{Var}(B)}{\text{Var}(B) + \text{Var}(W)} \tag{5.11}$$

Moreover, since the expected mean squares are related to $\text{Var}(B)$ and $\text{Var}(W)$ for twin data as follows

$$\left.\begin{array}{l} E[\text{MSB} - \text{MSW}] = 2\,\text{Var}(B) \\ E[\text{MSB} + \text{MSW}] = 2[\text{Var}(B) + \text{Var}(W)] \end{array}\right\} \tag{5.12}$$

The statistic

$$r = \frac{\text{MSB} - \text{MSW}}{\text{MSB} + \text{MSW}} \tag{5.13}$$

is an estimate of ρ. The results from one-way ANOVA for MZ and DZ twins can therefore be used to estimate the intraclass correlation for MZ twins (r_{MZ})

and for DZ twins (r_{DZ}). The hypothesis of a genetic contribution to X predicts a greater r_{MZ} than r_{DZ}. One simple but approximate method of testing r_{MZ} and r_{DZ} for equality is to use Fisher's z-transformation

$$z = \frac{1}{2} \ln \left[\frac{1+r}{1-r} \right] \tag{5.14}$$

A test statistic z_T for the difference between r_{MZ} and r_{DZ} is

$$z_T = \frac{z_{MZ} - z_{DZ}}{\left(\dfrac{1}{n_{MZ} - 2} + \dfrac{1}{n_{DZ} - 2} \right)^{1/2}} \tag{5.15}$$

which has approximately a standard normal distribution under the null hypothesis of equal intraclass correlations for MZ and DZ twins (Donner, 1986).

If there is evidence for a greater intraclass correlation among MZ than among DZ twins, then one may to proceed to obtain some measure of the relative importance of genetic to environmental factors. One early suggestion was Holzinger's H (Holzinger, 1929), defined as

$$H = \frac{r_{MZ} - r_{DZ}}{1 - r_{DZ}} \tag{5.16}$$

This statistic is now rarely used because it is not an estimate of *heritability*, which is technically defined as the proportion of phenotypic variance accounted for by genetic factors. In order to estimate heritability, it is necessary to consider the consequences of gene action on the correlations between relatives. This forms the basis of the biometrical genetic approach.

Example 5.3
Returning to the neuroticism data of Example 5.1 and using the analysis of variance output, the intraclass correlations for MZ and DZ twins are

$$r_{MZ} = \frac{MSB_{MZ} - MSW_{MZ}}{MSB_{MZ} + MSW_{MZ}} = 0.4623$$

$$r_{DZ} = \frac{MSB_{DZ} - MSW_{DZ}}{MSB_{DZ} + MSW_{DZ}} = 0.1931$$

The Z-test for equal intraclass correlations is

$$z = 4.0626$$

$$p = 0.000024$$

so that there is evidence for a genetic contribution to neuroticism. Finally, the statistic

$$\text{Holizinger's } H = \frac{r_{MZ} - r_{DZ}}{1 - r_{DZ}} = 0.33368$$

5.3 Biometrical genetics

The basis of the biometrical approach to the genetics of continuous characters is stated by the pioneers of biometrical genetics, Mather and Jinks (1977), as follows.

> If we accept that commonly we cannot distinguish any of the individual genes whose segregation contributes to continuous variation ... we must be content to deal with the relevant polygenic system as a whole. And since we cannot distinguish the segregant classes one from another, we cannot use a form of analysis based on class frequencies as in the classic Mendelian method. We can, however, recognize the biometrical properties of the frequency distributions of the phenotypes which are our raw material, and we can estimate the biometrical quantities, the means, variances, and so on, that characterize these distributions.... We shall thus be concentrating on the genetical information that can be derived from comparisons among the means, variances, and covariances of related families or groups of individuals. These we shall seek to interpret in terms of appropriate parameters representing the consequences of the various genetic phenomena in which we may be interested. Having defined these parameters, expectations are formulated in terms of them for the means, variances and covariances of the families or groups that our experiments yield. The means, etc observed are then related to these expectations in such a way as to yield estimates of the parameters and tests of their significance.

Biometrical genetics has its origin in a classic paper by Fisher (1918) entitled 'The correlation between relatives on the supposition of Mendelian inheritance' the purpose of which was:

> to interpret the well-established results of biometry in accordance with the Mendelian scheme of inheritance ... to make a more general analysis of the causes of human variability.

Interestingly, this paper introduced the term *variance* and the concept of *analysis of variance*:

> When there are two independent causes of variability capable to producing in an otherwise uniform population distributions with standard deviations σ_1 and σ_2 it is found that the distribution, when both causes act together, has a standard deviation of $\sqrt{(\sigma_1^2 + \sigma_2^2)}$. It is therefore desirable in analysing the causes of variability to deal with the square of the standard deviation as the measure of variability. We shall term this quantity the Variance of the normal population to which it refers, and we may wish now to ascribe to the constituent causes fractions or percentages of the total variance which they together produce.

This paper also planted the seeds for the subsequent invention of the factorial design in connection with agricultural experiments (Fisher, 1952):

> The factorial method of experimentation ... derives its structure, and its name, from the simultaneous inheritance of Mendelian factors.

5.3.1   Genetic components of variance

We now show how the total genetic variance of a trait can be partitioned for a one-locus system and a two-locus system, under the simplifying assumptions of random mating in a large population. These results generalize to multi-locus systems that are the concern of biometrical genetics (Kempthorne, 1957).

Single-locus model   We assume that the trait concerned, Y, is determined by a single biallelic locus under Hardy–Weinberg equilibrium. We denote the two alleles at the locus by A, a, with frequencies p_A, p_a, and the three genotypes by AA, Aa, aa, with means y_{AA}, y_{Aa}, y_{aa}. The residual variance in Y around these means is assumed to be environmental and the same for the three genotypes.

Since we are interested in a decomposition of variance, we can regard the genotypic means y_{AA}, y_{Aa}, y_{aa} as deviations from the overall mean, without loss of generality. The total genetic variance of Y is therefore a weighted average of the squares of these mean deviations, the weight of each genotypic mean being the frequency of the genotype in the population.

$$V_G = p_A^2 y_{AA}^2 + 2p_A p_a y_{Aa}^2 + p_a^2 y_{aa}^2 \qquad (5.17)$$

An additive model (M_3) considers each genotypic mean to be determined by the sum of the effects of the alleles present. Let μ_A and μ_a denote the effects of alleles A and a, we write

$$\left. \begin{array}{l} y_{AA} = 2\mu_A + \mu_{AA} \\ y_{Aa} = \mu_A + \mu_a + \mu_{Aa} \\ y_{aa} = 2\mu_a + \mu_{aa} \end{array} \right\} \qquad (5.18)$$

where μ_{AA}, μ_{Aa} and μ_{aa} are defined as residual *dominance deviations*, which should be small if the additive model is adequate. Exact additivity holds when y_{Aa} is the average of y_{AA} and y_{aa}, since then the three dominance deviations can be made to vanish by setting μ_A and μ_a equal to 0.5 y_{AA} and 0.5 y_{aa} respectively. When exact additivity does not hold, then the values of μ_A and μ_a should still be chosen to minimize the residual dominance variance, which is

$$\left. \begin{array}{l} V_D = p_A^2 (y_{AA} - 2\mu_A)^2 + 2p_A p_a (y_{Aa} - \mu_A - \mu_a)^2 + p_a^2 (y_{aa} - 2\mu_a)^2 \\ = p_A^2 \mu_{AA}^2 + 2p_A p_a \mu_{Aa}^2 + p_a^2 \mu_{aa}^2 \end{array} \right\} \qquad (5.19)$$

The difference between V_G and V_D is the additive variance, V_A

$$V_A = p_A^2 (2\mu_A)^2 + 2p_A p_a (\mu_A + \mu_a)^2 + p_a^2 (2\mu_a)^2 \qquad (5.20)$$

The minimization of V_D can be achieved by obtaining the partial derivatives of V_D with respect to μ_A and μ_a and setting these partial derivatives to zero.

Omitting mathematical details, it can be shown that the expressions for μ_A and μ_a, which minimize V_D, are

$$\left.\begin{array}{l} \mu_A = p_A y_{AA} + p_a y_{Aa} \\ \mu_a = p_A y_{Aa} + p_a y_{aa} \end{array}\right\} \qquad (5.21)$$

From these expressions, it is clear that the additive or *genic effect* of a specific allele is simply a weighted average of genotypic means, where the weight attached to a particular genotype is the probability that the second gene is the allele necessary to make up the genotype given that the first gene is the allele concerned. For example, in the case of μ_A, the weight given to y_{AA} is p_A because given that the first allele in a genotype is A, there is a probability p_A that the second allele is also A. This suggests writing μ_A as $y_{A.}$ where the dot at the second position represents a weighted summation over all alleles that can occupy that position.

Substituting the obtained expressions of the additive genic effects μ_A and μ_a back into V_D and simplifying, we obtain the dominance variance

$$V_D = p_A^2 p_a^2 (y_{AA} - 2y_{Aa} + y_{aa})^2 \qquad (5.22)$$

Similarly, the additive variance is obtained by substituting these expressions of μ_A and μ_a into V_A

$$V_A = 2p_A p_a [p_A (y_{AA} - y_{Aa}) + p_a (y_{Aa} - y_{aa})]^2 \qquad (5.23)$$

Example 5.4
Consider a trait under the influence of a single biallelic locus with allele frequencies $p_a = 0.99$, $p_A = 0.01$ and genotypic means $y_{aa} = 0$, $y_{Aa} = 1$, $y_{AA} = 1$, what are the values of the additive and dominance components of variance?
Using the above formulae

$$V_A = 0.019406$$
$$V_D = 0.000098$$

Alternatively, these components of variance may be obtained by a two-way analysis of variance using a standard statistical package. First, create a data file as follows

1	1	1	0.01	0.01
1	2	1	0.01	0.99
2	1	1	0.99	0.01
2	2	0	0.99	0.99

The first two columns represent the two alleles that make up a genotype (a value of 1 representing allele A, and a value of 2 representing allele a). Note that the genotype Aa is represented twice, once as (1, 2) and again as (2, 1). The third column gives the means for the four genotypes. The last two columns are the frequencies of the alleles in the first two columns. This dataset is then subjected to a two-way ANOVA. If the above data file is called 1locus.dat, then an appropriate command file for SPSS-PC is as follows

```
DATA LIST FILE '1locus.dat' FREE / A1 A2 y p1 p2.
compute f = (p1*p2)*1000.
weight by f.
anova /var y by A1 A2 (1,2) /option 10.
```

Option 10 specifies a hierarchical analysis. The output from the analysis is as follows.

Source of variation	Sum of squares
Main effects	19.406
A1	9.703
A2	9.703
2-way interactions	0.098
A1 A2	0.098
Explained	19.504
Residual	0.000
Total	19.504

Since each genotype was weighted by a factor of 1000 for the analysis, the sums of squares should be divided by 1000 in order to obtain variance components. Thus, the variance due to the main effects (i.e. the additive component) is 0.019406, and the variance due to two-way interactions (i.e. the dominance component) is 0.000098. These values are identical to those obtained by standard formulae.

Two-locus model The extension to two loci introduces the possibility of interactions between alleles at different loci, called *epistasis*. As for the one-locus system, we assume that each locus is in Hardy–Weinberg equilibrium. In addition, we also assume linkage equilibrium between the loci, so that the frequency of each joint genotype is the product of the frequencies of the marginal genotypes present. Let the alleles at the two loci be denoted as A, a and B, b, their frequencies be p_A, p_a and p_B, p_b, and the mean values of the nine joint genotypes be $y_{AABB}, y_{AABb}, y_{AAbb}, y_{AaBB}, y_{AaBb}, y_{Aabb}, y_{aaBB}, y_{aaBb}, y_{aabb}$. For each marginal genotype (i.e. AA, Aa, aa, BB, Bb, bb), a marginal genotypic mean is defined as the weighted average of the joint genotypic means, the weight attached to a particular joint genotype being the frequency of the genotype at the other locus that will, together with the marginal genotype being considered, make up the joint genotype. For example, the marginal genotypic mean for AA is

$$y_{AA.} = p_B^2 y_{AABB} + 2p_B p_b y_{AABb} + p_b^2 y_{AAbb} \tag{5.24}$$

Similarly, the marginal means of alleles A, a, B, b are defined as weighted averages of joint genotypic means. For example,

$$y_{A...} = p_A p_B^2 y_{AABB} + 2p_A p_B p_b y_{AABb} + p_A p_b^2 y_{AAbb}$$
$$+ p_a p_B^2 y_{AaBB} + 2p_a p_B p_b y_{AaBb} + p_a p_b^2 y_{Aabb} \tag{5.25}$$
$$= p_A y_{AA.} + p_a y_{Aa.}$$

These marginal means of the alleles can be shown to be the genic effects that maximize the additive genetic variance. We can therefore define the three weighted sums of squares:

$$
\begin{aligned}
SS_1 = \; & p_A^2 p_B^2 y_{AABB}^2 + 2p_A^2 p_B p_b y_{AABb}^2 \\
& + p_A^2 p_b^2 y_{AAbb}^2 + 2p_A p_a p_B^2 y_{AaBB}^2 \\
& + 4p_A p_a p_B p_b y_{AaBb}^2 \\
& + 2p_A p_a p_b^2 y_{Aabb}^2 + p_a^2 p_B^2 y_{aaBB}^2 \\
& + 2p_a^2 p_B p_b y_{aaBb}^2 + p_a^2 p_b^2 y_{aabb}^2 \\
SS_2 = \; & p_A^2 p_B^2 (y_{AA..} + y_{..BB})^2 + 2p_A^2 p_B p_b (y_{AA..} + y_{..Bb})^2 \\
& + p_A^2 p_b^2 (y_{AA..} + y_{..bb})^2 + 2p_A p_a p_B^2 (y_{Aa..} + y_{..BB})^2 \\
& + 4p_A p_a p_B p_b (y_{Aa..} + y_{..Bb})^2 \\
& + 2p_A p_a p_b^2 (y_{Aa..} + y_{..bb})^2 + p_a^2 p_B^2 (y_{aa..} - y_{..BB})^2 \\
& + 2p_a^2 p_B p_b (y_{aa..} + y_{..Bb})^2 + p_a^2 p_b^2 (y_{aa..} - y_{..bb})^2 \\
SS_3 = \; & p_A^2 p_B^2 (2y_{A...} + 2y_{..B.})^2 + 2p_A^2 p_B p_b (2y_{A...} + y_{..B.} + y_{...b})^2 \\
& + p_A^2 p_b^2 (2y_{A...} + 2y_{...b})^2 + 2p_A p_a p_B^2 (y_{A...} + y_{.a.} + 2y_{..B.})^2 \\
& + 4p_A p_a p_B p_b (y_{A...} + y_{.a.} + y_{..B.} + y_{...b})^2 \\
& + 2p_A p_a p_b^2 (y_{A...} + y_{.a.} + 2y_{...b})^2 + p_a^2 p_B^2 (2y_{.a.} + 2y_{..B.})^2 \\
& + 2p_a^2 p_B p_b (2y_{.a.} + y_{..B.} + y_{...b})^2 + p_a^2 p_b^2 (2y_{.a.} + 2y_{...b})^2
\end{aligned}
\tag{5.26}
$$

where the summations are over the nine joint genotypes. These three quantities represent, respectively, $V_A + V_D + V_I$, $V_A + V_D$ and V_A where V_I is defined as the *epistatic variance*. These components of variance are therefore obtained by

$$
\left.
\begin{aligned}
V_A &= SS_3 \\
V_D &= SS_2 - SS_3 \\
V_I &= SS_1 - SS_2
\end{aligned}
\right\}
\tag{5.27}
$$

It is possible to decompose the epistatic variance V_I further into three subcomponents. The first subcomponent represents the interactive effects of combinations of two alleles, one from each locus, and is denoted V_{AA} (*additive-additive* interactions). The second subcomponent represents the interactive effects of combinations of three alleles, one from one locus and two from the other, and is denoted V_{AD} (*additive-dominance* interactions). The third subcomponent represents the interactive effects of combinations of four alleles, two from each locus, and is denoted V_{DD} (*dominance-dominance* interactions). The derivation of these components involves the calculation of means for marginal genotypes containing alleles at different loci. For example, the mean of the marginal genotype AAB is

$$
y_{AAB.} = p_B y_{AABB} + p_b y_{AABb}
\tag{5.28}
$$

and the mean of the marginal genotype AB is

$$
y_{A.B.} = p_A p_B y_{AABB} + p_a p_B y_{AaBB} + p_A p_b y_{AABb} + p_a p_b y_{AaBb}
\tag{5.29}
$$

We then define quantities such as

$$
\left.
\begin{aligned}
\mu_A &= y_{A...} \\
\mu_{AA} &= y_{AA..} - 2\mu_A \\
\mu_{AB} &= y_{A.B.} - \mu_A - \mu_B \\
\mu_{AAB} &= y_{AAB.} - \mu_{AA} - 2\mu_{AB} - 2\mu_A - \mu_B \\
\mu_{AABB} &= y_{AABB} - 2\mu_{AAB} - 2\mu_{ABB} - 4\mu_{AB} - \mu_{AA} - \mu_{BB} - 2\mu_A - 2\mu_B
\end{aligned}
\right\}
\tag{5.30}
$$

The full array of such quantities for two biallelic loci is as follows

Genic effects: $\quad \mu_A, \mu_a, \mu_B, \mu_b$

Dominance interactions: $\quad \mu_{AA}, \mu_{Aa}, \mu_{aa}, \mu_{BB}, \mu_{Bb}, \mu_{bb}$

AA interactions: $\quad \mu_{AB}, \mu_{Ab}, \mu_{aB}, \mu_{ab}$

AD interactions: $\quad \mu_{AAB}, \mu_{AAb}, \mu_{AaB}, \mu_{Aab}, \mu_{aaB}, \mu_{aab}, \mu_{ABB},$
$\qquad\qquad\qquad \mu_{ABb}, \mu_{Abb}, \mu_{BB}, \mu_{aBb}, \mu_{abb}$

DD interactions: $\quad \mu_{AABB}, \mu_{AABb}, \mu_{AAbb}, \mu_{AaBB}, \mu_{AaBb}, \mu_{Aabb}, \mu_{aaBB}, \mu_{aaBb}, \mu_{aabb}$

Recalling that all genotypic means are deviations from the overall mean, it should be clear that V_A is the expectation of the squares of the genic effects for an individual in the population.

$$
\left.
\begin{aligned}
V_A &= p_A^2 p_B^2 (2\mu_A + 2\mu_B)^2 + 2p_A^2 p_B p_b (2\mu_A + \mu_B + \mu_b)^2 \\
&+ p_A^2 p_b^2 (2\mu_A + 2\mu_b)^2 + 2p_A p_a p_B^2 (\mu_A + \mu_a + 2\mu_B)^2 \\
&+ 4p_A p_a p_B p_b (\mu_A + \mu_a + \mu_B + \mu_b)^2 \\
&+ 2p_A p_a p_b^2 (\mu_A + \mu_a + 2\mu_b)^2 + p_a^2 p_B^2 (2\mu_a + 2\mu_B)^2 \\
&+ 2p_a^2 p_B p_b (2\mu_a + \mu_B + \mu_b)^2 + p_a^2 p_b^2 (2\mu_a + 2\mu_b)^2
\end{aligned}
\right\}
\tag{5.31}
$$

It also follows that V_D is the expectation of the squares of the dominance interactions

$$
\left.
\begin{aligned}
V_D &= p_A^2 p_B^2 (\mu_{AA} + \mu_{BB})^2 + 2p_A^2 p_B p_b (\mu_{AA} + \mu_{Bb})^2 \\
&+ p_A^2 p_b^2 (\mu_{AA} + \mu_{bb})^2 + 2p_A p_a p_B^2 (\mu_{Aa} + \mu_{BB})^2 \\
&+ 4p_A p_a p_B p_b (\mu_{Aa} + \mu_{Bb})^2 \\
&+ 2p_A p_a p_b^2 (\mu_{Aa} + \mu_{bb})^2 + p_a^2 p_B^2 (\mu_{aa} + \mu_{BB})^2 \\
&+ 2p_a^2 p_B p_b (\mu_{aa} + \mu_{Bb})^2 + p_a^2 p_b^2 (\mu_{aa} + \mu_{bb})^2
\end{aligned}
\right\}
\tag{5.32}
$$

V_{AA} is the expectation of the squares of the AA interactions

$$
\left.
\begin{aligned}
V_{AA} &= p_A^2 p_B^2 (4\mu_{AB})^2 + 2p_A^2 p_B p_b (2\mu_{AB} + 2\mu_{Ab})^2 \\
&+ p_A^2 p_b^2 (4\mu_{Ab})^2 + 2p_A p_a p_B^2 (2\mu_{AB} + 2\mu_{aB})^2 \\
&+ 4p_A p_a p_B p_b (\mu_{AB} + \mu_{Ab} + \mu_{aB} + \mu_{ab})^2 \\
&+ 2p_A p_a p_b^2 (2\mu_{Ab} + 2\mu_{ab})^2 + p_a^2 p_B^2 (4\mu_{aB})^2 \\
&+ 2p_a^2 p_B p_b (2\mu_{aB} + 2\mu_{ab})^2 + p_a^2 p_b^2 (4\mu_{ab})^2
\end{aligned}
\right\}
\tag{5.33}
$$

V_{AD} is the expectation of the squares of the AD interactions

$$
\left.
\begin{aligned}
V_{AD} &= p_A^2 p_B^2 (2\mu_{AAB} + 2\mu_{ABB})^2 + 2p_A^2 p_B p_b (2\mu_{ABb} + \mu_{AAB} + \mu_{AAb}) \\
&+ p_A^2 p_b^2 (2\mu_{AAb} + 2\mu_{Abb})^2 + 2p_A p_a p_B^2 (2\mu_{AaB} + \mu_{ABB} + \mu_{aBB}) \\
&+ 4p_A p_a p_B p_b (\mu_{AaB} + \mu_{Aab} + \mu_{ABb} + \mu_{aBb})^2 \\
&+ 2p_A p_a p_b^2 (2\mu_{Aab} + \mu_{Abb} + \mu_{abb})^2 + p_a^2 p_B^2 (2\mu_{aaB} + 2\mu_{aBB}) \\
&+ 2p_a^2 p_B p_b (\mu_{aaB} + \mu_{aab} + 2\mu_{aBb})^2 + p_a^2 p_b^2 (2\mu_{aab} + 2\mu_{abb})
\end{aligned}
\right\} \tag{5.34}
$$

V_{DD} is the expectation of the squares of the DD interactions

$$
\left.
\begin{aligned}
V_{DD} &= p_A^2 p_B^2 \mu_{AABB}^2 + 2p_A^2 p_B p_b \mu_{AABb}^2 + p_A^2 p_b^2 \mu_{AAbb}^2 \\
&+ 2p_A p_a p_B^2 \mu_{AaBB}^2 + 4p_A p_a p_B p_b \mu_{AaBb}^2 + 2p_A p_a p_b^2 \mu_{Aabb}^2 \\
&+ p_a^2 p_B^2 \mu_{aaBB}^2 + 2p_a^2 p_B p_b \mu_{aaBb}^2 + p_a^2 p_b^2 \mu_{aabb}^2
\end{aligned}
\right\} \tag{5.35}
$$

From this formulation, it is clear that the genic effects represent the effects of the individual genes. The dominance interactions represent the effects of combinations of two genes, both from the same locus, after the effects of the individual genes are discounted. The AA interactions represent the effects of combinations of two genes, one from each locus, after the effects of the individual genes are discounted, and so on. In general, each component consists of the effects of having certain combinations of genes after discounting the effects of all subcombinations of genes.

An important feature of this decomposition of variance is that if additive and dominance variances are obtained for the two loci separately, using the means of the marginal genotypes, then the sum of the additive variances is equal to the total additive variance, and the sum of the dominance variances is equal to the total dominance variance. This important result generalizes to multilocus systems, so that the total additive variance is the sum of the additive variances, and the total dominance variance is the sum of the dominance variances, of the contributory loci.

Another important feature of this decomposition, which is implicit in a hierarchical factorial analysis of variance, is that the components are orthogonal to each other. This feature simplifies the derivation of the genetic covariances and correlations between relatives, and will be discussed later. In summary, for two biallelic loci, the total genetic variance V_G can be partitioned as follows

$$
\left.
\begin{aligned}
V_G &= V_A + V_D + V_I \\
&= V_A + V_D + V_{AA} + V_{AD} + V_{DD}
\end{aligned}
\right\} \tag{5.36}
$$

Example 5.5
Consider a two-locus model with the following allele frequencies and phenotypic means

$$p_a = 0.99, \; p_A = 0.01$$

$$p_b = 0.90, \; p_B = 0.10$$

$$y_{AABB} = 1.0, \; y_{AaBB} = 1.0, \; y_{aaBB} = 0.0$$

$$y_{AABb} = 1.0, \; y_{AaBb} = 1.0, \; y_{aaBb} = 0.0$$

$$y_{AAbb} = 1.0, \; y_{Aabb} = 0.0, \; y_{aabb} 0.0$$

The overall mean is

$$y_{...} = 0.003862$$

The centred means are therefore,

$$y_{AABB} = 0.996138, y_{AaBB} = 0.996138, y_{aaBB} = -0.003862$$
$$y_{AABb} = 0.996138, y_{AaBb} = 0.996138, y_{aaBb} = -0.003862$$
$$y_{AAbb} = 0.996138, y_{Aabb} = -0.003862, y_{aabb} = -0.003862$$

Using the above formulae, the additive effects are

$$\mu_A = 0.194238, \mu_a = -0.001962, \mu_B = 0.016038, \mu_b = -0.001782$$

The dominance effects are

$$\mu_{AA} = 0.607662, \mu_{Aa} = -0.006138, \mu_{aa} = 0.000062$$
$$\mu_{BB} = -0.016038, \mu_{Bb} = 0.001782, \mu_{bb} = -0.000198$$

The AA interactions are

$$\mu_{AB} = 0.785862, \mu_{Ab} = -0.087318, \mu_{aB} = -0.007938, \mu_{ab} = 0.000882$$

The AD interactions are

$$\mu_{AAB} = -1.587762, \mu_{AAb} = 0.176418, \mu_{AaB} = 0.016038$$
$$\mu_{Aab} = -0.001782, \mu_{aaB} = -0.000162, \mu_{aab}0.000018$$
$$\mu_{ABB} = -0.785862, \mu_{ABb} = 0.087318, \mu_{Abb} = -0.009702$$
$$\mu_{ABB} = -0.785862, \mu_{aBb} = -0.000882, \mu_{abb} = 0.000098$$

The DD interactions are

$$\mu_{AABB} = 1.587762, \mu_{AABb} = -0.176418, \mu = 0.019602$$
$$\mu_{AaBB} = -0.016038, \mu_{AaBb} = 0.001782, \mu_{Aabb} = -0.000198$$
$$\mu_{aaBB} = 0.000162, \mu_{aaBb} = -0.000018, \mu_{aabb} = 0.000002$$

From these we obtain

$$V_A = 0.000819$$
$$V_D = 0.000041$$
$$V_{AA} = 0.002773$$
$$V_{AD} = 0.000211$$
$$V_{DD} = 0.000003$$

Alternatively, these components can be obtained by a factorial analysis of variance of the following data using SPSS.

1	1	1	1	1	0.01	0.01	0.1	0.1
1	1	1	2	1	0.01	0.01	0.1	0.9
1	1	2	1	1	0.01	0.01	0.9	0.1
1	1	2	2	1	0.01	0.01	0.9	0.9

1	2	1	1	1	0.01	0.99	0.1	0.1
1	2	1	2	1	0.01	0.99	0.1	0.9
1	2	2	1	1	0.01	0.99	0.9	0.1
1	2	2	2	0	0.01	0.99	0.9	0.9
2	1	1	1	1	0.99	0.01	0.1	0.1
2	1	1	2	1	0.99	0.01	0.1	0.9
2	1	2	1	1	0.99	0.01	0.9	0.1
2	1	2	2	0	0.99	0.01	0.9	0.9
2	2	1	1	0	0.99	0.99	0.1	0.1
2	2	1	2	0	0.99	0.99	0.1	0.9
2	2	2	1	0	0.99	0.99	0.9	0.1
2	2	2	2	0	0.99	0.99	0.9	0.9

Columns 1 and 2 represent the alleles at locus A. Columns 3 and 4 represent the alleles at locus B. Column 5 is the genotypic means. Column 6 and 7 are the frequencies of the alleles at locus A. Columns 8 and 9 are the frequencies of the alleles at locus B. If this data file is called 2loci.dat, then an appropriate command file for SPSS-PC is as follows:

```
DATA LIST FILE '210ci.dat' FREE / A1 A2 B1 B2 y
p1 p2 q1 q2.
compute f = (p1*p2*q1*q2)*1000.
weight by f.
ANOVA /VARIABLES Y BY A1 A2 B1 B2 (1,2) /OPTIONS
10.
```

Option 10 specifies a hierarchical analysis. The output from the analysis is as follows.

Source of variation	Sum of squares
Main effects	0.819
A1	0.381
A2	0.381
B1	0.029
B2	0.029
2-way interactions	2.813
A1 A2	0.038
A1 B1	0.693
A1 B2	0.693
A2 B1	0.693
A2 B2	0.693
B1 B2	0.003
3-way interactions	0.211
A1 A2 B1	0.029
A1 A2 B2	0.029
A1 B1 B2	0.077
A2 B1 B2	0.077
Explained	3.844
Residual	0.003
Total	3.847

Since each genotype was weighted by a factor of 1000 for the analysis, the sums of squares should be divided by 1000 in order to obtain variance components. Thus

$$V_A = 0.000819$$

$$V_D = 0.000038 + 0.000003 = 0.000041$$

$$V_{AA} = 0.002813 - 0.000041 = 0.002772$$

$$V_{AD} = 0.000211$$

$$V_{DD} = 0.000003$$

These values are identical to those obtained by standard formulae.

General multilocus models   In the general case of any arbitrary number of loci each with an arbitrary number of alleles, the principles of the above decomposition hold. The number of components due to the interaction between alleles increases with the number of loci. For example, with three loci, the additional components are V_{AAA}, V_{AAD}, V_{ADD} and V_{DDD}. In general, we have

$$\left.\begin{aligned} V_G &= V_A + V_D + V_I \\ &= V_A + V_D + V_{AA} + V_{AD} + V_{DD} + V_{AAA} + V_{AAD} + V_{ADD} + V_{DDD} + \ldots \end{aligned}\right\} \quad (5.37)$$

For any given set of population allele frequencies and genotypic means, the values of these variance components can be obtained using a hierarchical factorial analysis of variance, by SPSS or a similar software.

Decomposition of genetic variance with sample data   The above decomposition of genetic variance assumes full knowledge of the population allele frequencies and genotypic means. However, it can readily be adapted for use on sample data. Consider a random sample of the population for whom phenotypic and genotypic data are available. Suppose initially that only one biallelic locus is involved. There are thus three possible genotypes. The factorial analysis of variance, however, requires each individual to be assigned to one of four cells in a 2×2 table, i.e. $(1, 1)$, $(1, 2)$, $(2, 1)$, $(2, 2)$. It is unclear whether a heterozygous individual should be placed in $(1, 2)$ or $(2, 1)$. A simple solution is to duplicate each heterozygous observation, and place the first duplicate in $(1, 2)$, and the second duplicate in $(2, 1)$. All these duplicated observations are then given a weight of $1/2$. A simple hierarchical 2-way analysis of variance is then performed.

For k loci, the same principles apply. An observation that is heterozygous at k loci is made into 2^k duplicates and distributed to the appropriate 2^k cells. Each of these duplicate observations is then given a weight of 2^{-k} in the analysis. For two loci, for example, a doubly heterozygous individual is made into four duplicates and distributed to the four cells $(1, 2, 1, 2)$, $(1, 2, 2, 1)$, $(2, 1, 1, 2)$, $(2, 1, 2, 1)$, and each of these duplicate observations is given a weight of $1/4$. Whereas hypothesis testing is irrelevant in a theoretical partitioning of variance using population frequencies and means, F-tests should be performed in an analysis of variance of sample data in order to assess the statistical significance of the various genetic components, and to obtain the most parsimonious model consistent with the data.

Example 5.6
Genotypic and phenotypic data on 20 individuals were simulated under the following single locus genetic model

$$p_1 = p_2 = 0.5, \; \mu_{11} = \mu_{12} = 1, \; \mu_{22} = 0$$

with a residual variance (V_R) of 1. The population variance components can be calculated to be

$$V_A = 0.125, \; V_D = 0.0625, \; V_R = 1$$

The simulated data, with the heterozygous observations being duplicated and weighted by 0.5, are as follows.

OBS	Y	W	A_1	A_2
1	1.73501	1.0	1	1
2	1.19375	1.0	1	1
3	1.32509	1.0	1	1
4	1.37223	1.0	1	1
5	1.96093	1.0	1	1
6	-0.42765	1.0	1	1
7	0.96554	1.0	1	1
8	2.77968	1.0	1	1
9	1.35472	0.5	1	2
10	1.35472	0.5	2	1
11	1.26041	0.5	1	2
12	1.26041	0.5	2	1
13	1.82858	0.5	1	2
14	1.82858	0.5	2	1
15	0.08447	0.5	1	2
16	0.08447	0.5	2	1
17	0.66040	0.5	1	2
18	0.66040	0.5	2	1
19	0.59135	0.5	1	2
20	0.59135	0.5	2	1
21	1.55433	0.5	1	2
22	1.55433	0.5	2	1
23	0.47725	0.5	1	2
24	0.47725	0.5	2	1
25	1.55933	0.5	1	2
26	1.55933	0.5	2	1
27	0.16300	1.0	2	2
28	0.59306	1.0	2	2
29	-0.57894	1.0	2	2

Here Y is the phenotypic trait value, W is the weight, and A_1 and A_2 are the two alleles that make up the genotype of the observation. Although only 20 observations were generated, the nine heterozygous observations were duplicated, giving a total of 29 rows of data.

The results of a two-way factorial hierarchical ANOVA on this dataset using SPSS are as follows.

Source of variation	Sum of squares	DF	Mean square	F	Sig of F
Main effects	3.233	2	1.616	2.728	0.096
A1	1.681	1	1.681	2.837	0.111
A2	1.552	1	1.552	2.619	0.125
2-way interactions	0.483	1	0.483	0.815	0.380
A1 A2	0.483	1	0.483	0.815	0.380
Explained	3.716	3	1.239	2.091	0.142
Residual	9.479	16	0.592		
Total	13.195	19	0.694		

The sums of squares can be divided by the sample size, 20, to obtain sample estimates of the various components of variance. These sample estimates (denoted as S) are

$$S_A = 0.162, \; S_D = 0.0241, \; S_R = 0.474$$

These sample estimates are not very close to the population values due to the small sample size.

5.3.2   Genetic covariance and correlation between relatives

In order to derive the predicted genetic covariance between relatives of a certain kind (e.g. parent–offspring, siblings) from first principles, it is necessary to consider the joint probability distribution of the two relatives, and evaluate a weighted sum of the products of the genotypic means for all possible combinations of genotypes, each combination being weighted by its joint probability. This is a tedious procedure, especially when several loci are considered. Fortunately, there is a simpler method based on the components of genetic variance, when the assumption of random mating in a large population is reasonable (Kempthorne, 1957).

This simple procedure for obtaining the genetic covariance between two relatives requires the definition of some coefficients that characterize the nature of the relationship between the pair of relatives. These coefficients are based on the concept of *identity-by-descent* (IBD). Two genes are defined to be identical-by-descent if they are descended from and are therefore replicates of the same ancestral gene. We assume that the two genes at the same locus of any individual are not IBD, or, in other words, that the two parents of any individual are unrelated. Under this assumption, two individuals may have either 0, 1 or 2 genes IBD at each locus. The probabilities of these three events at any locus provide important information about how closely two individuals are related. We denote these *IBD probabilities* as p_0, p_1 and p_2. The values of these IBD probabilities for some simple relationships can be deduced quite easily from the nature of the relationship. The *coefficient of relationship* for two individuals, which we denote as r_A, is defined as the expected proportion of genes of the two individuals that are

Table 5.2 IBD probabilities and coefficient of relationship for simple relationships

Relationship	p_0	p_1	p_2	r_A
MZ twins	0	0	1	1
DZ twins	1/4	1/2	1/4	1/2
Parent–offspring	0	1	0	1/2
Full siblings	1/4	1/2	1/4	1/2
Grandparent–grandchild	1/2	1/2	0	1/4
Half siblings	1/2	1/2	0	1/4
Uncle–nephew	1/2	1/2	0	1/4
First cousins	3/4	1/4	0	1/8

IBD, i.e.

$$r_A = \frac{1}{2} p_1 + p_2 \qquad (5.38)$$

Alternatively, r_A can be thought of as the probability that a gene drawn at random from one individual is IBD to one of the two genes at the same locus in the other individual. The coefficient of relationship is sometimes confused with the *coefficient of kinship*, which is defined as the probability that two genes at the same locus, drawn at random, one from each person, will be IBD. The coefficient of the relationship is twice the coefficient of kinship in non-inbred populations.

Recalling that each genetic component of variance is due to the effects of having certain combinations of alleles after discounting the effects of all subcombinations, it is clear that the correlations between these components of two individuals are determined by the probabilities of sharing various combinations of alleles. Moreover, the different components are defined in such a way that the correlation between any two components is 0. The covariance between two individuals, including variance components due to interactions of up to two loci, is therefore

$$\text{Cov}_G = r_A V_A + p_2 V_D + r_A^2 V_{AA} + r_A p_2 V_{AD} + p_2^2 V_{DD} \qquad (5.39)$$

In general, the correlation between two relatives for the additive effects is r_A, the correlation for the dominance deviations is p_2, the correlation for epistatic effects associated with combinations of $(u + 2v)$ alleles consisting of one allele from each of u distinct loci and two alleles from each of another v distinct loci, is $r_A^u p_2^u$.

Having obtained the genetic covariance, the *genetic correlation* is simply the genetic covariance divided by the total genetic variance, i.e.

$$\text{Corr}_G = \text{Cov}_G / V_G \qquad (5.40)$$

In particular the genetic correlation of MZ twins is

$$\text{Corr}_G = 1 \qquad (5.41)$$

while, ignoring epistatic effects between more than two loci, the genetic correlation for full siblings (and DZ twins) is

$$\text{Corr}_G = \frac{\dfrac{V_A}{2} + \dfrac{V_D}{4} + \dfrac{V_{AA}}{4} + \dfrac{V_{AD}}{8} + \dfrac{V_{DD}}{16}}{V_A + V_D + V_{AA} + V_{AD} + V_{DD}} \tag{5.42}$$

and the genetic correlation between parent and offspring is

$$\text{Corr}_G = \frac{\dfrac{V_A}{2} + \dfrac{V_{AA}}{4}}{V_A + V_D + V_{AA} + V_{AD} + V_{DD}} \tag{5.43}$$

A greater correlation between siblings than between parent and offspring would therefore suggest the presence of dominance or epistatic interactions, although it could also arise from a greater similarity of the environments experienced by siblings than by parent and offspring.

Example 5.7
For the genetic model specified in Example 5.5, what are the phenotypic correlations between MZ twins, full siblings, and parent–offspring, in the absence of any environmental variance?
The allele frequencies and genotypic means are

$$p_a = 0.99, \qquad p_A = 0.01$$

$$p_b = 0.90, \qquad p_B = 0.10$$

$$y_{AABB} = 1.0, \qquad y_{AaBB} = 1.0, \qquad y_{aaBB} = 0.0$$

$$y_{AABb} = 1.0, \qquad y_{AaBb} = 1.0, \qquad y_{aaBb} = 0.0$$

$$y_{AAbb} = 1.0, \qquad y_{Aabb} = 0.0, \qquad y_{aabb} = 0.0$$

for which the variance components are

$$V_A = 0.000819$$

$$V_D = 0.000041$$

$$V_{AA} = 0.002773$$

$$V_{AD} = 0.000211$$

$$V_{DD} = 0.000003$$

and the total phenotypic variance is

$$V_T = 0.003847$$

The phenotypic correlations are therefore

$\text{Corr}_M = 1$

$\text{Corr}_S = (0.0004095 + 0.0007035 + 0.000026375 + 0.000000187)/(0.003847)$
$\qquad = 0.2962$

$\text{Corr}_O = (0.0004095 + 0.00069325)/(0.003847) = 0.2867$

Recurrence risk of diseases in relatives   For an all-or-none trait such as a disease, the decomposition of genetic variance leads to a simple method for determining the recurrence risk of the trait in the relatives of affected individuals (James, 1971). Let the disease status of an individual be represented by the dichotomous random variable T, so that $T = 1$ indicates that the individual is affected, and $T = 0$ indicates that the individual is unaffected. The probability that a randomly selected individual from the population is affected (i.e. the population frequency of the disease, denoted as K) is

$$P(T = 1) = K \qquad (5.44)$$

This quantity is also equal to the expectation of T, denoted as $E(T)$. Now consider two relatives whose disease states are denoted by T_1 and T_2. Let the conditional probability $P(T_2 = 1 \mid T_1 = 1)$ be K_R. The probability that both members of the relative pair are affected is therefore

$$KK_R = E(T_1 T_2) = K^2 + \text{Cov}(T_1, T_2) \qquad (5.45)$$

so that the recurrence risk K_R is given by

$$K_R = K + \frac{\text{Cov}(T_1, T_2)}{K} \qquad (5.46)$$

$\text{Cov}(T_1, T_2)$ is calculated from the variance components of the trait and the IBD coefficients between the relatives.

Example 5.8
Suppose that the genotypic means in Example 5.5 are in fact the penetrances of a disease, what are the recurrence risks of the disease in an MZ twin, a full sibling, and an offspring of an affected individual according to this two-locus model?
The penetrances and allele frequencies of the two-locus disease model are

$$p_a = 0.99, \qquad p_A = 0.01$$
$$p_b = 0.90, \qquad p_B = 0.10$$

$$y_{AABB} = 1.0, \qquad y_{AaBB} = 1.0, \qquad y_{aaBB} = 0.0$$
$$y_{AABb} = 1.0, \qquad y_{AaBb} = 1.0, \qquad y_{aaBb} = 0.0$$
$$y_{AAbb} = 1.0, \qquad y_{Aabb} = 0.0, \qquad y_{aabb} = 0.0$$

for which the overall prevalence is the mean penetrance

$$K = 0.003862$$

The covariances for MZ twins, full siblings, and parent–offspring are

$$\text{Cov}_M = 0.003847$$
$$\text{Cov}_S = (0.0004095 + 0.0007035 + 0.000026375 + 0.000000187) = 0.0011396$$
$$\text{Cov}_P = (0.0004095 + 0.00069325) = 0.0011028$$

The recurrence risks are therefore

$$K_M = 0.003862 + (0.003847/0.003862) = 1$$
$$K_S = 0.003862 + (0.0011396/0.003862) = 0.2989$$
$$K_O = 0.003862 + (0.0011028/0.003862) = 0.2894$$

5.3.3   Estimating heritability using the classical twin design

The concept of *heritability* was introduced in order to measure the importance of genetics in relation to other factors in causing the variability of a trait in a population. However, there are two different measures that are both often referred to as *heritability*. The first is called *broad heritability*, or *coefficient or genetic determination*, and is the proportion of total phenotypic variance accounted for by all genetic components (i.e. additive, dominance and epistasis). The second is called *narrow heritability*, or just *heritability*, and is the proportion of phenotypic variance accounted for by the additive genetic component.

Analysis of variance   The classical twin method is based on the partition of genetic variance into additive and dominance components, and the partition of environmental variance into shared and non-shared components (Jinks and Fulker, 1970; Eaves, 1977). Furthermore, the method assumes that MZ and DZ twins do not differ in total environmental variance, or in the proportion of environmental variance that is common to members of the same twin-pairs (the *equal environment assumption*). In other words, one can define a component of variance, V_C, that represents the common environmental variance for MZ and DZ twin-pairs, and another component of variance, V_E, that represents the remaining, non-shared, environmental variance. The method ignores epistatic genetic effects, and models the total phenotypic variance, V_P, as

$$V_P = V_A + V_D + V_C + V_E \qquad (5.47)$$

The relationships between these variance components and the intraclass correlations for MZ and DZ twins are as follows

$$\left.\begin{aligned} \rho_{MZ} &= \frac{V_A + V_D + V_C}{V_A + V_D + V_C + V_E} \\[2ex] \rho_{DZ} &= \frac{\dfrac{1}{2}V_A + \dfrac{1}{4}V_D + V_C}{V_A + V_D + V_C + V_E} \end{aligned}\right\} \qquad (5.48)$$

Recalling the relationship between intraclass correlation and expected mean squares, it can be shown that expected mean squares from one-way ANOVA of MZ and DZ twin data are related to the variance components as follows

$$\left.\begin{aligned} E(\mathrm{MSW_{MZ}}) &= V_E \\[1ex] E(\mathrm{MSB_{MZ}}) &= 2V_A + 2V_D + 2V_C + V_E \\[1ex] E(\mathrm{MSW_{DZ}}) &= \frac{1}{2}V_A + \frac{3}{4}V_D + V_E \\[1ex] E(\mathrm{MSB_{DZ}}) &= \frac{3}{2}V_A + \frac{5}{4}V_D + 2V_C + V_E \end{aligned}\right\} \qquad (5.49)$$

Since we are interested in the proportions of the variance components, we can set the total phenotypic variance, V_P, to 1 with no loss of generality. We are then attempting to estimate the values of three unknown parameters (V_A, V_D, V_C) with the two statistics (r_{MZ}, r_{DZ}) and so there is no unique solution. We note, however, that this model requires that the ratio of ρ_{MZ} to ρ_{DZ} (the true correlations) takes values between 1 (when $V_C > 0$, $V_A = V_D = 0$) and 4 (when $V_D > 0$ and $V_A = V_C = 0$). Moreover, $\rho_{MZ}/\rho_{DZ} = 2$ when $V_A > 0$ and $V_C = V_D = 0$, $\rho_{MZ}/\rho_{DZ} < 2$ when $V_A > 0$, $V_C > 0$ and $V_D = 0$, and $\rho_{MZ}/\rho_{DZ} > 2$ when $V_A > 0$, $V_D > 0$ and $V_C = 0$. Hence, when $r_{MZ}/r_{DZ} < 1$ or $r_{MZ}/r_{DZ} > 4$, we conclude that the model is inappropriate. When $1 \leqslant r_{MZ}/r_{DZ} \leqslant 2$, we set $V_D = 0$ and estimate V_A and V_C as

$$\left.\begin{aligned}\hat{V}_A &= 2r_{MZ} - 2r_{DZ} \\ \hat{V}_C &= 2r_{DZ} - r_{MZ}\end{aligned}\right\} \tag{5.50}$$

and when $2 < r_{MZ}/r_{DZ} \leqslant 4$, we set $V_C = 0$ and estimate V_A and V_D as

$$\left.\begin{aligned}\hat{V}_A &= 4r_{DZ} - r_{MZ} \\ \hat{V}_D &= 2r_{MZ} - 4r_{DZ}\end{aligned}\right\} \tag{5.51}$$

This procedure does not imply that V_C and V_D cannot coexist, but merely that they cannot be jointly estimated with the data available. An estimate of broad heritability is therefore

$$H^2 = \hat{V}_A + \hat{V}_D \tag{5.52}$$

and an estimate of narrow heritability is

$$h^2 = \hat{V}_A \tag{5.53}$$

Since these heritability estimates are linear combinations of intraclass correlations estimates, their approximate standard errors can be obtained by considering the sampling variances of the intraclass correlations. The variance of the intraclass correlation, r, estimated from data on n twin-pairs is approximately

$$\mathrm{Var}(r) = \frac{(1-\rho^2)^2}{n} \tag{5.54}$$

where ρ is the true intraclass correlation (Donner, 1986). When $1 \leqslant r_{MZ}/r_{DZ} \leqslant 2$, for example, narrow heritability is estimated by

$$h^2 = \hat{V}_A = 2r_{MZ} - 2r_{DZ} \tag{5.55}$$

so that its standard error is approximately

$$\mathrm{SE}(h^2) = 2\left(\frac{(1-r_{MZ}^2)^2}{n_{MZ}} + \frac{(1-r_{DZ}^2)^2}{n_{DZ}}\right)^{1/2} \tag{5.56}$$

This method can be used to obtain approximate standard errors of h^2 and H^2 for the different ranges of values of the r_{MZ}/r_{DZ} ratio.

Example 5.9.
Returning to the twin data on neuroticism in Example 5.1 and using the intraclass

correlations estimated in Example 5.3, the MZ:DZ ratio in intraclass correlations is

$$r_{MZ}/r_{DZ} = 2.3946123986$$

Since this is between 2 and 4, a model including additive genetic effects and dominance is selected. The components of variance are then obtained by using the above formulae as:

$$V_A = 0.3099$$

$$V_D = 0.1524$$

$$V_E = 0.5377$$

Finally, the broad heritability estimate is

$$H^2 = 0.4623$$

$$SE(H^2) = 0.0344$$

and the narrow heritability estimate is

$$h^2 = 0.3099489195$$

$$SE(h^2) = 0.2360174398$$

The large standard error for narrow heritability is due to the partial confounding between additive genetic effects and dominance. In other words, although the total genetic contribution can be estimated quite precisely, there is much more uncertainty about the relative contributions of additive genetic effects and dominance.

Linear regression   There is a simpler method of estimating heritability from twin data based on *linear regression* (DeFries and Fulker, 1985). This method requires only a single analysis of the entire dataset, instead of separate analyses on MZ and DZ twins. The heritability is estimated by a regression coefficient, so that its standard error is easily obtained. The method is applicable when the MZ and DZ twin-pairs are random samples from a population, and also when the twin-pairs are ascertained through proband twins selected to be over-representative of certain ranges of trait values.

We first describe the method for the situation where the twins have been selected at random from a population (e.g. from a population twin register). This sampling procedure is also assumed by the classical method using one-way ANOVA. Recall that the intraclass correlation is the proportion of trait variance due to a random effect shared by members of the same class, and that it can be estimated from the values of mean squares from a one-way ANOVA. For twin data, the intraclass correlation is also the covariance of the trait between twins divided by the variance of the trait. In order to estimate this without arbitrarily assigning a member of each twin-pair as variable 1 and the other as variable 2, we can simply duplicate the data of each twin-pair so that the order of assignment is reversed in the two duplicates. Since the sample size has been inflated by a factor of 2, the standard error of the correlation estimated from the duplicated data must be inflated by a factor of $\sqrt{2}$.

Since the two variables in the duplicated data must have the same variance, their correlation is equal to the regression coefficient of either variable on the other. An estimate of the intraclass correlation can therefore be obtained by a linear regression analysis on the duplicated data. However, since the apparent sample size is twice the real sample size, the estimated standard error should be inflated by a factor of $\sqrt{2}$. Alternatively, each observation should be given the weight of half an observation in the analysis (using, for example, the weight command in SPSS).

For MZ twins, the theoretical value of the intraclass correlation, and hence the regression coefficient, is $(V_A + V_D + V_C)$. The regression equation for MZ twins can therefore be written as

$$X_C = K_M + (V_A + V_D + V_C)X_P + E_M \tag{5.57}$$

where X_C and X_P are the trait values of the cotwin and the proband twin, respectively, K_M is a constant, and E_M is a random 'error term'. In a duplicated dataset, proband and cotwin status is entirely arbitrary, so that the expected trait values for proband and cotwins are equal. Let the mean trait value be m, then the constant K_M is $(1 - V_A - V_D - V_C)m$, so that the regression equation for MZ twins can be rewritten as

$$X_C - m = V_A(X_P - m) + V_D(X_P - m) + V_C(X_P - m) + E_M \tag{5.58}$$

Similarly, the regression equation for DZ twins is

$$X_C = K_D + \left(\frac{V_A}{2} + \frac{V_D}{4} + V_C\right)X_P + E_D \tag{5.59}$$

which can be rewritten as

$$X_C - m = \frac{1}{2} V_A(X_P - m) + \frac{1}{4} V_D(X_P - m) + V_C(X_P - m) + E_D \tag{5.60}$$

These equations suggest a regression analysis of MZ and DZ twins together, through the origin, with $X_C - m$ as a dependent variable, and with three 'dummy' independent variables, A, D and C, coded as

	A	D	C
MZ	$X_P - m$	$X_P - m$	$X_P - m$
DZ	$\dfrac{X_P - m}{2}$	$\dfrac{X_P - m}{4}$	$X_P - m$

However, this single regression analysis assumes a single 'error term' for both MZ and DZ twins. This is unrealistic, as DZ twins are expected to have a greater residual variance than MZ twins, in the presence of a genetic component. This potential violation of model assumption is often ignored, and the regression coefficients of A, D and C taken as estimates for V_A, V_D and V_C respectively. However, taking appropriate account of the possible difference in error variance between MZ and DZ twins is expected to improve the precision of the parameter estimates.

Regardless of the treatment of the error variance, the complete model for the fixed effects might be denoted as (A, D, C, E) to represent the three dummy variables A, D and C, and the error term E. However, the three variables A, D

and C are related by the equation

$$C - 3A + 2D = 0 \qquad (5.61)$$

so that they cannot all be entered into a single regression model. Moreover, if the regression coefficients are unconstrained, the three submodels, (A, D, E), (A, C, E), (D, C, E), will fit the observed data equally well, so that it is impossible to choose a submodel on the basis of goodness-of-fit. However, the (D, C, E) model is usually discarded because the presence of dominance interactions in the absence of additive genetic effects is considered extremely unlikely. The choice between the submodels (A, D, E) and (A, C, E) is then made by considering the signs of the estimated regression coefficients; the submodel with positive regression coefficients is selected. Whichever submodel is selected, it can be subjected to a backward elimination procedure to obtain a final model. The aim of the analysis is to assess the compatibility of the data with the alternative models (A, D, E), (A, C, E), (A, E), (D, E), (C, E) and (E), and to obtain the parameter estimates of the best supported model.

Great care must be taken in assessing the significance of a variable since the data have been duplicated for the analysis. The simplest method is to use a statistical package (such as SPSS) which has a procedure for assigning a fractional weight to an observation, so that all the duplicated observations can be assigned a weight of $1/2$. The results of such an analysis will require no adjustment. Alternatively, if an unadjusted analysis is performed on the duplicated sample, then the results will need to be corrected for the artificial inflation of the sample size. Duplicating the data has the effect of doubling all the sums of squares and increasing the residual degrees of freedom by the actual sample size, n. A reasonable adjustment is therefore to halve all the sums of squares, and to reduce the residual degrees of freedom by n. Revised values for the mean squares and the F-statistics can be calculated from these adjusted sums of squares and degrees of freedom. Similarly, in assessing the regression coefficient of a variable, its standard error based on the duplicated data should be multiplied by a factor of $\sqrt{2}$ to give an adjusted standard error.

Example 5.10
The linear regression approach for estimating heritability from twin data is illustrated by the twin neuroticism data of Example 5.1. First, all neuroticism scores are adjusted by subtracting the mean score, which is 10.23. Then the independent variables A and D are defined as above. The observations are duplicated, so that each twin acts as a proband twin in one duplicate and as the cotwin in the other. All observations are given a weight of $1/2$. The results of linear regression analyses with the (A, D, E) and the (A, E) models, using SPSS-WIN are as follows.

(A, D, E) model
Parameter estimates

Variable	B	SE B	Beta	T	Sig T
A	0.303547	0.22427	0.260323	1.353	0.1763
D	0.158051	0.23508	0.129308	0.672	0.5016

Analysis of variance

	DF	Sum of squares	Mean square
Regression	2	2143.54334	1071.77167
Residual	792	12068.16926	15.23759

$F = 70.33736$ Signif $F = 0.0000$

(*A, E*) model

Parameter estimates

Variable	*B*	SE *B*	Beta	*T*	Sig *T*
A	0.452124	0.038168	0.387743	11.846	0.0000

Analysis of variance

	DF	Sum of squares	Mean square
Regression	1	2136.65606	2136.65606
Residual	793	12075.05654	15.22706

$F = 140.31970$ Signif $F = 0.0000$

The best-supported model is therefore (A, E), with a heritability estimate of 0.4521 (SE 0.038168). These analyses do not take account of the potentially greater residual variance of DZ twins as compared with MZ twins. The heteroscedasticity was taken into account by an appropriate specification of random effects in the MLN program. However, as there is no appropriate weight function in MLN, the output is adjusted to take account of the artificial doubling of the sample size. The standard errors are multiplied by a factor of $\sqrt{2}$, and the -2 log-likelihoods are multiplied by a factor of $1/2$.

(*A, D, E*) model

Parameter	Estimates	SE	Adjusted SE
A	0.3029	0.1699	0.2403
D	0.1587	0.1764	0.2495

Unadjusted -2 log(likelihood) = 8816.7
Adjusted -2 log(likelihood) = 4408.35

(*A, E*) model

Parameter	Estimate	SE	Adjusted SE
A	0.4539	0.0261	0.0369

Unadjusted -2 log(likelihood) = 8817.5
Adjusted -2 log(likelihood) = 4408.75

Again, the (A, E) model is best-supported, with a heritability estimate of

0.4539. As expected, the standard error of this heritability estimate is slightly smaller than that obtained from SPSS.

When twin-pairs are ascertained through a sample of proband twins who may be selected for particular ranges of values of the trait, the same principles apply except that the twin-pair need not be duplicated unless both members of the pair are probands. Where there is only one proband in a pair, the non-proband member is treated as the dependent variable, and the proband member as the independent variable. The analysis proceeds as before, although the results should be adjusted for the ascertainment procedure and the duplication of some twin-pairs. Using software which allows fractional weightings for observations, each twin-pair in the regression analysis can be assigned a weight of n/N, where n is the actual number of twin-pairs, and N is the total number of pairs in the regression analysis (including the duplicated pairs). If an unadjusted analysis is performed, then all sums of squares should be multiplied by n/N, and the residual degrees of freedom reduced by $N - n$. Similarly, standard errors should be increased by a factor of $(N/n)^{1/2}$. An alternative approach is to use bootstrap methods to obtain empirical sampling distributions of F statistics and regression coefficient estimates.

Example 5.11
The application of the linear regression approach to selected data is illustrated by the neuroticism data of Example 5.1. The selection criterion is that all twin-pairs in which at least one member has a neuroticism score of 16 or above are included, while all the others are excluded, from the analysis. This procedure results in the selection of 108 MZ twin-pairs and 66 DZ twin-pairs. Of the 108 MZ twin-pairs, 85 were singly ascertained because one member of the pair scored above the threshold of 15, and 23 were doubly ascertained because both members of the pair scored above the threshold of 15. Doubly ascertained twin-pairs were duplicated, so that $85 + 2(23) = 131$ MZ observations were subjected to the analysis. Similarly, the numbers of singly and doubly ascertained DZ twin-pairs were 57 and 9 respectively, so that $57 + 2(9) = 75$ DZ observations were subjected to the analysis. Using SPSS, a weight of $(108 + 66)/(131 + 75) = 0.845$ was assigned to all observations, and a linear regression was carried out, with all scores being measured as deviations from the population mean, and the constant term restricted to 0. The output is as follows

(*A*, *D*, *E*) model

Parameter estimates

Variable	*B*	SE *B*	Beta	*T*	Sig *T*
A	0.37349	0.304888	0.450112	1.225	0.2222
D	0.086413	0.320246	0.099147	0.270	0.7876

Analysis of variance

	DF	Sum of squares	Mean square
Regression	2	1272.62209	636.31105
Residual	172	2964.78251	17.23711

$F = 36.91519$ Signif $F = 0.0000$

(*A, E*) model

Parameter estimates

Variable	*B*	SE *B*	Beta	*T*	Sig *T*
A	0.454511	0.052781	0.547754	8.611	0.0000

Analysis of variance

	DF	Sum of squares	Mean square
Regression	1	1271.36705	1271.36705
Residual	173	2966.03755	17.14473

$F = 74.15499$ Signif $F = 0.0000$

The best-supported model is therefore (A, E), with a heritability estimate of 0.4545 (SE 0.05278). These results are similar to those obtained from the complete sample, although the standard errors are larger. Using MLN, the results are:

(*A, D, E*) model

Parameter	Estimates	SE	Adjusted SE
A	0.3722	0.3144	0.3421
D	0.0877	0.3247	0.3533

Unadjusted $-2 \log(\text{likelihood}) = 1163.69$
Adjusted $-2 \log(\text{likelihood}) = 983.32$

(*A, E*) model

Parameter	Estimate	SE	Adjusted SE
A	0.4562	0.04503	0.0490

Unadjusted $-2 \log(\text{likelihood}) = 1163.76$
Adjusted $-2 \log(\text{likelihood}) = 983.38$

To adjust for the inflated sample size, standard errors are multiplied by a factor of $1/\sqrt{0.845}$, and the -2 log-likelihoods are multiplied by a factor of 0.845. Again, the (A, E) model is best-supported, with a heritability estimate of 0.4562. As expected, the standard error of this heritability estimate is slightly smaller than that obtained from SPSS.

A final advantage of the regression approach is that covariates, such as zygosity, sex and age, can be easily included into the analysis. The interaction between these covariates and C, A and D can also be included, and such terms may represent differences in the relative importance of these variance components according to the values of the covariates. The interpretation of such models, however, requires great care.

5.4   Scale

The genetic analysis of a trait is sometimes simplified by a suitable transformation of scale. A transformation may help to normalize the distribution of the trait in the population, it may reduce heteroscedasticity (e.g. a correlation between pair-differences and pair-means), and the need for interaction terms (e.g. dominance, epistasis, gene–environment interaction and shared–nonshared environment interaction) in an analysis of variance. For example, if gene action is multiplicative on the original scale of a variable, then an analysis of variance on the original scale would lead to significant dominance and epistasis. However, multiplicative action on the original scale translates to additive effects on a logarithmic scale, so that interactions will be absent in an analysis of variance of the logarithm of the original variable. Similarly, when the trait is a function of an area or a volume of a structure, but gene action is additive on the linear dimension of the structure, then an additive model will fit the data after a square root or a cube root transformation, but not the raw data on the original scale.

Even in the absence of a theoretical rationale, a transformation may still be justified on empirical grounds if it reduces non-additivity. A transformation that normalizes the variable often has other desirable effects, such as removing the correlation between pair-differences and pair-means and the interaction terms in the analysis of variance. If this is not the case, then other transformations should be tried in order to find one that produces data compatible with an additive model.

The usefulness of scale transformation in the genetic analysis of continuous characters is a matter of some disagreement among experts. The more negative view, expressed by Falconer and Mackay (1996), is that:

> Transformations of scale, however, should not be used without good reason. The first purpose of experimental observations is the description of the genetic properties of the population, and a scale transformation obscures rather than illuminates this description. If epistasis, for example, is found, this is an essential part of the description and it is better labelled as such than a scale effect.

Others, such as Mather and Jinks (1977), hold a more positive view

> the justification for using a transformed scale is not theoretical but empirical ... while we must recognise that it is not always possible to find a transformation which in effect removes non-additivity when this is present in the direct measurements, the search for such a transformation is always well-while.

There is some validity in both points of view. There is no doubt that transformations can sometimes reduce the complexity of the genetic model necessary for providing an adequate description of the data. However, great care must be taken when drawing conclusions from such analyses, in that the simpler description applies to the transformed and not the original scale. For example, if an additive genetic model offers an adequate description of the cube root of body weight, this implies that an adequate genetic model for weight itself will probably include dominance and epistatic components. The simpler model based on the cube root transformation is more appealing from a statistical point of view, but the model based on the original scale may still be relevant, for example, if the risk of heart disease is more directly related to body weight itself rather than its cube root.

5.5 Quasi-continuous characters

Characters that are determined by the action of alleles at a single locus are necessarily discontinuous, because of the discrete nature of the alleles. However, the converse is not true, in that not all discrete traits demonstrate Mendelian segregation. Many discrete traits in animals (e.g. the number of sternopleural chaetae in fruit flies, the number of toes in guinea pigs, and the number of vertebrae in mice) appear to be inherited in a fashion similar to continuous characters. Such traits, sometimes referred to as 'quasi-continuous' (Gruneberg, 1952), may therefore be under the influence of multiple genetic loci. In humans, the notion that multiple loci are involved in common diseases, such as congenital malformations, ischaemic heart disease and diabetes mellitus, has gained wide acceptance (Crittenden, 1961; Falconer, 1965; Carter, 1969; Edwards, 1969).

5.5.1 Liability-threshold model

There are many ways of modelling the relationship between multiple genetic and environmental factors and the presence or absence of a discrete characteristic such as a common disease. In epidemiology, the standard method of analysis is based on the logistic regression model, where the presence or absence of the disease is treated as a binary response variable, and potential risk factors as predictor variables. In genetics, however, it is common to assume the *liability-threshold model*, introduced by Pearson and Lee (1901), as a natural extension of biometrical models for quantitative traits.

> If we take a problem like that of coat-colour in horses, it is by no means difficult to construct an order of intensity of scale. The variable on which it depends may be the amount of pigment in the hair ... we may reasonably argue that, if we could find the quantity of pigment, we should be able to form a continuous curve of frequency ... Now if we take any line parallel to the axis of frequency and dividing the curve, we divide the total frequency into two classes, which, so long as there is a quantitative order of tint or colour, will have their relative frequency unchanged.

The liability-threshold model postulates an underlying continuous variable called *liability*, X, that has, or can be transformed to have, a normal distribution with mean 0 and variance 1, in the general population. The disease is assumed to be present in all individuals whose liability is above a certain *threshold* value, t, and to be absent in all other individuals. The value of the threshold t can be estimated from the *population frequency* of the disease, p. Let Φ be the standard normal distribution function, then the value of the threshold t is such that

$$\Phi(t) = 1 - p \qquad (5.62)$$

which is equivalent to

$$t = \Phi^{-1}(1 - p) \qquad (5.63)$$

where Φ^{-1} is the inverse standard normal distribution (i.e. probit) function.

The notion of an abrupt threshold has been criticized on biological grounds, and an alternative model has been proposed that relates risk of illness to liability by a probit function (Curnow and Smith, 1975). This model is, however, mathematically equivalent to the liability-threshold model (Figure 5.1).

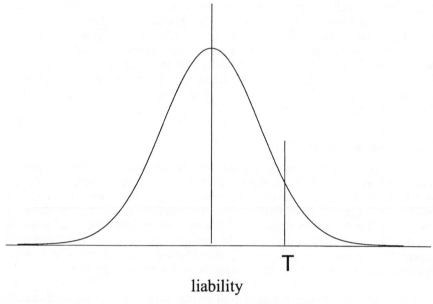

liability

Figure 5.1   Distribution of liability in general population with threshold T.

Example 5.12
Consider the neuroticism data of Example 5.1. Suppose that the neuroticism is measured as a dichotomous rather than a continuous trait, with those scoring 15 or less being classified as low and those scoring 16 or more being classified as high. For MZ twins, this divides the sample into 132 high scorers and 914 low scorers, so that the frequency of high scorers is 0.126. For DZ twins, the numbers of high and low scorers are 76 and 470, respectively, giving a frequency of high scorers of 0.139. Assuming a liability-threshold model, the thresholds of the liability to having a high neuroticism score (>15) are therefore

$$t_{MZ} = \Phi^{-1}(1 - 0.126) = \Phi^{-1}(0.874) = 1.145$$
$$t_{DZ} = \Phi^{-1}(1 - 0.139) = \Phi^{-1}(0.861) = 1.084$$

5.5.2   Relationship between mean liability and risk

Suppose that a population is stratified into subgroups according to the presence or absence of risk factors that may be genetic or environmental. Assuming that the distribution of liability in subgroup i, denoted as X_i, is normal with mean μ_i

and variance 1, then the risk of disease in this stratum, p_i, is

$$p_i = P(X_i > t) \\ \left. \begin{aligned} &= P[(X_i - \mu_i) > (t - \mu_i)] \\ &= 1 - \Phi(t - \mu_i) \end{aligned} \right\} \quad (5.64)$$

This relationship has implications for the joint effect of risk factors on the risk of disease, when the effects of the factors are additive on liability. Suppose that there are two risk factors, denoted as F_1 and F_2, which occur independently of each other at frequencies f_1 and f_2 in the population. The presence or absence of these two factors divide the population into four groups: $(F_1 = 0, F_2 = 0)$, $(F_1 = 0, F_2 = 1)$, $(F_1 = 1, F_2 = 0)$ and $(F_1 = 1, F_2 = 1)$, with relative frequencies $(1 - f_1)(1 - f_2)$, $(1 - f_1)f_2$, $f_1(1 - f_2)$ and $f_1 f_2$, respectively. Let the mean liabilities of these groups be μ_{00}, μ_{01}, μ_{10} and μ_{11} respectively. Under an additive model for liability, we define the effects of the two factors as

$$\left. \begin{aligned} e_1 &= \mu_{10} - \mu_{00} \\ e_2 &= \mu_{01} - \mu_{00} \end{aligned} \right\} \quad (5.65)$$

and then the joint effect of having both factors is $e_1 + e_2$, so that

$$\mu_{11} = \mu_{00} + e_1 + e_2 \quad (5.66)$$

In other words, the four group means can be written as μ_{00}, $\mu_{00} + e_1$, $\mu_{00} + e_2$ and $\mu_{00} + e_1 + e_2$. The mean of these group means must be 0, so that

$$(1 - f_1)(1 - f_2)\mu_{00} + (1 - f_1)f_2(\mu_{00} + e_2) \\ + f_1(1 - f_2)(\mu_{00} + e_1) + f_1 f_2(\mu_{00} + e_1 + e_2) = 0 \quad (5.67)$$

This equation can be rearranged to express the 'baseline liability' μ_{00} in terms of the effect sizes e_1 and e_2 and the frequencies f_1 and f_2.

$$\mu_{00} = -(f_1 e_1 + f_2 e_2) \quad (5.68)$$

The four group means are therefore

$$\left. \begin{aligned} \mu_{00} &= -(f_1 e_1 + f_2 e_2) \\ \mu_{01} &= -(1 - f_2)e_2 - f_1 e_1 \\ \mu_{10} &= -(1 - f_1)e_1 - f_2 e_2 \\ \mu_{11} &= -(1 - f_1)e_1 + (1 - f_2)e_2 \end{aligned} \right\} \quad (5.69)$$

Thus the risks of disease in the four groups are

$$\left. \begin{aligned} p_{00} &= 1 - \Phi[t + (f_1 e_1 + f_2 e_2)] \\ p_{01} &= 1 - \Phi[t - (1 - f_2)e_2 + f_1 e_1] \\ p_{10} &= 1 - \Phi[t - (1 - f_1)e_1 + f_2 e_2] \\ p_{11} &= 1 - \Phi[t - (1 - f_1)e_1 - (1 - f_2)e_2] \end{aligned} \right\} \quad (5.70)$$

The effects of the two factors on risk of disease for any set of values of t, f_1, f_2, e_1 and e_2, can be found by substituting the values into the above expressions for risk of disease. If the results are such that

$$p_{11} = p_{01} + p_{10} - p_{00}$$ (5.71)

then the effects of the factors on risk are described by an additive model. On the other hand, if the results are such that

$$p_{11} = \frac{p_{01} p_{10}}{p_{00}}$$ (5.72)

then the effects of the factors on risk are described by a multiplicative model. The properties of the standard normal distribution function are such that small additive effects on liability are often translated approximately to multiplicative effects on the risk of disease, especially if the disease is common. This approximate correspondence provides a conceptual link between the liability-threshold models frequently used in genetics and the risk models favoured by epidemiologists.

Example 5.13
Consider two factors that have additive effects on the liability of disease that has a population frequency of 1%. If the frequencies of the two factors are 0.01 and 0.10, and their effects on liability are 1.0 and 0.1 units, what is the pattern of effects of these factors on the risk of the disease?
   The threshold liability is

$$t = \Phi^{-1}(0.99) = 2.326$$

The four levels of risks are

$$p_{00} = 1 - \Phi[2.326 + 0.01 + 0.01] = 1 - \Phi[2.346] = 0.0095$$

$$p_{01} = 1 - \Phi[2.326 - 0.09 + 0.01] = 1 - \Phi[2.246] = 0.0124$$

$$p_{10} = 1 - \Phi[2.326 - 0.99 + 0.01] = 1 - \Phi[1.346] = 0.0892$$

$$p_{11} = 1 - \Phi[2.326 - 0.99 - 0.09] = 1 - \Phi[1.246] = 0.1064$$

Under an additive model, the risk associated with the two factors occurring jointly is expected to be $(0.0124 + 0.0892 - 0.0095) = 0.0921$. Under a multiplicative model, the risk associated with the two factors occurring jointly is expected to be $(0.0124)(0.0892)/(0.0095) = 0.1164$. The actual risk of 0.1064 is somewhat closer to the value implied by a multiplicative model than the value implied by an additive model. Under these assumptions, an additive model on the liability scale corresponds to a model that is intermediate between additive and multiplicative in terms of risk.

5.5.3   Multi-threshold models for ordered polychotomous traits

The liability-threshold model can be generalized to *ordered polychotomous traits* by the introduction of multiple thresholds. An ordered polychotomy is a trait with three or more categories that can reasonably be arranged in a linear sequence. It is not uncommon, for example, for medical conditions to be categorized as severe, moderate and mild, or as definite, probable and possible.

Let there be k ordered categories $c_1, c_2, ..., c_k$ of an ordered polychotomy, with frequencies $p_1, p_2, ..., p_k$ in the population, then a standard normal liability is defined with $k - 1$ thresholds t_1, t_2, t_{k-1} such that

$$t_i = \Phi^{-1}(p_1 + p_2 + \cdots p_i) \qquad (5.73)$$

A factor that increases liability will increase the probability that an individual will belong to a higher category.

Example 5.14
Returning to the neuroticism data of Example 5.1. Suppose that neuroticism is measured as three categories, low (0–6), medium (7–15) and high (16–21). The distributions of MZ and DZ twins in terms of these these categories are:

	Neuroticism			
	Low	Medium	High	Total
MZ	237	676	131	1044
DZ	124	345	75	544

From these frequency distributions, the thresholds in liability are

	t_1	t_2
MZ	−0.75	1.15
DZ	−0.75	1.09

5.5.4 Correlation in liability between relatives

Under a liability-threshold model, the recurrence risk of an illness in a relative of a proband with the illness depends not only on the correlation in liability between proband and relative, but also on the position of the threshold for illness along the continuum of liability. It is convenient to assume that the threshold is fixed, and consider the genetics of the continuous liability. The aim is to estimate the correlations in liability between different classes of relatives, as well as the proportions of variance in liability due to different genetic and environmental components. Historically, the problem of estimating the correlation in liability between relatives was first considered by Pearson (1900), who introduced the term *tetrachoric correlation*. Pearson proposed that the tetrachoric correlation should be used as a general measure of association in 2×2 contingency tables, but this recommendation failed to gain wide acceptance, because the assumption of an underlying continuous liability is thought by many to be unrealistic and unnecessary for many categorical variables (Yule, 1912; Pearson and Heron, 1913). For the genetic analysis of common diseases, however, the liability-threshold model has remained popular, because of its link with biometrical genetic models for continuous traits.

5.5.5   Tetrachoric correlation from population data

Since liability is not directly measurable, the correlation in liability between relatives must be estimated from the observed categorical data, which, for example, may consist of the affection (i.e. disease) status of a random sample of relative-pairs of a certain class (e.g. parent–offspring pairs) from the population. Let the affection status of the two relatives be Y_1 and Y_2, each coded as 0 (unaffected) and 1 (affected), then there are four possible combinations of trait values: $(Y_1 = 0, Y_2 = 0)$, $(Y_1 = 0, Y_2 = 1)$, $(Y_1 = 1, Y_2 = 0)$ and $(Y_1 = 1, Y_2 = 1)$. The data can be summarized by the counts of these four categories of observations, which can be denoted as n_{00}, n_{01}, n_{10} and n_{11}, respectively, in a 2×2 contingency table. The marginal totals of such a table are denoted as $n_{0.}$, $n_{1.}$, $n_{.0}$ and $n_{.1}$, and the grand total as $n_{..}$.

Y_1	Y_2		
	0	1	
0	n_{00}	n_{01}	$n_{0.}$
1	n_{10}	n_{11}	$n_{1.}$
	$n_{.0}$	$n_{.1}$	$n_{..}$

Assuming that the liabilities underlying Y_1 and Y_2, denoted as X_1 and X_2, are each standard normal, then their threshold values, t_1 and t_2, can be estimated by referring the marginal proportions

$$\left. \begin{aligned} p_{0.} &= \frac{n_{0.}}{n_{..}} \\ p_{.0} &= \frac{n_{.0}}{n_{..}} \end{aligned} \right\} \tag{5.74}$$

to the inverse normal distribution function

$$\left. \begin{aligned} t_1 &= \Phi^{-1}(p_{0.}) \\ t_2 &= \Phi^{-1}(p_{.0}) \end{aligned} \right\} \tag{5.75}$$

The correlation between X_1 and X_2 can be estimated by equating the observed proportion of one of the four cells of the contingency table (e.g. $p_{11} = n_{11}/n_{..}$) to the expected proportion given that (X_1, X_2) is bivariate normal with correlation ρ and thresholds t_1 and t_2

$$p_{11} = P(X_1 > t_1, X_2 > t_2) \tag{5.76}$$

Pearson's method for estimating ρ was to expand the expression $P(X_1 > t_1, X_2 > t_2)$ into the so-called tetrachoric series, and solve the resulting equation for ρ. An estimate of ρ obtained in this way is known as a tetrachoric correlation, r. Pearson (1901) suggested several approximations for r, the simplest of which is

$$r = \frac{n_{00} n_{11} - n_{01} n_{10}}{n_{00} n_{11} + n_{01} n_{10}} \quad (5.77)$$

also known as Yule's *coefficient of association* (Yule, 1912). A more accurate approximation for r is

$$r = \sin\left[\left(\frac{\pi}{2}\right)c\right] \quad (5.78)$$

where

$$c = \frac{(n_{00} n_{11})^{1/2} - (n_{01} n_{10})^{1/2}}{(n_{00} n_{11})^{1/2} + (n_{01} n_{10})^{1/2}} \quad (5.79)$$

is Yule's *coefficient of colligation*.

Hamdan (1970) showed that the tetrachoric correlation is equivalent to the maximum likelihood estimate of ρ, and hence derived the approximate sampling variance

$$V(r) = \frac{\left(\dfrac{1}{n_{00}} + \dfrac{1}{n_{01}} + \dfrac{1}{n_{10}} + \dfrac{1}{n_{11}}\right)}{n\,f(t_1, t_2; r)} \quad (5.80)$$

where $f(t_1, t_2; r)$ is the bivariate standard normal density function with correlation r, evaluated at (t_1, t_2). More accurate estimates of r than the above approximations can also be obtained by iterative procedures based on maximum likelihood (Froemel, 1971; Kirk, 1973).

It is important to note that, while a liability-threshold model can be fitted to a 2×2 table, this involves the estimation of three parameters: two thresholds and a tetrachoric correlation. This guarantees a perfect fit to the data, leaving no degree of freedom to test the validity of the liability-threshold model itself.

Example 5.15
Returning to the neuroticism data of Example 5.1 and the dichotomous definition of high (H) and low (L) scorers in Example 5.14. Suppose that twin-pairs are classified into those with two high scorers (HH), those with one high scorer and one low scorer (HL), and those with two low scorers (LL). The distributions of these three groups among the MZ and DZ twins are as follows:

	LL	LH	HH
MZ	414	85	23
DZ	206	57	9

Using Pearson's approximation

$$r = \sin\left[\frac{\pi}{2}\, \frac{(n_{00}\,n_{11})^{1/2} - (n_{01}\,n_{10})^{1/2}}{(n_{00}\,n_{11})^{1/2} + (n_{01}\,n_{10})^{1/2}}\right]$$

and Hamdan's formula for the sampling variance on the 2×2 tables:

MZ	L	H
L	414	42.5
H	42.5	23

DZ	L	H
L	206	28.5
H	28.5	9

we obtain

$$r_{MZ} = 0.579,\ SE(r_{MZ}) = 0.089$$

$$r_{DZ} = 0.314,\ SE(r_{DZ}) = 0.106$$

Using the PRELIS program on these same 2×2 tables gives the more exact results

$$r_{MZ} = 0.491,\ SE(r_{MZ}) = 0.084$$

$$r_{DZ} = 0.252,\ SE(r_{DZ}) = 0.134$$

These values are not far from the estimates obtained from the original continuous data ($r_{MZ} = 0.462$, $r_{DZ} = 0.193$).

5.5.6   Tetrachoric correlation from proband-ascertained data

The above methods for estimating ρ are applicable for 2×2 tables that represent a random sample of the general population. However, this situation is rare in genetic studies of human diseases, where it is more usual to study relatives of a sample of affected *probands* to obtain an estimate of the recurrence risk, q, and to compare this recurrence risk with the population risk p. The reason is that, for rare diseases, a random sample of relative-pairs from the population will consist mostly of normal–normal pairs and very few normal–affected or affected–affected pairs. The inclusion of the relatives of affected individuals but not the relatives of normal individuals can be viewed as a form of *censoring*. Only two of the four cells of the 2×2 contingency table are filled.

In order to estimate the correlation in liability, ρ, from censored data it is usual to assume that an accurate estimate of the population risk, p, is available, which allows the threshold t to be specified as

$$t = \Phi^{-1}(1 - p) \tag{5.81}$$

An estimate for p may then be obtained by equating the predicted recurrence risk with the observed recurrence risk q

$$q = P(X_2 > t \mid X_1 > t) \qquad (5.82)$$

where (X_1, X_2) is bivariate standard normal with correlation p and thresholds t. Falconer (1965) derived an estimate for p from the proportion q, for a given value of p. This estimate is based on an approximation of the conditional distribution of X_2 given $X_1 > t$. It can be shown that the expected value of X_1 given that $X_1 > t$, i.e. the mean deviation of the probands from the population mean, is

$$E(X_1 \mid X_1 > t) = \frac{\phi(t)}{1 - \Phi(t)} \qquad (5.83)$$

where ϕ is the standard normal density function. Denoting this mean deviation of the probands as a, then the expected value of X_2, given that $X_1 > t$, i.e. the mean deviation of the relatives from the population mean, is approximately

$$E(X_2 \mid X_1 > t) = pa \qquad (5.84)$$

Falconer assumed further that, conditional on $X_1 > t$, the distribution of X_2 remains normal with variance 1. An approximation of the probability that $X_2 > t$, given that $X_1 > t$, is then

$$P(x_2 > t \mid X_1 > t) = 1 - \Phi(t - pa) \qquad (5.85)$$

An estimate, r (of p), is obtained by equating this to the observed recurrence risk q

$$q = 1 - \Phi(t - ra) \qquad (5.86)$$

which can be rearranged to give

$$r = \frac{t - \Phi^{-1}(1 - q)}{a} \qquad (5.87)$$

Assuming that p, and therefore $t = \Phi^{-1}(1 - p)$, is known to a high degree of accuracy, Falconer derived an approximate standard error for r by the delta method

$$\text{SE}(r) = \frac{1}{a^2 r} \left(\frac{1 - q}{qN} \right)^{1/2} \qquad (5.88)$$

where N is the number of proband-relative pairs in the analysis. In the case of multiple ascertainment, proband-relative pairs that have been doubly ascertained can be duplicated in the analysis, treating each affected member as proband in turn. The standard error of r obtained should then be inflated by a factor of $(N/n)^{1/2}$ where N is the number of pairs in the analysis including the duplicates, and n is the actual number of pairs in the sample.

Reich *et al.* (1972) proposed a more accurate estimate of p, based on a better approximation of the variance of X_2 conditional on $X_1 > t$. The conditional variance of X_1 given that $X_1 > t$ can be shown to be

$$\text{Var}(X_1 \mid X_1 > t) = 1 + at - a^2 \qquad (5.89)$$

Using the formulae by Aitken (1934) on the effect of selection on a subset of variables in a multivariate normal distribution, the conditional variance of $X_2 > t$ given that $X_1 > t$ is approximately

$$\text{Var}(X_2 \mid X_1 > t) = 1 + \rho^2(at - a^2) \tag{5.90}$$

Retaining the approximation that X_2 is normal conditional on $X_1 > t$, an estimate of ρ is obtained by equating the observed with the predicted recurrence risk in relatives

$$q = 1 - \Phi\left(\frac{t - ra}{[1 + r^2(at - a^2)]^{1/2}}\right) \tag{5.91}$$

Solving this equation for r gives

$$r = \frac{t - d\left(1 - (t^2 - d^2)\left(1 - \dfrac{t}{a}\right)\right)^{1/2}}{a + d^2(a - t)} \tag{5.92}$$

where d is an abbreviation for $\Phi^{-1}(1 - q)$.

The inability to test the validity of the liability-threshold model applies also to recurrence risk data. One parameter, the tetrachoric correlation, is estimated, and this guarantees a perfect fit to the recurrence risk data.

Example 5.16
Returning to the neuroticism data of Example 5.1 and the dichotomous definition of high (H) and low (L) scorers in Example 5.15. Suppose that all high scorers in the sample are ascertained as probands. The frequencies of high scorers among MZ and DZ cotwins are as follows:

	MZ	DZ
Concordance	46/131	18/75

Assuming that the frequencies of H among MZ and DZ twins are known, then application of Falconer's approximation leads to the following estimates for the MZ and DZ tetrachoric correlations.

	N	n	t	a	r	SE(r)
MZ	131	108	1.15	1.64	0.464	0.104
DZ	75	66	1.08	1.59	0.237	0.364

These estimated intraclass correlations are not far from the those obtained from the complete data including the LL twin-pairs ($r_{MZ} = 0.491$, $r_{DZ} = 0.252$), although their standard errors are larger. If Reich's slightly more accurate approximation is used, then the estimated tetrachoric correlations are $r_{MZ} = 0.488$, $r_{DZ} = 0.248$.

5.5.7   Polychoric correlations

Under a multi-threshold liability model, the correlation between the liabilities of two ordered polychotomous variables is known as a *polychoric correlation*. Data from a random sample of relative-pairs can be arranged in a $k \times k$ table, and can be used to estimate the polychoric correlation and the $k - 1$ thresholds. If only the relatives of certain categories of probands are included, then some of the cells of the contingency table will be empty, and the data can be considered as being censored.

Maximum likelihood estimates of the polychoric correlation can be obtained by algorithms involving the numerical integration of the bivariate normal density function (Schervish, 1984). Each set of parameter values (i.e. thresholds and correlation) produces, through numerical integration, a set of probabilities for the cells of the contingency table. If the cells of the contingency table are labelled by the subscript j, then the log-likelihood of a set of parameter values is simply $\sum_j n_j \log(p_j)$, where p_j is the probability under the set of parameter values, and n_j is the count, of cell j. This log-likelihood can be maximized with respect of the parameter values using iterative numerical methods. Such algorithms have been implemented in computer programs such as PRELIS (Joreskog and Sorbom, 1988) and Mx (Neale, 1993); the latter is able to handle censored data if thresholds values are specified. These programs can be used to estimate tetrachoric correlations, since these can be regarded as polychoric correlations with $k = 2$. If available, these programs should be used to estimate tetrachoric correlations, instead of the approximations described in Sections 5.5.5 and 5.5.6.

Unlike the single-threshold case, the multi-threshold models allow the assumption of bivariate normality to be tested. For complete data in a $k \times k$ table (e.g. of parent–offspring pairs), the multi-threshold liability model is parameterized by $2(k - 1)$ thresholds (e.g. $k - 1$ thresholds for parents and $k - 1$ thresholds for offspring) and one correlation, whereas the unrestricted or saturated model has $k^2 - 1$ parameters. Twice the difference between the maximum log-likelihoods of the saturated and the multi-threshold liability model is therefore chi-squared with $(k^2 - 1) - (2k - 1) = k(k - 2)$ degrees of freedom, if the multi-threshold liability model is true. For censored data, the degrees of freedom in the saturated model are reduced by the number of censored cells in the table. The number of thresholds estimated from the data may also be reduced.

Example 5.17
Returning to the neuroticism data of Example 5.1 and the definition of the trichotomy in Example 5.14, i.e. low (0–6), medium (7–15) and high (16–21), the contingency tables of the categories in MZ and DZ twin-pairs are

MZ

	Low	Medium	High
Low	56	59.5	3
Medium	59.5	239	39.5
High	3	39.5	23

DZ

	Low	Medium	High
Low	13	42.5	6.5
Medium	42.5	108	22
High	6.5	22	9

Using the program PRELIS the polychoric correlations are estimated to be

$$r_{MZ} = 0.489,\ SE(r_{MZ}) = 0.047$$
$$r_{DZ} = 0.092,\ SE(r_{DZ}) = 0.079$$

The estimated tetrachoric correlation for DZ is quite far (although still within two standard errors) from that obtained from the original continuous data ($r_{DZ} = 0.193$).

PRELIS also provides a chi-squared test for the assumption of bivariate normality. With three degrees of freedom, the chi-squared statistics for MZ and DZ twins are 0.786 and 2.926, respectively, giving the non-significant *P*-values of 0.853 and 0.403, respectively. The assumption of multivariate normality is therefore not rejected.

5.5.8   Estimating the heritability of liability

The estimated correlations in liability between relatives can be equated to their expectations according to biometrical genetic models, in order to quantify genetic and environmental sources of variation in liability in the population. For example, the additive genetic correlation between parent and offspring is $V_A/2$, where V_A is the proportion of phenotypic variance due to additive genetic effects (i.e. *heritability in the narrow sense*). An estimate of narrow heritability is therefore twice the tetrachoric or polychoric correlation between parent and offspring. However, this ignores dominance interactions and a common family environment. Heritability is therefore often estimated using the twin method, which assumes that the environment is equally similar for MZ and DZ twins.

The standard method for obtaining a twin sample in order to study a rare disease is to identify proband twins among a large series of affected cases, and then study their cotwins for the presence or absence of the disease. The recurrence risk of the disease among the cotwins of the probands is known as a *probandwise concordance rate*. Twin-pairs in which both members are probands are double counted in the calculation of the probandwise concordance rate, as in the proband method for estimating a segregation ratio (Chapter 2). Under a liability-threshold model, the probandwise concordance rate is the conditional probability that a cotwin exceeds the threshold, given that the proband exceeds the threshold. The correlation in liability between MZ and DZ twins can therefore be estimated by the methods described in Section 5.5.6.

Another method for obtaining a twin sample in order to study a rare disease is to identify affected individuals in a population (or a volunteer) twin register, for example, by direct interviews, postal questionnaires, or by record linkage to a disease register. This procedure will produce counts for the number of normal–normal pairs, affected–normal pairs, and affected–affected pairs. Since this represents complete ascertainment, the proband method of analysis involves duplicating all pairs so that each member is considered as a proband in one observation and cotwin in another. This generates a full 2×2 contingency table. The correlation in liability between MZ and DZ twins can then be estimated by the methods described in Section 5.5.5, although care must be taken to double the sampling variance of the estimate obtained from the duplicated data.

Having obtained estimates for MZ correlation (r_{MZ}) and DZ correlation (r_{DZ}) in liability, one can proceed to estimate the proportions of liability variance explained by additive genetic effects (V_A), dominance (V_D) and common family environment (V_C) by solving the simultaneous equations:

$$r_{MZ} = \hat{V}_A + \hat{V}_D + \hat{V}_C$$
$$r_{DZ} = \frac{1}{2} \hat{V}_A + \frac{1}{4} \hat{V}_D + \hat{V}_C \qquad (5.93)$$

The total variance in liability is assumed to be 1. Not all three components can be estimated simultaneously. The usual procedure is to set $V_D = 0$, and estimate V_A and V_C as

$$\left. \begin{array}{l} \hat{V}_A = 2(r_{MZ} - r_{DZ}) \\ \hat{V}_C = 2r_{DZ} - r_{MZ} \end{array} \right\} \qquad (5.94)$$

when the $r_{MZ} : r_{DZ}$ ratio is between 1 and 2, and set $V_C = 0$ and estimate V_A and V_D as

$$\left. \begin{array}{l} \hat{V}_A = 4r_{DZ} - r_{MZ} \\ \hat{V}_D = 2(r_{MZ} - 2r_{DZ}) \end{array} \right\} \qquad (5.95)$$

when the $r_{MZ} : r_{DZ}$ ratio is between 2 and 4. The variance component $\hat{V}_A$ is an estimate of narrow heritability, while the sum of the components $\hat{V}_A + \hat{V}_D$ is an estimate of the broad heritability. Since these estimates are linear combinations of the tetrachoric correlations, their standard errors can be obtained quite simply from the standard errors of the tetrachoric correlations.

Example 5.18
From the tetrachoric correlations in Example 5.16

$$r_{MZ} = 0.488, \ SE(r_{MZ}) = 0.104$$
$$r_{DZ} = 0.248, \ SE(r_{DZ}) = 0.364$$

The estimates for V_A and V_C are

$$V_A = 0.480, \ SE(V_A) = 0.758$$
$$V_C = 0.008, \ SE(V_C) = 0.736$$

The very large standard errors means that neither component is statistically significant. Indeed, the MZ and DZ concordances of $46/131$ and $18/75$ (from

which the MZ and DZ tetrachoric correlations were derived) are not significantly different from each other (chi-squared = 2.75, degrees of freedom = 1,
$P = 0.097$).

As an aside, another measure of twin similarity for a dichotomous trait is the
so-called *pairwise concordance rate*, which is defined as the proportion of twin-
pairs with both members affected, in a sample of twin-pairs where each pair has
at least one affected member. In effect, only one member of each concordant
pair is treated as a proband. This is only appropriate under single ascertainment,
or if the probability of ascertainment is proportional to the number of affected
members in a twin-pair. Under this situation, the pairwise concordance rate is an
estimate of the recurrence risk in the cotwin of an affected individual (i.e. it is the
same as the probandwise concordance rate). When ascertainment is complete,
however, the probability of ascertainment will be the same for doubly as for
singly affected twin-pairs, so that the pairwise concordance rate (but not the
probandwise concordance rate) will under-estimate the recurrence risk in cotwins
of affected twins. It is therefore inappropriate to use the pairwise concordance
rate for a sample ascertained through probands. For a sample ascertained from a
population twin register, the assumption of complete ascertainment is reasonable,
but the pairwise concordance is identical to the probandwise concordance
obtained by regarding only one member of each concordant pair as proband. The
pairwise concordance rate is therefore inappropriate.

As a second aside, the ratio of the MZ concordance rate to the DZ concordance rate is sometimes used as an index to the genetic contribution to the trait
(e.g. Farmer *et al.*, 1987). This index, however, does not take account of the
population risk, and has no direct interpretation in terms of the
liability–threshold model, except that a ratio of greater than 1 indicates that the
heritability of the underlying liability is greater than 0.

5.6   Path analysis and structural equation models

The biometrical genetic approach to the analysis of polygenic traits developed
by Mather and Jinks (1977) was concerned mostly with characteristics in plants
and animals:

> The analysis of variation in a population becomes possible by experimen-
> tal means in species where we can use controlled matings and raise the
> progenies in such a way that we can determine the impact on them of the
> effects of the non-inheritable sources of variability.

This approach focuses on the nature of gene action on a trait, i.e. the number of
alleles involved, their main effects and interactions. In humans, however, the
inability to perform controlled matings severely limits the power to resolve
genetic components. Moreover, cultural factors transmitted from parents to
offspring in humans are not traditionally included in biometrical genetic
analysis.

Recognizing that in human genetics it is not usually possible to isolate one
causal relationship by the experimental control of other factors, Wright (1921)

developed the *'method of path coefficients'* with the aim of interpreting the empirical correlations between a set of variables in terms of an *a priori* model of the causal relations between the variables.

> In the biological sciences, especially, one often has to deal with a group of characteristics or conditions which are correlated because of a complex of interacting, uncontrollable, and often obscure causes. The degree of correlation between two variables can be calculated by well-known methods, but when it is found it gives merely the resultant of all connecting paths of influence. ... The present paper is an attempt to present a method of measuring the direct influence along each separate path in such a system and thus of finding the degree to which variation of a given effect is determined by each particular cause. The method depends on the combinations of knowledge of the degrees of correlations among the variables in a system with such knowledge as may be possessed of the causal relations. In cases in which the causal relations are uncertain, the method can be used to find the logical consequences of any particular hypotheses in regard to them.

Example 5.19
Suppose that there are good scientific reasons for believing that an observed variable X_3 is under the direct influences of two other observed variables X_1 and X_2, as well as a collection of unobserved variables denoted as U, assumed to be uncorrelated with X_1 and X_2. Given the correlations between the three observed variables X_1, X_2 and X_3 (r_{12}, r_{13}, r_{23}), how do we assess the relative contributions of X_1 and X_2 to X_3?

The first step of a path analysis is to construct a path diagram according to prior knowledge. In this case an appropriate diagram is shown in Figure 5.2.

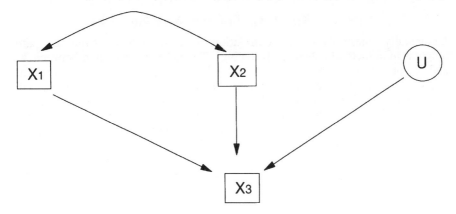

Figure 5.2 A simple path model.

In classical path analysis, it is customary to measure all variables (observed as well as unobserved) in terms of standard deviation units from the mean. The parameters of the path model are then:

(1)   the correlation between the predictor variables X_1 and X_2 (r_{12});
(2)   the regression (path) coefficient from X_1 to X_3 (b_{31});
(3)   the regression (path) coefficient from X_2 to X_3 (b_{32}).

The regression coefficient from U to X_3 (b_{3u}) is not an independent parameter since it is determined by the three parameters r_{12}, b_{31} and b_{32} by

$$V(X_3) = b_{31}^2 V(X_1) + b_{32}^2 V(X_2) + 2b_{31}b_{32}\,\mathrm{Cov}(X_1, X_2) + b_{3u}^2 V(U)$$
$$= b_{31}^2 + b_{32}^2 + 2b_{31}b_{32}r_{12} + b_{3u}^2$$
$$= 1$$

The model can be written in terms of a linear equation, and a set of correlations, as follows:

$$X_3 = b_{31}X_1 + b_{32}X_2 + b_{3u}U$$
$$r(X_1, X_2) = r_{12}$$
$$r(X_1, U) = r(X_2, U) = 0$$

The next step of the analysis is to write down the correlations between the observed variables in terms of the parameters of the model. The correlation between the 'predictor variables' X_1 and X_2, namely r_{12}, is already a parameter of the model. The correlation between a 'predictor variable' and a 'predicted variable' is more complex. Taking X_1 and X_3, the correlation can be decomposed as

$$r_{13} = r(X_1, X_3) = r(X_1, b_{31}X_1 + b_{32}X_2) = b_{31} + b_{32}r_{12}$$

In other words, the correlation between the predicted variable X_3 and the predictor variable X_1 is made up of a direct component (b_{31}) and an indirect component due to the correlation between X_1 with the other predictor variable, namely X_2 ($b_{32}r_{12}$). Similarly, the correlation between X_2 and X_3 is

$$r_{23} = r(X_2, X_3) = r(X_2, b_{31}X_1 + b_{32}X_2) = b_{31}r_{12} + b_{32}$$

Incidentally, these theoretical correlations can be deduced from the path diagram by a method called 'path tracing'. To find the correlation between X_1 and X_3, one starts from the predicted variable and traces back to the predictor variable through the two possible routes. The direct route contains just one path coefficient, b_{31}. The indirect route through X_2 contains a path coefficient b_{32} and a correlation r_{12}, which are multiplied to give $b_{32}r_{12}$. The contributions from the direct and indirect routes are then summed to give $b_{31} + b_{32}r_{12}$. Although path tracing is unnecessary in this simple example, it is a convenient tool in more complex models.

    The model can be written in terms of a theoretical correlation matrix of the observed variables, as follows.

$$\mathrm{Corr}(X_1, X_2, X_3) = \begin{bmatrix} 1 & r_{12} & b_{31} + b_{32}r_{12} \\ r_{12} & 1 & b_{31}r_{12} + b_{32} \\ b_{31} + b_{32}r_{12} & b_{31}r_{12} + b_{32} & 1 \end{bmatrix}$$

The final step of the path analysis is to express the path coefficients in terms of the observed correlations. This involves equating the observed correlations to the theoretical correlations. For this example, this leads to the simultaneous linear equations

$$r_{13} = b_{31} + b_{32}r_{12}$$
$$r_{23} = b_{31}r_{12} + b_{32}$$

The solutions of which are

$$b_{31} = \frac{r_{13} - r_{12}r_{23}}{1 - r_{12}^2}$$

$$b_{32} = \frac{r_{23} - r_{12}r_{13}}{1 - r_{12}^2}$$

These are equal to the partial correlation coefficients between X_3 and X_1, and between X_3 and X_2. Path analysis is therefore equivalent to multiple linear regression in this simple example. The common aim is, of course, to isolate the direct influences of X_1 on X_3, and of X_2 on X_3, assuming that X_1 and X_2 may be correlated, but that other determinants of X_3 are uncorrelated with X_1 or X_2.

Another notable point of this example is that the three observed correlations (r_{12}, r_{13}, r_{23}) are consistent with just one set of values of the model parameters (r_{12}, b_{31}, b_{32}). When this occurs a perfect fit between the data and the model is guaranteed, and there is no room in the data to check the adequacy of the assumptions of the model. Under these circumstances we say that the model is identified but not over-identified.

This example shows that a causal model can be specified not only in the form of a path diagram, but also as a set of linear equations (which can be written in matrix notation), or as a matrix of predicted correlations. Nevertheless, the path diagram is useful as a visual representation of the model. In this example, the causal model consists of just two layers of variables: the independent variables X_1, X_2 and U, and the dependent variables X_3. In general, path diagrams can be much more complicated, as described by Wright (1968):

> every included variable, measured or hypothetical, is represented by arrows as either completely determined by certain others, which may in turn be represented as similarly determined, or as an ultimate variable. Each ultimate factor in the diagram must be connected by lines with arrow heads at both ends with each of the other ultimate factors, to indicate possible correlations through still more remote, unrepresented factors, except in cases in which it can be safely assumed that there is no correlation ... the strict validity of the method depends on the properties of formally complete systems of unitary variables.

In modern statistical methodology, path analysis is part of a more general approach to the analysis of linear relationships between variables known as structural equation models (Bentler, 1986; Bollen, 1989). Structure equation models are more general than path analysis is several respects. First, the variables are not necessarily standardized, so that the data are summarized in terms of the variances and covariances (rather than the correlations) of the variables. This stemmed from the development of variance components models (Searle *et al.*, 1992). Secondly, unobserved (i.e. latent) variables are no longer restricted to be 'residual errors' of observed variables; they are allowed to be correlated with, to be influenced by, and to have influences on, other variables. This stemmed from the development of confirmatory factor analysis and measurement error models (Joreskog, 1969, 1971). Thirdly, estimation and the hypothesis testing of model parameters are performed using likelihood-based (or related) methods, usually under the assumption of multivariate normality. This stemmed from the theoretical work on the analysis of covariance structures (Joreskog, 1970).

5.6.1   Model-fitting and model-selection procedures

The consistency of sample data with a particular structural equation model (denoted as M_1) can be assessed by the degree of discrepancy between the sample covariance matrix and the theoretical covariance matrix predicted by the model. Let the sample covariance matrix of the p observed variables be S, and the predicted covariance matrix be Σ. The elements in the matrix Σ are functions of the q free parameters (denoted as θ) of the model M_1. Assuming that the observed variables are multivariate normal, then under the model M_1, the log-likelihood of a set of multivariate observations $x_1, x_2, \ldots, x_n$, is

$$
\begin{aligned}
\ln L_1 &= -\frac{n}{2} \ln(2\pi |\Sigma|) - \frac{1}{2} \sum_i (x_i - \mu)^{\mathrm{T}} \Sigma^{-1} (x_i - \mu) \\[2mm]
&= -\frac{n}{2} \ln(2\pi |\Sigma|) - \frac{n}{2} (m - \mu)^{\mathrm{T}} \Sigma^{-1} (m - \mu) \\[2mm]
&\quad - \frac{1}{2} \sum_i (x_i - m)^{\mathrm{T}} \Sigma^{-1} (x_i - m) \\[2mm]
&= -\frac{n}{2} \ln(2\pi |\Sigma|) - \frac{n}{2} (m - \mu)^{\mathrm{T}} \Sigma^{-1} (m - \mu) \\[2mm]
&\quad - \frac{n}{2} \operatorname{tr}(\Sigma^{-1} S) \\[2mm]
&= -\frac{n}{2} [\ln(2\pi) + \ln|\Sigma| + (m - \mu)^{\mathrm{T}} \Sigma^{-1} (m - \mu) \\[2mm]
&\quad + \operatorname{tr}(\Sigma^{-1} S)]
\end{aligned} \tag{5.96}
$$

where μ and m are vectors of theoretical and sample means of the p observed variables, respectively. When interest is focused on the covariances between variables, the variables can be assumed to be mean-centred, so that the term concerning the observed means m and the predicted means μ can be ignored. The log-likelihood is then simply

$$\ln L_1 = -\frac{n}{2}\left[\ln(2\pi) + \ln|\Sigma| + \mathrm{tr}(\Sigma^{-1}S)\right] \tag{5.97}$$

Under a saturated model (denoted M_0) in which each element of Σ is an independent parameter, a perfect fit between Σ and S is ensured, and the log-likelihood is simply

$$
\left.
\begin{aligned}
\ln L_0 &= -\frac{n}{2}\left[\ln(2\pi) + \ln|S| + \mathrm{tr}(S^{-1}S)\right] \\[2mm]
&= -\frac{n}{2}\left[\ln(2\pi) + \ln|S| + p\right]
\end{aligned}
\right\} \tag{5.98}
$$

The adequacy of the submodel M_1, in relation to the saturated model M_0, can therefore be assessed by the statistic

$$2(\ln L_0 - \ln L_1) = n\left[\ln|\Sigma| - \ln|S| + \mathrm{tr}(\Sigma^{-1}S) - p\right] \tag{5.99}$$

The value of this statistic depends on the values of the q free parameters (θ) of M_1. If the function

$$f(\theta) = \ln|\Sigma| - \ln|S| + \mathrm{tr}(\Sigma^{-1}S) - p \tag{5.100}$$

is minimized with respect to θ, and the minimum value of the function denoted as f_1, then $F_1 = nf_1$ has asymptotically a chi-squared distribution with degrees of freedom equal to $[p(p+1)/2] - q$, if the model M_1 is true. The chi-squared statistic F_1 is thus commonly used as an index of the goodness-of-fit between the model M_1 and the data.

It is not necessary for all observations to have the same predicted covariance matrix. If the population consists of k groups, with predicted and sample covariance matrices $\Sigma_1, \Sigma_2, \ldots \Sigma_k$ and $S_1, S_2, \ldots, S_k$, respectively, then the overall fit function of the model is

$$f(\theta) = \sum_{i=1}^{k}\frac{n_i}{n}\left[\ln|\Sigma_i| - \ln|S_i| + \mathrm{tr}(\Sigma_i^{-1}S_i) - p\right] \tag{5.101}$$

where n_i is the sample size of group i, and n is the total sample size. The chi-squared goodness-of-fit index of the model, F, is n times the minimum value of this fit function.

Comparison between two models, say M_1 and M_2, can be performed by a chi-squared test if the two models are nested in the sense that one of the models can be obtained by fixing or imposing certain constraints on the parameters of the other model. Suppose that M_2 (with q_2 free parameters) is a submodel of M_1 (with q_1 free parameters). If the goodness-of-fit indices of M_1 and M_2 are

F_1 and F_2 respectively, then the statistic

$$F = F_2 - F_1 \tag{5.102}$$

has a chi-squared distribution with $q_1 - q_2$ degrees of freedom.

If the two models are not nested, then chi-squared asymptotic theory does not apply. A common procedure is then to modify the F index to take account of the number of free parameters in the model (i.e. the degree of parsimony of the model). One popular index is the Akaike information criterion (AIC), which (for model i) is defined as

$$\text{AIC}_i = F_i + 2q_i \tag{5.103}$$

The model with the smallest AIC is then considered to represent the best compromise between goodness-of-fit and parsimony.

Several programs are available for fitting structural equation models, including LISREL, EQS and Mx. The Mx program is particularly flexible for genetic applications.

5.6.2   Structural equation models for continuous twin data

Although regression analysis offers a convenient way of estimating various genetic and environmental components from twin data, there are advantages in using the more general framework of structural equation models (Martin and Eaves, 1977). While the hypothetical causal relationships are implicit in the regression model, they can be made explicit in a structural equation model. Thus, a causal model for the phenotypic trait X of a twin can be written as shown in Figure 5.3 where A, D, C, E are latent variables that represent additive genetic effects, dominance, environment shared with cotwin, and environment not shared with cotwin, respectively. This model can also be written as

$$X = aA + dD + cC + eE \tag{5.104}$$

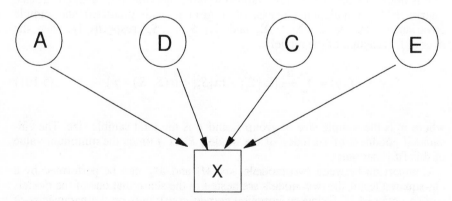

Figure 5.3   Path model for the phenotype of an individual.

Since A, D, C, E are latent variables, they can be assumed to be standard normal. Furthermore, the parameters of the model, the path coefficients a, d, c, e, can be defined to be non-negative. The path diagram can be extended for MZ twin pairs as shown in Figure 5.4. The perfect correlations between A_1 and A_2, and between D_1 and D_2 are the consequences of the genetic identity between MZ twins. The perfect correlation between C_1 and C_2 and the zero correlation between E_1 and E_2, arise from the definition that C is the shared environment, and E the unique environments, of the two twins. The path diagram for DZ twin pairs is identical except that the correlation between A_1 and A_2 is $1/2$ instead of 1, and the correlation between D_1 and D_2 is $1/4$ instead of 1 (see Figure 5.5). These correlations are consequences of biometrical genetic theory.

If it is further assumed that the values of the four unknown parameters a, d, c, and e are equal for MZ and DZ twins, then the model will predict the

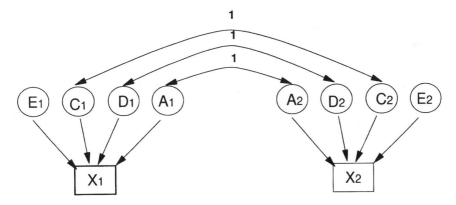

Figure 5.4   Path model for the phenotypes of an MZ twin pair.

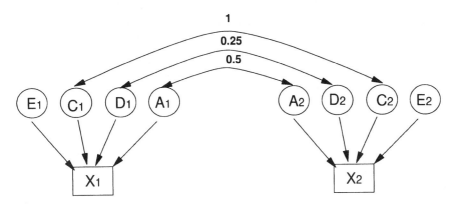

Figure 5.5   Path model for the phenotypes of a DZ twin pair.

covariance matrices

$$
\Sigma_{MZ} = \begin{pmatrix} a^2 + d^2 + c^2 + e^2 & a^2 + d^2 + c^2 \\ a^2 + d^2 + c^2 & a^2 + d^2 + c^2 + e^2 \end{pmatrix}
$$

$$
\Sigma_{DZ} = \begin{pmatrix} a^2 + d^2 + c^2 + e^2 & a^2/2 + d^2/4 + c^2 \\ a^2/2 + d^2/4 + c^2 & a^2 + d^2 + c^2 + e^2 \end{pmatrix}
$$

(5.105)

which can be fitted to the two sample covariance matrices

$$
S_{MZ} = \begin{pmatrix} s^2_{MZ} & c_{MZ} \\ c_{MZ} & s^2_{MZ} \end{pmatrix}
$$

$$
S_{DZ} = \begin{pmatrix} s^2_{DZ} & c_{DZ} \\ c_{DZ} & s^2_{DZ} \end{pmatrix}
$$

(5.106)

provided that at most one of the two latent variables C and D is included in any one model.

Example 5.20
Returning to the neuroticism data of Example 5.1, the MZ and DZ covariance matrices can be calculated to be

$$
S_{MZ} = \begin{pmatrix} 17.640 & 8.142 \\ 8.142 & 17.640 \end{pmatrix}
$$

$$
S_{DZ} = \begin{pmatrix} 18.460 & 3.350 \\ 3.530 & 18.460 \end{pmatrix}
$$

based on the sample sizes of $n_{MZ} = 522$ and $n_{DZ} = 272$ pairs, respectively. The symmetry of these matrices is due to the arbitrariness of the order of the two twins in a twin-pair, which mean that the MZ variance should be estimated from all 1044 MZ twins, and the DZ variance from all 544 DZ twins.

When these data were fitted to simple genetic models by Mx, the following results were obtained.

Model	a^2	d^2	c^2	e^2	F	q	df	AIC
ADE	0.279	0.188	(0)	0.533	0.34	3	1	6.34
ACE	0.460	(0)	0	0.540	1.00	3	1	7.00
AE	0.460	(0)	(0)	0.540	1.00	2	2	5.00
DE	(0)	0.472	(0)	0.528	1.78	2	2	5.78
CE	(0)	(0)	0.366	0.634	21.2	2	2	25.2
E	(0)	(0)	(0)	1	135.3	1	3	141.3

Parameters in brackets are fixed rather than estimated, and therefore do not contribute to the number of free parameters, q. The fit function may nevertheless maximize at a boundary of a free parameter. The data have a maximum of four degrees of freedom (df), because there are two variances and two covariances. The degrees of freedom of a model is this total (4) minus the number of free parameters, q. For ease of interpretation, the parameters a^2, d^2, c^2 and e^2 have been standardized so that they sum to 1.

The ADE model has the smallest value of F and is therefore the best-fitting model. It does not allow the MZ and DZ variances to be different from each other, and is therefore not saturated. The AE model has the smallest AIC and therefore represents the best compromise between goodness-of-fit and parsimony.

The only models that can be rejected by a chi-squared test are CE and E, which represent the absence of any genetic effect and the absence of any familial effect, respectively, on neuroticism. Although the AE model is the most preferred model according to AIC, the alternative models AD, ADE, and ACE cannot be considered excluded. The predicted covariance matrices of the AE model are

$$\Sigma_{MZ} = \begin{pmatrix} 17.969 & 8.264 \\ 8.264 & 17.969 \end{pmatrix}$$

$$\Sigma_{DZ} = \begin{pmatrix} 17.969 & 4.132 \\ 4.132 & 17.969 \end{pmatrix}$$

If the twin sample is not representative of the population but is selected for certain ranges of trait values, then it may be necessary to make allowance for the process of ascertainment by adjusting the likelihood function. Suppose that the twins in a population are screened for a trait value of above a certain threshold t. The twins identified by the screening process are called probands, and their cotwins are then measured and included into the sample. If there are N probands, the data can be summarized in a matrix with N rows and two columns, one column for the proband's trait value, and another for the cotwin's trait value. Twin-pairs in which both members are probands are entered twice in the data matrix. If there are b doubly ascertained twin-pairs in the sample, then the actual number of twin-pairs is $n = N - b$.

The log-likelihood of a proband–cotwin pair with trait values $x = (x_1, x_2)^T$, conditional on ascertainment (i.e. $x_1 > t$) and assuming bivariate normality, is

$$\ln L = -\frac{1}{2} [\ln(2\pi|\Sigma|) + (x - \mu)^T \Sigma^{-1}(x - \mu)] - \ln(A) \qquad (5.107)$$

where μ and Σ are the mean vector and covariance matrix of x. The adjustment term $\ln(A)$, is the logarithm of the probability of ascertainment (i.e. of $x_1 > t$). Writing a bivariate normal density with mean vector μ and covariance matrix Σ as $f(x_1, x_2)$, the ascertainment probability A is

$$A = 1 - \int_{-\infty}^{t} \int_{-\infty}^{\infty} f(x_1, x_2)\, dx_2\, dx_1 = 1 - \Phi\left(\frac{t - \mu_1}{\sigma_1}\right) \qquad (5.108)$$

where μ_1 and σ_1 are the mean and standard deviation of x_1, and Φ is the standard normal distribution function. If the population values of μ_1 and σ_1 are known, then they can be specified as fixed constants for the analysis. The adjustment term $\ln(A)$ is then independent of the model parameters, so that it need not be included in the analysis. On the other hand, if μ_1 and σ_1 are unknown parameters to be estimated from the data, then the adjustment term $\ln(A)$ will vary according to these parameters, and so its inclusion is necessary. In either case, the overall log-likelihood of the sample is the sum of the adjusted log-likelihoods of the proband–cotwin pairs, multiplied by the factor n/N to allow for the duplication of doubly ascertained pairs.

Example 5.21
Consider the same data as in Example 5.20 but with complete ascertainment such that all twins with a neuroticism score of 16 or more are selected as probands. Twin-pairs where both members have a score of 15 or below are therefore excluded. This ascertainment scheme identifies 85 singly ascertained MZ twin-pairs and 23 doubly ascertained MZ twin-pairs, so that the number of MZ proband–cotwin pairs is $85 + 46 = 131$. Similarly, 57 singly ascertained DZ twin-pairs and nine doubly ascertained DZ twin-pairs are identified, so that the number of DZ proband–cotwin pairs is $57 + 18 = 75$. The total number of proband–cotwin pairs is therefore $N = 131 + 75 = 206$, when the actual number of twin-pairs is $n = 108 + 66 = 174$. The ratio n/N is therefore 0.84466.

Two analyses using Mx are performed, both using an appropriate adjustment for ascertainment. In the first analysis, the mean and variance of neuroticism are specified as the approximately correct values of 10.23 and 18.00. The results, with $-2 \ln L$ being adjusted by a factor of 0.8466, are as follows.

Model	a^2	d^2	c^2	e^2	$-2 \ln L$	q	AIC
ADE	0.295	0.166	(0)	0.539	1500.23	3	1506.23
ACE	0.452	(0)	0	0.548	1500.55	3	1506.55
AE	0.452	(0)	(0)	0.548	1500.55	2	1504.55
DE	(0)	0.468	(0)	0.532	1501.26	2	1505.26
CE	(0)	(0)	0.352	0.648	1510.89	2	1514.89
E	(0)	(0)	(0)	1	1573.32	1	1575.32

Instead of F, the likelihood ratio statistic, Mx gives $-2 \ln L$ because the fit function is user-defined. The results are remarkably similar to those obtained from the complete data in Example 5.20. Models CE and E can be rejected, and model AE is the best as judged by AIC.

The second analysis is performed with the mean and variance as free parameters. The results are as follows

Model	μ_1	σ_1^2	a^2	d^2	c^2	e^2	$-2 \ln L$	q	AIC
ADE	9.16	16.99	0.518	0	(0)	0.482	1494.23	3	1500.23
ACE	7.77	19.19	0.405	(0)	0.180	0.415	1493.67	3	1499.67
AE	9.16	16.99	0.518	(0)	(0)	0.482	1494.23	2	1498.23
DE	10.39	15.17	(0)	0.434	(0)	0.566	1496.56	2	1500.50
CE	8.21	18.78	(0)	(0)	0.483	0.517	1505.89	2	1509.89
E	12.14	12.86	(0)	(0)	(0)	1	1518.47	1	1520.47

Despite not making any assumptions about the mean and variance, the results are still quite similar to those obtained from the complete data in Example 5.20. Models CE and E can be rejected, and model AE is the best as judged by AIC. Moreover, the estimates of the mean and variance for the AE model are fairly close to the correct values of 10.23 and 18.00.

Thus, if accurate estimates of population parameters such as mean and variance are available, then the analysis can be conducted with the parameters fixed at their estimated values. On the other hand, if accurate estimates of population parameters are not available, then these parameters should be estimated from the data, with ascertainment being taken into account in the log-likelihood function.

5.6.3 Structural equation models for quasi-continuous twin data

Twin data on quasi-continuous traits can be subjected to structural equation modelling under the assumption of a liability-threshold model. In contrast to twin data on continuous traits which can be summarized by covariance matrices, twin data on quasi-continuous traits are summarized as contingency tables. A structural equation model can be fitted to contingency tables indirectly, by first converting the contingency tables to tetrachoric or polychoric correlation matrices, and then subjecting these matrices to an analysis of covariance structure. This is the usual approach implemented by the combined use of the programs PRELIS and LISREL (Joreskog and Sorbom, 1986, 1988; Neale *et al.*, 1989; Neale and Cardon, 1992). However, it is now possible to fit structural equation models (with additional threshold parameters) directly to contingency tables by maximum likelihood, using the Mx program.

For the simplest case of a quasi-continuous trait with two categories, the status of a twin-pair can be summarized into four indicator functions, I_{00}, I_{01}, I_{10}, I_{11}, where the first subscript indicates the affection status of twin 1 ($0 = $ unaffected, $1 = $ affected) and the second subscript indicates the affection status of twin 2. The indicator function is 1 if the twin-pair is of the status specified by the two subscripts, and 0 otherwise. The log-likelihood of a twin-pair is therefore

$$\ln L = \sum_{i=0}^{1} \sum_{j=0}^{1} I_{ij} \ln (p_{ij}) \tag{5.109}$$

Under a liability-threshold model, the probabilities p_{ij} are determined by the correlation in liability between twin 1 and twin 2, and the thresholds in liability for twin 1 and twin 2. Each probability is the volume under a bivariate normal density function, bounded by the appropriate thresholds, and can be found by numerical integration if the correlation and the thresholds are known. For example, the probability p_{00} is given by

$$p_{00} = \int_{-\infty}^{t_2} \int_{-\infty}^{t_1} \phi(x_1, x_2) \, dx_1 \, dx_2 \tag{5.110}$$

The limits t_1 and t_2 are the thresholds in liability for twin 1 and twin 2. The variables x_1 and x_2 are the liabilities of twin 1 and twin 2, and $\phi(x_1, x_2)$ is the bivariate normal density function with zero means, unit variances and correlation r. The correlation in liability, r, is $a^2 + d^2 + c^2$ for MZ twins, and $a^2/2 + d^2/4 + c^2$ for DZ twins. The log-likelihood is therefore ultimately a function of the thresholds and the parameters of the structural equation model. The overall log-likelihood of the sample, which is simply the sum of the log-likelihoods of the individual twin-pairs, can therefore be maximized with respect to the parameters a^2, d^2, c^2, e^2, t_1 and t_2.

Example 5.22

Returning to the dichotomized neuroticism data of Example 5.15:

	LL	LH	HH
MZ	414	85	23
DZ	206	57	9

The data can be fitted to a liability-threshold model directly by Mx by providing the contingency tables.

MZ

	Twin 2	
Twin 1	L	H
L	414	42.5
H	42.5	23

MZ

	Twin 2	
Twin 1	L	H
L	206	28.5
H	28.5	9

The results are as follows.

Model	t	a^2	d^2	c^2	e^2	F	q	df	AIC
ADE	1.13	0.495	0	(0)	0.505	0.41	4	1	8.41
ACE	1.13	0.492	(0)	0.003	0.505	0.41	4	1	8.41
AE	1.13	0.495	(0)	(0)	0.505	0.41	3	2	6.41
DE	1.13	(0)	0.506	(0)	0.494	1.26	3	2	7.26
CE	1.13	(0)	(0)	0.412	0.588	2.98	3	2	8.98
E	1.13	(0)	(0)	(0)	1	30.52	2	3	34.52

where F is the likelihood ratio chi-squared statistic, q is the number of estimated parameters, and df is the number of degrees of freedom. Because of the symmetry of the tables, the total number of degrees of freedom is $6 - 1 = 5$, and there is only one threshold parameter. The number of degrees of freedom of a model is therefore $5 - q$. The AE model represents the best compromise between goodness-of-fit and parsimony, according to the AIC. The heritability estimate obtained from the AE model, of 0.495, is not far from that obtained from the original continuous data (0.460). No model other than E can be rejected by a formal test of significance. As the CE model cannot be rejected, the presence of a genetic component is not firmly established. This represents a drop in power, as compared with the results obtained from the original continuous data in Example 5.20.

An adjustment for ascertainment can also be built into the analysis of quasi-continuous data. Assuming that ascertainment is through probands with the disease, the probability of ascertainment is

$$A = 1 - \int_{-\infty}^{t} \int_{-\infty}^{\infty} f(x_1, x_2) \, dx_2 \, dx_1 = 1 - \Phi(t) \qquad (5.111)$$

where x_1 and x_2 are liabilities whose marginal distributions are standard normal, and t is the threshold for the disease and is assumed to be known from the population risk of the disease. Since twin 1 (the proband) is certain to be affected, the adjusted log-likelihood of a proband–cotwin pair as

$$\ln L = I_{10} \ln(p_{10}) + I_{11} \ln(p_{11}) - \ln(A) \qquad (5.112)$$

The inclusion of the ascertainment adjustment is unnecessary if the threshold t is set at a fixed value in the analysis (because in this situation the adjustment term is constant). If the number of proband–cotwin pairs is N and the number of actual twin-pairs is n, then the overall log-likelihood is just the sum of the adjusted log-likelihoods of the proband–cotwin pairs, multiplied by the factor n/N.

Example 5.23
Returning to the data of Example 5.22. Suppose that the data were subjected to complete ascertainment for the disease. This would produce 131 MZ probands and 75 DZ probands, with the following distribution for the affection status of the cotwins.

	Cotwin unaffected	Cotwin affected
MZ	85	46
DZ	57	18

The total number of proband–cotwin pairs is $N = 131 + 75 = 206$, when the actual number of twin-pairs is $n = 108 + 66 = 174$. The ratio n/N is therefore 0.84466. Adjusted for this ratio, and with the threshold fixed at 1.13, the results from Mx are as follows.

Model	t	a^2	d^2	c^2	e^2	F	q	df	AIC
ADE	(1.13)	0.490	0	(0)	0.510	0.68	3	0	6.68
ACE	(1.13)	0.420	(0)	0.063	0.516	0.00	3	0	6.00
AE	(1.13)	0.490	(0)	(0)	0.510	0.68	2	1	4.68
DE	(1.13)	(0)	0.500	(0)	0.500	1.71	2	1	5.71
CE	(1.13)	(0)	(0)	0.413	0.587	2.38	2	1	6.38
E	(1.13)	(0)	(0)	(0)	1	41.16	1	2	43.16

Again the only model that can be rejected is E, although AE remains the most favoured model according to AIC.

5.6.4   More complex structural equation models

Structural equation models for twin data are not only easy to interpret, they can also be generalized to deal with additional complexities. One simple addition is reciprocal sibling interaction, where the trait value of one twin can have an effect on the trait value of the cotwin. As discussed in Section 5.2.3, reciprocal sibling interaction leads to a difference between the MZ phenotypic variance and the DZ phenotypic variance. Let the effect of one twin on the other twin be b, then the reciprocal interaction between the trait values of two twins (X_1 and X_2) can be added to the basic biometrical genetic model as follows

$$\left. \begin{array}{l} X_1 = bX_2 + aA_1 + dD_1 + cC_1 + eE_1 \\ X_2 = bX_1 + aA_2 + dD_2 + cC_2 + eE_2 \end{array} \right\} \tag{5.113}$$

In matrix form, this can be written more simply as

$$X = BX + YH \tag{5.114}$$

where

$$\left. \begin{array}{c} B = \begin{pmatrix} 0 & b \\ b & 0 \end{pmatrix} \\[2mm] X = (X_1 \quad X_2)^T \\[2mm] Y = \begin{pmatrix} A_1 & D_1 & C_1 & E_1 \\ A_2 & D_2 & C_2 & E_2 \end{pmatrix} \\[2mm] H = (a \quad d \quad c \quad e)^T \end{array} \right\} \tag{5.115}$$

This can be rearranged as

$$\left. \begin{array}{r} X - BX = YH \\ (I - B)X = YH \\ X = (I - B)^{-1}YH \end{array} \right\} \tag{5.116}$$

With the interest being on covariance structure, the variables can be assumed to be mean centred, so that the covariance matrix of X is

$$E(XX^T) = (I - B)^{-1} E(YHH^T Y^T)(I - B)^{-1} \qquad (5.117)$$

The effect of sibling interaction is therefore to pre-multiply and post-multiply the simple genetic covariance structure by the matrix $(I - B)^{-1}$. This can be implemented very simply in Mx.

Another generalization is to allow for the effect of a covariate, such as age, on the trait. The inclusion of age (denoted as V) introduces an additional observed variable, so that each vector of observation consists of the three variables (X_1, X_2, V). The observed covariance matrix is therefore 3×3. The basic genetic model can be modified to take account of Y as follows

$$\left. \begin{aligned} X_1 &= sG + aA_1 + dD_1 + cC_1 + eE_1 \\ X_2 &= sG + aA_2 + dD_2 + cC_2 + eE_2 \\ V &= gG \end{aligned} \right\} \qquad (5.118)$$

where G can be thought of as a 'dummy' latent variable introduced for convenience. The implied covariance matrix of this model can be easily specified in Mx and fitted to a set of twin data with age.

It is also possible to allow for the effect of sex or other dichotomous factors. A twin can be classified as male (M) or female (F), so that there are five groups of twins, MZ-MM, MZ-FF, DZ-MM, DZ-FF, DZ-MF. Suppose that the model for a male twin is

$$X_m = a_m A_m + d_m D_m + c_m X_m + e_m E_m \qquad (5.119)$$

In order to allow for sex differences in all four components, the model for a female twin can be written as

$$X_f = a_{fm} A_m + d_{fm} D_m + c_{fm} C_m + a_f A_f + d_f D_f + c_f C_f + e_f E_f \qquad (5.120)$$

where the first three terms represent components shared with males, and the last four terms represent components specific to females. The phenotypic covariances under this model for the five classes of twin-pairs are as follows

$$\left. \begin{aligned} \text{Cov}_{MZ-MM} &= a_m^2 + d_m^2 + c_m^2 \\ \text{Cov}_{MZ-FF} &= a_{fm}^2 + d_{fm}^2 + c_{fm}^2 + a_f^2 + d_f^2 + c_f^2 \\ \text{Cov}_{DZ-MM} &= \frac{a_m^2}{2} + \frac{d_m^2}{4} + c_m^2 \\ \text{Cov}_{DZ-FF} &= \frac{a_{fm}^2}{2} + \frac{d_{fm}^2}{4} + c_{fm}^2 + \frac{a_f^2}{2} + \frac{d_f^2}{4} + c_f^2 \\ \text{Cov}_{DZ-MF} &= \frac{a_m a_{fm}}{2} + \frac{d_m d_{fm}}{4} + c_m c_{fm} \end{aligned} \right] \qquad (5.121)$$

As usual, either dominance (D) or common environment (C), but not both, can be entered simultaneously into a model. Even then, there still remain six parameters in the five covariances, so that it is necessary to fix at least one additional parameter to 0, or to impose at least one constraint on the parameters.

If there are sex differences, then the path coefficients a_{fm}, d_{fm}, c_{fm} for the shared components may be smaller than the path coefficients a_m, d_m, c_m for the total male components, and the path coefficients a_f, d_f, c_f for the female-specific components may be non-zero. The absence of sex differences is specified by the restrictions $a_m = a_{fm}$, $d_m = d_{fm}$, $c_m = c_{fm}$, $a_f = d_f = c_f = 0$. Any of these restrictions can be relaxed to see if the goodness-of-fit of the model to the data is significantly improved. This type of model is called 'sex-limitation', because the effects of the different components are dependent on (or limited by) the sex of the individual.

A similar model can be constructed for a dichotomous variable such as the presence (1) or absence (0) of an environmental exposure. The only difference is that six groups are now possible, namely MZ-00, MZ-11, MZ-01, DZ-00, DZ-11, DZ-01. With six groups and therefore six covariances, it is possible to estimate six parameters. This type of model is called 'gene–environment interaction'.

Structural equation models can also be easily generalized for multivariate data. In the simplest situation, the same underlying character is measured multiple times under almost identical conditions. Suppose that the underlying character of twin i, denoted by X_i, is measured by two observed variables denoted by Z_{i1} and Z_{i2}, then a reasonable 'measurement model' may be

$$\left.\begin{array}{l} Z_{11} = mX_1 + R_{11} \\ Z_{12} = mX_1 + R_{12} \\ Z_{21} = mX_2 + R_{21} \\ Z_{22} = mX_2 + R_{22} \end{array}\right\} \tag{5.122}$$

where R_{11}, R_{12}, R_{21}, R_{22} are independent, identically distributed 'measurement errors'. The latent variables X_1 and X_2 are in turn determined by the usual genetic model

$$\left.\begin{array}{l} X_1 = aA_1 + dD_1 + cC_1 + eE_1 \\ X_2 = aA_2 + dD_2 + cC_2 + eE_1 \end{array}\right\} \tag{5.123}$$

The measurement model and the genetic model together constitute an overall model. The implied covariance structure of this model for the observed variables (i.e. Z_{11}, Z_{12}, Z_{21}, Z_{22}) can be fitted to the observed covariance matrix in order to obtain estimates of the model parameters. The use of multiple measurements can potentially separate out measurement errors from 'true' environmental influences. This gives improved heritability estimates that reflect more accurately the importance of the genetic component in relation to the 'stable' phenotypic variance.

If multiple measures of the same character are taken at regular time intervals, then a 'repeated measures' model may be used to examine the changes in the genetic structure of the character over time. It is possible, for example, that the genetic component is constant, but different sets of environmental influences are involved at different times. Assuming that the usual genetic model applies for the trait values X_j at time-point j, i.e.

$$X_j = a_j A_j + d_j D_j + c_j X_j + e_j E_j \tag{5.124}$$

then the phenotypic covariances between consecutive measurements of the trait for the twin-pairs can be modelled by linear relationships between consecutive values of the underlying genetic and environmental components

$$
\left.\begin{array}{l}
A_j = b_{aj}A_{j-1} + A_{sj} \\
D_j = b_{dj}D_{j-1} + D_{sj} \\
C_j = b_{cj}C_{j-1} + C_{sj} \\
E_j = b_{ej}E_{j-1} + E_{sj}
\end{array}\right\} \tag{5.125}
$$

Taking the additive genetic component for example; the component operating at time j (A_j) is determined by a linear combination of the component at time $j-1$ (A_{j-1}) and a fresh component (A_{sj}). At time 1, there is no previously measured component, so that $A_1 = A_{s1}$. The twin correlation of A_1 can be specified as usual (i.e. 1 for MZ and $1/2$ for DZ). For time 2 onwards, it is necessary to specify twin correlations for the fresh components (i.e. A_{s2}, A_{s3}, ...) only, as this fixes the twin correlations between the total components (i.e. A_2, A_3, ...) to the values predicted by biometrical genetic theory. As usual, however, some of the components (i.e. either dominance or shared environment, or both) will have to be omitted to ensure that the model is identified.

Another multivariate extension of the simple genetic model concerns two or more variables that represent entirely different constructs rather than repeated measures of the same construct. A number of questions may be of interest, depending on how much is known about the biological basis of the variables. The hypothesis may be that two traits share the same genetic component, but have different environmental influences, or it may be that one trait has a direct causal effect on another trait. For two traits, X and Y, a multivariate genetic model may be written as

$$
\left.\begin{array}{l}
X = a_{sx}A_s + d_{sx}D_s + c_{sx}C_s + e_{sx}E_s + a_xA_x + d_xD_x + c_xC_x + e_xE_x \\
Y = a_{sy}A_s + d_{sy}D_s + c_{sy}C_s + e_{sy}E_s + a_yA_y + d_yD_y + c_yC_y + e_yE_y
\end{array}\right\} \tag{5.126}
$$

where A_s, D_s, C_s, E_s are components shared by X and Y, A_x, D_x, C_x, E_x are components unique to X, and A_y, D_y, C_y, E_y are components unique to Y. This model is sometimes said to have 'independent pathways' because the path coefficients a_{sx}, d_{sx} c_{sx}, e_{sx} from the shared factors to X are independent of the path coefficients a_{sy}, d_{sy}, c_{sy}, e_{sy} from the shared factors to Y. However, with just two variables the path coefficients a_{sx}, d_{sx}, c_{sx}, e_{sx} cannot be identified separately from the path coefficients a_{sy}, d_{sy}, c_{sy}, e_{sy}, since the expected covariance matrix will remain unchanged as long as the products $a_{sx}a_{sy}$, $d_{sx}d_{sy}$, $c_{sx}c_{sy}$, $e_{sx}e_{sy}$ are unchanged. It is therefore convenient to fix $a_{sx} = d_{sx} = c_{sx} = e_{sx} = 1$, so that parameters a_{sy}, d_{sy}, c_{sy}, e_{sy} will alone determine the extent of shared genetic and environmental components of the two traits.

If an intermediate latent variable is introduced between the shared factors and the observed variables X and Y, then the resulting model is said to have a 'common pathway'. In this model, the path coefficient from A_s to X is constrained to be equal to the product of the path coefficient from A_s, to the intermediate variable and the path coefficient from the intermediate variable to

X. Denoting the intermediate variable by Z, the model can be rewritten as

$$\left.\begin{aligned} X &= z_{xz}Z + a_xA_x + d_xD_x + c_xC_x + e_xE_x \\ Y &= z_{yz}Z + a_yA_y + d_yD_y + c_yC_y + e_yE_y \\ Z &= a_{zs}A_s + d_{zs}D_s + c_{zs}C_s + e_{zs}E_s \end{aligned}\right\} \tag{5.127}$$

As usual, some of the components (dominances or common environment, or both) must be omitted in order to ensure that the model is identified.

Another submodel of the general independent pathways model is the so-called 'reciprocal causation model' Here, direct causal paths are specified between the two traits

$$\left.\begin{aligned} X &= b_{xy}Y + a_xA_x + d_xD_x + c_xC_x + e_xE_x \\ Y &= b_{yx}X + a_yA_y + d_yD_y + c_yC_y + e_yE_y \end{aligned}\right\} \tag{5.128}$$

If this model compares favourably with the general independent pathways model, then each of the paths b_{xy} and b_{yx} can be set to 0 in order to assess the evidence for reciprocal causation as against unidirectional causation (Heath *et al.*, 1993).

The standard twin model can be extended to include parents. This allows more elaborate models involving assortative mating, gene–environment correlation and cultural transmission to be identified and tested (Rao *et al.*, 1974, 1976; Rice *et al.*, 1978; Cloninger *et al.*, 1979). An example of such a model for DZ twins (or full siblings) is shown in Figure 5.6

Although the path diagram in Figure 5.6 is highly complex, the general principles of the analysis remain the same. A set of linear equations is used to describe the hypothetical causal relationships, together with a set of hypothetical correlations between the ultimate independent variables (i.e. variables which are not determined by any other variables within the model), and certain constraints on the path coefficients, correlations or variances. The expected covariance matrix is a function of the model parameters (path coefficients, correlations and variances), and can be fitted to an observed covariance matrix by maximum likelihood.

The problem of phenotypic assortative mating is, however, worth mentioning separately. Phenotypic assortative mating refers to the situation where individuals prefer to mate with other individuals who are similar (or dissimilar) in phenotype. This leads to a correlation between the phenotypes of mates which cannot be explained by common causes nor by reciprocal causal interaction. Moreover, classical path analysis does not allow explicit correlations to be specified between dependent variables. In order to resolve this problem, the methods of reverse paths and copaths were introduced. However, a more elegant solution has been suggested by Fulker (1988). Suppose that the expected covariance matrix in the absence of phenotypic assortment is

$$\Sigma = \begin{pmatrix} \Sigma_P & \Sigma_C \\ \Sigma_C^T & \Sigma_O \end{pmatrix} \tag{5.129}$$

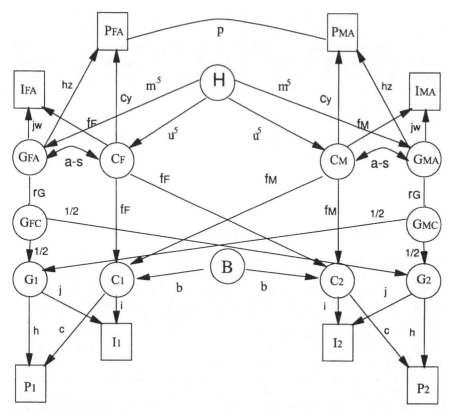

Figure 5.6   Path diagram for nuclear family data.

where Σ_P is the covariance matrix of the parental phenotypes, Σ_O is the covariance matrix of the offspring phenotypes, and Σ_C contains the covariances between parental and offspring phenotypes. In the absence of assortment, the elements in Σ_P for the covariances between the two parents are zero. With assortment, these covariances may become non-zero. In the presence of correlations between the assorted variables (i.e. the parental phenotypes) and the other variables (i.e. the offspring phenotypes), the change in Σ_P will distort the rest of the covariance matrix, according to the formula of Aitken (1934). This formula states that, if the assortment alters the covariance matrix of the parental phenotypes from Σ_P to D, then the overall covariance matrix is distorted to

$$\Sigma_A = \begin{pmatrix} D & D\Sigma_P^{-1}\Sigma_C \\ \Sigma_C^T\Sigma_P^{-1}D & \Sigma_O - \Sigma_C^T(\Sigma_P^{-1} - \Sigma_P^{-1}D\Sigma_P^{-1})\Sigma_C \end{pmatrix} \tag{5.130}$$

Thus, instead of fitting the data to the covariance matrix Σ, which assumes no phenotypic assortment, the data can be fitted to the more general covariance matrix Σ_A, which does allow for phenotypic assortment between mates and its consequences for the covariances between other observed variables. In addition to phenotypic assortment, the Aitken formula may also be used to allow for ascertainment-induced distortion of the covariance matrix. This requires identifying the variables involved in the ascertainment process, and possibly an estimate of the covariance matrix of these variables prior to selection (i.e. in the general population).

Structural equation models can be extended further to relatives of other degrees and to relatives separated by adoption. The latter design is a power-ful alternative to the twin method for the separation of genetic from environmental factors. The reader is referred to Neale and Cardon (1992) for a more detailed exposition of the use of structural equation models in human genetics.

5.6.5   The interpretation of structural equation models

Path analysis and structural equation models have been criticized by some geneticists and statisticians for a number of reasons. One philosophical criticism concerns the interpretation of the results from a structural equation model as causal relationships. Although path analysis is designed to isolate a causal relation when experimental control of potential confounding factors is not possible, the interpretation of the results as a true causal system is only justified if all possible confounding factors are included and modelled correctly. This is, of course, seldom possible. It is often the case that several alternative models are almost equally consistent with the data. Moreover, the set of models being considered by the investigator is almost never exhaustive. The 'true model' is probably not even identified with the data available. An example of this in the analysis of twin data is the obligatory exclusion of either dominance or common environment, even though it is possible for the 'true model' to contain both dominance and common environment. The casual interpretation of the path coefficients in a model as a set of causal relationships is therefore potentially hazardous.

Other criticisms of structural equation models concern the restrictiveness of some of the assumptions such as linearity, additivity and multivariate normality. New methods are being developed which relax some of these assumptions. Some of these methods are based on higher order moment matrices of the variables (means are first-order moments, variances and covariances are second-order moments). However, it is probably simpler to transform the data to approximate normality whenever possible and, failing this, to polychotomize the data into a number of ordered categories (and assume an underlying normal liability). In either case, the resulting data can be fitted to structural equation models using Mx.

5.7   Complex segregation analysis

Classical segregation analysis is concerned with the detection of Mendelian segregation ratios in sibship data. For complex traits, the segregation ratios are not expected to be Mendelian, even if a locus of major effect is involved, because of the influence of other genetic and environmental factors. The detection of a major locus effect requires a more sophisticated set of statistical methods known as *complex segregation analysis*. The main distinction between classical and complex segregation analysis is that the former is concerned with segregation ratios in specific types of sibships, whereas the latter is based on a population genetic model of the trait involving allele frequencies, penetrances and other parameters.

5.7.1 Commingling

For a quantitative trait, the presence of a locus of major effect may result in a multimodal population frequency distribution. For instance, if the three genotypic means at a biallelic locus are sufficiently separated in relation to the variation within a genotype, then the three genotypic classes may form a trimodal distribution. Moreover, under random mating the proportions of the three component distributions are expected to be in Hardy–Weinberg equilibrium. If the residual phenotypic distributions within the three genotypes can be assumed to be normal with equal variance, then it is possible to attempt to infer the presence of a major locus by 'commingling analysis'. A mixture of three normal distributions, with different means but the same variance, and under Hardy–Weinberg proportions, is fitted to the data. Denoting the allele frequency as q, the genotypic means as m_1, m_2, m_3, and the residual variance as s^2, then the likelihood function for the model, given a single observation with trait value x ascertained at random from the population, is

$$L(q,m_1,m_2,m_3,s^2; x) = q^2 f(x; m_1,s^2) + 2q(1-q)f(x; m_2,s^2)$$
$$+ (1-q)^2 f(x; m_3,s^2) \qquad (5.131)$$

where $f(x; m,s^2)$ is a normal density function with mean m and variance s^2, i.e.

$$f(x; m, s^2) = \frac{1}{\sqrt{2\pi}s} \exp\left(-\frac{(x-m)^2}{2s^2}\right) \qquad (5.132)$$

Given a sample of independent observations, the overall likelihood of this mixture model is simply the product of the likelihoods of the individual observations. The maximum likelihood of this model can be compared with that of the null model, which consists of a single normal distribution, for a test of the major locus effect. Denoting the maximum log-likelihood of the mixture model as $\ln L_1$, and the maximum log-likelihood of the null model as $\ln L_0$, then it may appear that the likelihood ratio statistic, $2(\ln L_1 - \ln L_0)$, is chi-squared with three degrees of freedom, since the mixture model has five parameters (three means, one variance, one allele frequency) and the null model has just two parameters (one mean, one variance). This is unfortunately not the case, because the boundary of the parameter space containing the null model is degenerate. Thus, when the allele frequency is 0 or 1, the three genotypic means become redundant; and conversely when the three genotypic means are equal, the allele frequency is irrelevant. It is therefore necessary to estimate the statistical significance of the likelihood ratio statistic by simulation.

The power of this test based on commingling analysis is limited, especially when the allele frequency is near 0 or 1, and when the separations between the genotypic means are small relative to the residual variance. Moreover, the test is sensitive to violations of the normality assumption, so that skewness and kurtosis may give rise to the erroneous inference of a major locus effect. The specificity of the test depends also on the detection of Hardy–Weinberg ratios, as mixtures of distributions may arise from the inward migration of a population with a different mean, or the presence of a major environmental factor in a subset of the population.

5.7.2   The mixed model

Commingling analysis does not, strictly speaking, constitute a segregation analysis, which must consider genetic transmission from parent to offspring, as well as population frequency distributions. The assumptions of normality and equal residual variance of commingling analysis are also made in the complex segregation analysis of quantitative traits. In addition, alternative models of parent–offspring transmission must be considered, in order to test the hypothesis of a major locus effect.

The most 'natural' alternative to major locus transmission is perhaps polygenic inheritance. Under a polygenic model, each individual's phenotype is determined additively by a polygenic value and an environmental residual (which may consist of familial and non-familial components). In the population, the polygenic value is assumed to be normally distributed with variance V. The polygenic value of an offspring is determined additively by contributions from the two parents. Under random mating, the contribution from a parent with polygenic value G is normally distributed with mean $G/2$ and variance $V/4$. The distribution of the polygenic component in an off-spring with parental polygenic values G_f and G_m (the subscripts f and m referring to father and mother) is therefore normal with mean $(G_f + G_m)/2$ and variance $V/2$. In the population of offspring, the variance of the polygenic component is thus $[V(G_f) + V(G_m)]/4 + V/2 = V/2 + V/2 = V$. The population variance of the polygenic component is therefore maintained at a constant level (i.e. V) from generation to generation. Half of this variance is due to variations in parental polygenic values, and the other half is due to Mendelian segregation.

The so-called *mixed model* contains both a major locus and a polygenic component. With the overall mean being fixed, the major locus component has three parameters: one allele frequency (q) and two free genotypic means (since the three genotypic means m_1, m_2, m_3 are constrained by the overall mean) while the polygenic component has just one parameter: the polygenic variance (V). A *polygenic model* can be regarded as a submodel of the mixed model without the major locus component. Similarly, a *single locus model* can be regarded as a submodel of the mixed model without the polygenic component. If the maximum log-likelihood of the mixed model is denoted as $\ln L_1$, and the maximum log-likelihood of the polygenic model is denoted as $\ln L_0$, then a likelihood ratio test for the presence of a major locus is provided by the statistic $2(\ln L_1 - \ln L_0)$. This statistic may appear to be chi-squared with three degrees of freedom, but unfortunately this is not so because the null hypothesis can be specified by either $q = 0$ or $q = 1$, in which case the genotypic means are redundant, or by $m_1 = m_2 = m_3$, in which case the allele frequency is redundant.

In addition to having a non-standard distribution for the likelihood ratio statistic, the mixed model also has a likelihood function involving a multi-variate normal integral that can be extremely laborious to compute and maximize, particularly for multigenerational pedigrees. The Elston–Stewart algorithm for evaluating pedigree likelihoods is not easily applicable, as each individual can take an infinite number of unknown polygenic values. One possible solution is to restrict the unit of analysis to nuclear families; any multi-generational pedigree can be broken down into its constituent nuclear families which are then considered as independent observations. The likelihood calculation can be simplified further by considering the mean of the two parental polygenic values (the 'midparental breeding value') instead of the two parental polygenic values separately. This is the approach adopted by Morton and MacLean (1974) and by Lalouel and Morton (1981), and implemented in the POINTER program.

An alternative solution to the computational problem for the mixed model is to use an approximation to the likelihood that avoids multiple integration. Hasstedt (1982, 1991, 1993) suggested approximating an N-variate normal integral by the product of N univariate normal integrals, by repeated uses of the Pearson–Aitken formula (Pearson, 1903b; Aitken, 1934). This algorithm for approximating the likelihood of a mixed model has been implemented in the PAP program.

5.7.3 The general transmission model

The computational problems of the mixed model have led to an alternative approach for testing the hypothesis of the major locus effect, one that does not incorporate a polygenic component. The idea is to construct a general model of parent–offspring transmission which includes Mendelian segregation as a submodel (Elston and Stewart, 1971). Under Mendelian segregation, the conditional probability of transmitting allele A_1, given the parental genotypes A_1A_1, A_1A_2 and A_2A_2 are 1, 1/2 and 0, respectively. A general model of transmission can be obtained by treating these conditional probabilities not as fixed values, but as free *transmission parameters*. The biological rationale for introducing free transmission parameters is that familial factors other than a major locus are not expected to follow Mendelian segregation. If the maximum log-likelihood over transmission and the other model parameters is denoted as $\ln L_1$, and the maximum log-likelihood over the other model parameters only (with the transmission parameters fixed at the Mendelian values of 1, 1/2, 0) is denoted as $\ln L_0$, then the likelihood ratio statistic $2(\ln L_1 - \ln L_0)$ has asymptotically a chi-squared distribution with three degrees of freedom, and provides a test for Mendelian transmission. An advantage of this *transmission test* is that the likelihood calculations can be performed using the Elston–Stewart algorithm.

5.7.4 The unified model

The mixed model and the general transmission model have been combined into the so-called unified model. This model has been implemented in the

POINTER program (Lalouel *et al.*, 1983). The most general model contains a polygenic component as well as a major locus with free transmission parameters. Various restrictions can be imposed on this general model, in order to evaluate the decrease in log-likelihood, and hence the adequacy of the restricted model in relation to the full model. It is customary to fit a series of models, and to compare them using likelihood ratio chi-squared tests (for nested models) or the Akaike information criterion (minus twice the maximum log-likelihood plus twice the number of free parameters).

The generalized transmission, mixed and unified models for quantitative traits can also be applied to diseases (or other dichotomous or polychotomous traits). For the transmission test, this can be achieved simply by introducing penetrances (i.e. the conditional probabilities of affection given the different possible genotypes) to replace genotypic means. For the mixed model, it is necessary to postulate a liability-threshold model. The underlying liability is modelled in exactly the same way as an observed quantitative trait. The liability is above threshold for individuals with the disease, and below threshold for individuals without the disease.

5.7.5   Regressive models

The unified model suffers from the same computational difficulties as the mixed model. The difficulty arises from pedigree members having latent polygenic values which are assumed to be multivariate normal with a particular correlational structure implied by additive Mendelian inheritance. Any particular set of phenotypic values is consistent with an infinite number of sets of latent polygenic values, so that the evaluation of the likelihood of the pedigree requires the numerical integration of multivariate normal distributions.

Bonney (1984) argued that the role of the polygenic component is merely to provide a background of residual correlations between relatives against which the presence of a major locus can be tested. Instead of introducing an explicit polygenic component, he suggested that such background correlations could be modelled more simply by introducing an autogressive model structure. The basic requirement of this regressive approach is that the pedigree members are considered in some order, so that the probability distribution of the phenotype of a relative (conditional on the major genotype) can be modelled as a linear function of the phenotypic values of the preceding relatives. The likelihood can be calculated using the Elston–Stewart algorithm, with the penetrance parameters being modified successively to take account of the phenotypic values of the preceding relatives.

The simplest (Class A) regressive model specifies that, excluding major locus effects, sibling resemblance is due entirely to the regression of offspring phenotype on parental phenotypes. In other words, the siblings are conditionally independent, given the parental phenotypes (plus their own major genotypes). This specification results in equal parent–offspring and sib–sib correlations. The correlational structure of Class A models is therefore identical to that predicted by a polygenic component.

A more general (Class D) model regresses the phenotype of each offspring on the phenotypes of the older siblings, as well as the phenotypes of the parents. This specification has the effect that sib–sib correlations are greater than parent–offspring correlations. This type of correlational structure can arise from dominance or shared sibling environment.

The idea of introducing an autoregressive model to allow for residual familial resemblance has been generalized to dichotomous and polychotomous traits (Bonney, 1986; Bonney *et al.*, 1989). In these so-called regressive logistic models, the probability of affection (i.e. the penetrance) is related to a linear predictor by a logistic link function, where the linear predictor is modelled in the same way as a continuous phenotype (i.e. with major locus and autoregressive components).

The relationship between the regressive model and the mixed model has been discussed by Bonney (1992). Both models are currently used by genetic epidemiologists. The various forms of the regressive model have been implemented in the SAGE program package.

5.7.6   Covariates

The traditional mixed model and the newer regressive model differ in the treatment of covariates such as age, sex and other personal characteristics. In POINTER, the effects of covariates on the phenotype must be specified prior to the analysis. In the case of a quantitative phenotype, a regression analysis may be performed in order to obtain residuals which are independent of the covariates. These residuals may then be subjected to an analysis by POINTER for evidence of a major locus. For dichotomous traits (such as diseases), covariates are used to define liability classes, each of which is assigned an overall risk. These class-specific risks are used by POINTER to calculate class-specific thresholds (in the framework of a liability-threshold model), which are used in the likelihood calculations.

In regressive models, covariates can be included as part of the linear combination (in addition to the major genotype and the autoregressive term) which determines phenotype. This gives the option of estimating the effect of covariates together with, rather than before, the genetic effects.

5.7.7   Ascertainment

The selection of families for complex segregation analysis is usually phenotype-dependent. Ensuring that all families will have at least one member with an extreme phenotype (an affected individual in the case of a disease) can be achieved by the proband method of ascertainment, as described in Chapter 2. However, for complex segregation analysis, it is usual to extend the family beyond the spouse and first degree relatives of the proband, in order to obtain multigenerational pedigrees that are potentially more informative in revealing major gene action. The phenotypic data collected reflect, to some extent, the rules that govern ascertainment, as well as the underlying genetic mechanisms. For this reason, some adjustment for ascertainment is necessary in complex segregation analysis.

It turns out that ascertainment correction is far more difficult for pedigree than for sibship data. Two broad approaches have been adopted. In the more traditional approach (Cannings and Thompson, 1977; Elston and Sobel, 1979; Lalouel and Morton, 1981), an explicit model of the ascertainment mechanism is built into the analysis, and the parameters of this model may be specified prior to the analysis, or estimated jointly with the genetic parameters in the analysis. The most popular model is that the probands constitute a simple random sample of affected individuals in the population. The parameter of this model is the ascertainment probability, which is assumed to be the same for all affected individuals in the population. The alternative approach (Ewens and Shute, 1986) does not require an ascertainment model to be explicitly formulated. It involves conditioning the likelihood of the pedigrees on the part of the data relevant to ascertainment.

When the ascertainment mechanism is fairly well characterized the traditional approach is potentially more powerful than the model-free method. It is often convenient to estimate the ascertainment parameters from the data on proband status within the sample, prior to the segregation analysis. In practice, this procedure does not appear to result in much loss in information, relative to the more exact and computationally demanding procedure of jointly estimating ascertainment and genetic parameters.

The robust model-free method is applicable to situations where the ascertainment mechanism is ill-defined. It is perhaps most useful in the situation where family members have been added to an existing pedigree sample, so that the conditioning involves simply dividing the likelihood of the entire data set by the likelihood of the original data.

Vieland and Hodge (1995) have pointed out that both these approaches to ascertainment correction make the implicit assumption that the pedigree structure is independent of phenotypic information (except in the case of single ascertainment when this assumption can be relaxed). Otherwise it would be necessary to condition on the pedigree structure itself, against other possible pedigree structures (which are unobserved). Vieland and Hodge therefore concluded that the problem of ascertainment correction in pedigree data is inherently intractable. They suggested that further work is necessary to develop approximate methods of ascertainment correction. It is interesting that the POINTER program (which implements the unified model) already uses an approximate ascertainment correction which involves breaking up pedigrees into nuclear families, each containing a proband or a 'pointer' (defined as an affected pedigree member outside the nuclear family who led to the ascertainment of the family).

Ascertainment therefore remains an unresolved problem in segregation analysis. If the trait is very common or quantitative, then it may be feasible to sample families without regard to phenotype, in which case the ascertainment problem is irrelevant. Otherwise the investigator might design an ascertainment procedure that approximates single ascertainment, or apply an approximation such as that used in POINTER.

5.7.8   Violation of model assumptions

Violations of model assumptions in complex segregation analysis may lead to erroneous evidence of a major locus when it is absent, or to the erroneous rejection of a major locus when it is present. For instance, the presence of skewness and kurtosis may be misinterpreted as evidence for a major locus (MacLean *et al.*, 1975). It may be possible to remove skewness and kurtosis by transforming the phenotype prior to segregation analysis, but this runs the risk of reducing the evidence for a major locus when the skewness and kurtosis have actually resulted from the effect of a major locus rather than a violation of the normality assumption. The ideal solution may be to build the transformation into the model itself, so that transformation and genetic parameters can be estimated and tested jointly. However, this has been implemented only in the simple case of commingling analysis (MacLean *et al.*, 1976).

Another crucial set of assumptions in complex segregation analysis regards ascertainment. It is easy to see that misspecification of the ascertainment model may lead to erroneous conclusions. As an extreme example, suppose that the ascertainment of a family requires an affected parent–child pair. If the usual assumption of multiple independent ascertainment is adopted for data collected in this fashion, then one might well obtain erroneous evidence for a dominant model of inheritance.

There may also be methodological artefacts or biological phenomena that are not built into the segregation model, and which may lead to erroneous conclusions. For instance, a cohort effect with a greater risk of illness in younger than in older generations may appear as a greater recurrence risk among siblings than among parents, and this may be interpreted as evidence for a recessive gene (although most current segregation analysis programs do allow sib–sib correlation to differ from parent–child correlation). Other thorny problems include assortative mating and differential fertility, which are not usually accommodated into the analysis. Such complicating factors can have unpredictable and potentially undesirable effects on the analysis.

5.7.9 Statistical power

Complex segregation analysis has very disappointing power for the detection of major loci in dichotomous traits. Edwards (1960) has shown how the predictions of the polygenic model on the familial patterns of illness can be very similar to those of single locus models. The power of segregation analysis for complex disorders is so poor that, if one obtains highly significant evidence for a major locus, then one should search very carefully for any violation of model assumptions that might have led to such a result.

For quantitative and polychotomous traits segregation analysis is potentially more powerful. As a rough rule, the minimum effect size (measured in terms of the ratio of the displacement between the two homozygous genotypic means to the standard deviation of the residual variation), to give a realistic chance of detection, is about 1 for an additive locus with allele frequencies 0.1 and 0.9 (MacLean *et al.*, 1975).

5.8 Quantitative trait loci (QTL) linkage analysis

Recent advances in molecular genetics have made feasible attempts to localize and identify the individual loci that make up the genetic component of a quantitative trait. The loci are called *quantitative trait loci* (QTL), to distinguish them from rare mutations which have a major effect on the risk of disease. Current methods of QTL linkage analysis are derived from the integration of quantitative genetic methods concerning correlation between relatives and non-parametric linkage methods based on allele-sharing. It is possible that, in future, QTL linkage analysis will also incorporate variations of parametric methods of linkage analysis. The LINKAGE program can deal with a quantitative phenotype that is assumed to be multivariate normal but it requires the mean vectors and the covariance matrices of the phenotype, for the three genotypes at the trait locus, to be fully specified prior to the analysis. In addition, LINKAGE makes no allowance for residual familial correlations. For these reasons, the LINKAGE program is seldom used in QTL linkage analysis. Instead, researchers are currently using methods that attempt to correlate phenotypic similarity and local genetic similarity of pairs of relatives.

5.8.1 Genetic identity-by-descent (IBD)

The concept of genetic identity-by-descent has been described in Chapter 3. At every position of the genome, a pair of relatives may share 0, 1 or 2 alleles IBD. The proportion of alleles IBD at a locus is conventionally denoted as π. As shown in Chapter 3, the proportions of alleles IBD at two loci separated by recombination fraction θ have a correlation coefficient of $2\Psi - 1$, where $\Psi = \theta^2 + (1 - \theta)^2$.

Nearly all current methods measure the genetic similarity between two relatives at a given chromosomal location by π, the proportion of alleles identical-by-descent at that chromosomal location. Information about π at a particular location can be obtained from the genotypes of polymorphic genetic markers at or around that location. When information is complete at a given location, it will be known whether the pair of relatives share 0, 1 or 2 alleles IBD at that location, so that the estimate of π is either 0, 0.5 or 1. Incomplete information can be summarized by the conditional probabilities of sharing 0, 1 or 2 alleles IBD, given the marker genotype data. These conditional probabilities are conventionally denoted as π_0, π_1 and π_2. The expected proportion of alleles IBD is then $\hat{\pi} = \pi_1/2 + \pi_2$.

Several methods have been proposed for calculating π_0, π_1 and π_2 from marker genotype data. The most general of these that are applicable to general pedigrees and to multipoint data are based on the Elston–Stewart algorithm (Curtis and Sham, 1994) or the Lander–Green algorithm (Kruglyak and Lander, 1995b; Kruglyak *et al.*, 1996). The latter algorithm is particularly efficient for the small pedigrees usually collected for QTL linkage analysis. As a result of the application of this algorithm, it is possible to obtain a series of values of π_0, π_1 and π_2 for a series of chromosomal locations, for every pair of relatives in the sample. If the marker genotype data for a relative pair are nearly complete at a certain location, then one of π_0, π_1 and π_2 should be close to 1, and the other two close to 0.

5.8.2 The Haseman–Elston regression method

The earliest method of relating the values of π_0, π_1 and π_2 at a chromosomal location to the values of a quantitative phenotype in a sample of sib-pairs was suggested by Haseman and Elston (1972). Let the quantitative trait values of a sib-pair be X_1 and X_2. Haseman and Elston's method is to regress $(X_1 - X_2)^2$ onto the expected proportion of alleles IBD, $\hat{\pi} = \pi_1/2 + \pi_2$, at the locus. A regression coefficient significantly less than 0 is considered as evidence for linkage.

It is intuitively easy to see why the regression coefficient of $(X_1 - X_2)^2$ on $\hat{\pi}$ should be 0 when the QTL and the marker locus are unlinked, but negative when they are linked. The theoretical expectation of the regression coefficient of $(X_1 - X_2)^2$ on $\hat{\pi}$ can be derived by first expanding $(X_1 - X_2)^2$ and considering its conditional expectation given π_1 and π_2 ($\hat{\pi}$ being $\pi_1/2 + \pi_2$)

$$
\begin{aligned}
E[(X_1 - X_2)^2 \mid \pi_1, \pi_2] &= E[(X_1^2 + X_2^2 - 2X_1 X_2) \mid \pi_1, \pi_2] \\
&= \mathrm{Var}(X_1) + \mathrm{Var}(X_2) - 2\mathrm{Cov}(X_1, X_2 \mid \pi_1, \pi_2)
\end{aligned}
\tag{5.133}
$$

Assuming that the variance of the trait is made up of the orthogonal components V_{QA} (additive variance due to QTL), V_{QD} (dominance variance due to QTL), V_{RA} (residual additive genetic variance), V_{RD} (residual dominance variance), V_C (shared family environment) and V_E (unique environment), then the variances of X_1 and X_2, which are independent of π_1 and π_2, are given by

$$
\mathrm{Var}(X_1) = \mathrm{Var}(X_2) = V_{QA} + V_{QD} + V_{RA} + V_{RD} + V_C + V_E
\tag{5.134}
$$

The covariance between X_1 and X_2 due to the QTL is, however, dependent on π_1 and π_2. When the recombination fraction between the QTL and the marker locus is 0, the covariance due to the QTL additive variance is $\pi_1 V_{QA}/2 + \pi_2 V_{QA}$ (i.e. $\hat{\pi} V_{QA}$), and the covariance due to the QTL dominance variance is $\pi_2 V_{QD}$. The overall covariance between X_1 and X_2 is therefore

$$
\mathrm{Cov}(X_1, X_2 \mid \pi_1, \pi_2) = \hat{\pi} V_{QA} + \pi_2 V_{QD} + r_A V_{RA} + p_2 V_{RD} + V_C
\tag{5.135}
$$

where r_A is the coefficient of the relationship between the two relatives, and p_2 is the probability that the two relatives share two alleles IBD, without considering the marker genotype data (see Section 5.3.2). For sib-pairs, $r_A = 1/2$ and $p_2 = 1/4$, so that

$$
\mathrm{Cov}(X_1, X_2 \mid \pi_1, \pi_2) = \hat{\pi} V_{QA} + \pi_2 V_{QD} + (1/2)V_{RA} + (1/4)V_{RD} + V_C
\tag{5.136}
$$

The conditional expectation of $(X_1 - X_2)^2$ given π_1 and π_2, when the QTL and the marker locus are extremely tightly linked ($\theta = 0$), is therefore

$$
\begin{aligned}
E[(X_1 &- X_2)^2 \mid \pi_1, \pi_2] \\
&= 2(V_{QA} + V_{QD} + V_{RA} + V_{RD} + V_C + V_E) \\
&\quad - 2(\hat{\pi} V_{QA} + \pi_2 V_{QD} + V_{RA}/2 + V_{RD}/4 + V_C) \\
&= 2V_E + V_{RA} + 3V_{RD}/2 + 2V_{QA} + 2V_{QD} - 2V_{QA}\hat{\pi} - 2V_{QD}\pi_2
\end{aligned}
\tag{5.137}
$$

It is usual to assume an additive model, so that V_{QD} and V_{RD} are both 0. In this case, the regression coefficient of $(X_1 - X_2)^2$ on π is simply $-2V_{QA}$. Moreover, when the recombination fraction (θ) between the QTL and the marker is not 0, the regression coefficient is simply $-2V_{QA}(2\Psi - 1)$, where $\Psi = \theta^2 + (1 - \theta)^2$, and $(2\Psi - 1)$ is the correlation between the proportion of alleles IBD at the QTL and the proportion of alleles IBD at the marker locus.

In summary, the Haseman–Elston method regresses $(X_1 - X_2)^2$ on $\hat{\pi}$ and tests whether the regression coefficient is less than 0. The regression coefficient is an estimate of $-2V_{QA}(2\Psi - 1)$.

5.8.3 Likelihood methods

Despite its simplicity, the regression of $(X_1 - X_2)^2$ on $\hat{\pi}$ suffers from problems of non-normality and heteroscedasticity, which may reduce statistical power under the alternative hypothesis (Amos *et al.*, 1989). Kruglyak and Lander (1995b) suggested that the presence of a QTL can be tested more adequately by considering the likelihood of the the sib-pair difference $(X_1 - X_2)$. For a normally distributed quantitative trait, this difference is normal with mean 0 and variance

$$\text{Var}(X_1 - X_2) = \text{Var}(X_1) + \text{Var}(X_2) + 2\text{Cov}(X_1, X_2) \qquad (5.138)$$

Let the number of alleles IBD between a sib-pair at the QTL be i, then the conditional variance of $(X_1 - X_2)$ given i is, assuming that the QTL is additive

$$\text{Var}[(X_1 - X_2)|i] = 2(V_{QA} + V_{RA} + V_C + V_E) + 2(iV_{QA}/2 + V_{RA}/2 + V_C) \quad (5.139)$$

Let the conditional variances of $(X_1 - X_2)$ given $i = 0,1,2$ be V_0, V_1 and V_2, then the above result implies the constraint $V_0 + V_2 = 2V_1$. The likelihood for a sib-pair is

$$L(V_0, V_1, V_2) = \sum_{i=0}^{2} \pi_i f[(X_1 - X_2)|V_i] \qquad (5.140)$$

where $f[(X_1 - X_2)|V_i]$ is the normal density function with mean 0 and variance V_i. The overall likelihood for a sample of independent sib-pairs is simply the product of these likelihoods. If the maximum log-likelihood subject to the constraint $V_0 + V_2 = 2V_1$ is denoted as $\ln L_1$, and the maximum log-likelihood subject to the constraint $V_0 = V_1 = V_2$ is denoted as $\ln L_0$, then the likelihood ratio statistic $2(\ln L_1 - \ln L_0)$ has a chi-squared distribution with one degree of freedom, and provides a test for the presence of an additive QTL.

Instead of using the likelihood of the sib-pair difference $(X_1 - X_2)$, Fulker and Cherny (1997) suggested that a more powerful test can be obtained by considering the likelihood of (X_1, X_2) as a bivariate observation. The distribution of (X_1, X_2) is assumed to be bivariate normal, and under an additive model, has variances

$$\text{Var}(X_1) = \text{Var}(X_2) = V_{QA} + V_{RA} + V_C + V_E \qquad (5.141)$$

and covariance

$$\text{Cov}(X_1, X_2 | i) = (i/2)V_{QA} + V_{RA}/2 + V_C \qquad (5.142)$$

where i denotes the number of alleles IBD for the sib-pair. With sib-pair data, it is not possible to estimate the parameters V_{RA}, V_C and V_E. Instead, these components need to be repartitioned into a shared component $V_S = V_{RA}/2 + V_C$, and a non-shared component $V_N = V_{RA}/2 + V_E$. The covariance matrix of (X_1, X_2) is therefore written as

$$\Sigma_i = \begin{bmatrix} V_{QA} + V_S + V_N & (i/2)V_{QA} + V_S \\ (i/2)V_{QA} + V_S & V_{QA} + V_S + V_N \end{bmatrix} \qquad (5.143)$$

for $i = 0, 1, 2$. The likelihood of a sib-pair is then

$$L(V_{QA}, V_S, V_N) = \sum_{i=0}^{2} \pi_i f_2 [(X_1, X_2) | \mu, \Sigma_i] \tag{5.144}$$

where $f_2[(X_1, X_2) | \mu, \Sigma_i]$ is the bivariate normal density function with mean vector μ and covariance matrix Σ_i. The elements of μ may be assumed to be constant, but may also be modelled to take account of covariates. In any case, the overall likelihood of a sample of independent sib-pairs is simply the product of the these likelihoods. If the maximum log-likelihood of the model is denoted as $\ln L_1$, and the maximum log-likelihood of the model with the restriction $V_{QA} = 0$ is denoted as $\ln L_0$, then the likelihood ratio test $2(\ln L - \ln L_0)$ is distributed as a 50:50 mixture of 0 and a chi-squared random variable with one degree of freedom (because the null hypothesis $V_{QA} = 0$ lies on a boundary of the parameter space). Fulker and Cherny (1997) showed that a test based on this statistic has greater power to detect a QTL than the test based on sib-pair differences.

Fulker and Cherny also showed that, under usual circumstances, very little information is lost by conditioning the covariance matrix on the expected proportion of alleles IBD, $\hat{\pi}$ instead of on the distribution of the number of alleles IBD. The likelihood function of a sib-pair is then

$$L(V_{QA}, V_s, V_N) = f_2[(X_1, X_2) | \mu, \Sigma_{\hat{\pi}}] \tag{5.145}$$

where the covariance matrix conditional on $\hat{\pi}$ is

$$\Sigma_{\hat{\pi}} = \begin{bmatrix} V_{QA} + V_S + V_N & \hat{\pi} V_{QA} + V_S \\ \hat{\pi} V_{QA} + V_S & V_{QA} + V_S + V_N \end{bmatrix} \tag{5.146}$$

This variance components approach has the advantage of being easily extended to more complex situations involving multivariate phenotypic traits, larger families, and multiple QTLs (Goldgar, 1990; Schork, 1993; Amos, 1994). Adding phenotypic traits and family members increases the dimension of the covariance matrix, while adding QTLs increases the number of terms in the variances and covariances.

5.8.4 QTL linkage analysis using selected sib-pairs

The informativeness of a sib-pair for QTL analysis depends on the trait values (X_1, X_2) of the pair. Since the test for a QTL is based primarily on deviations of $\hat{\pi}$ from its expectation under the null hypothesis (i.e. $1/2$), a reasonable measure of the informativeness of a sib-pair is the difference between the conditional expectation of $\hat{\pi}$ given the trait values (X_1, X_2) in the presence of a QTL, and the null hypothesis value of $1/2$. The conditional expectation of $\hat{\pi}$ given (X_1, X_2) is

$$E(\hat{\pi} | X_1, X_2) = \sum_{i=0}^{2} \frac{i}{2} p(i | X_1, X_2) \tag{5.147}$$

where $i = 0, 1, 2$ is the number of alleles IBD. The conditional probability of i

given (X_1, X_2) under an addictive model is given by Bayes theorem as

$$P(i \mid X_1, X_2) = \frac{P(i) f_2(X_1, X_2 \mid i)}{\sum_{j=0}^{2} P(j) f_2(X_1, X_2 \mid j)} \tag{5.148}$$

where $P(i)$, the prior probability of i, is 0.25, 0.5 and 0.25 for values of i of 0, 1 and 2, and $f_2(X_1 X_2 \mid i)$ is the bivariate normal density function with zero mean and covariance matrix

$$\Sigma_i = \begin{bmatrix} V_{QA} + V_S + V_N & (i/2)V_{QA} + V_S \\ (i/2)V_{QA} + V_S & V_{QA} + V_S + V_N \end{bmatrix} \tag{5.149}$$

This makes the simlifying assumption that the QTL effect is normally distributed. These formulae allow the conditional expectation of $\hat{\pi}$ given (X_1, X_2), under any particular set of hypothetical values of V_{QA}, V_S and V_N, to be calculated. If these conditional expectations are calculated for each pair of siblings in a sample, then those pairs where the expected $\hat{\pi}$ deviate the most from $1/2$ can be selected for genotyping.

Risch and Zhang (1995, 1996) have derived the conditional expectation for a biallelic QTL. This involves partitioning the conditional IBD distribution further to take account of all possible combinations of QTL genotypes of the sib-pair. They concluded that extreme discordant sib-pairs (i.e. sib-pairs where one member occupies one phenotypic extreme and the other occupies the other phenotypic extreme) are informative for the detection of a QTL regardless of allele frequency and dominance. On the other hand, among extreme concordant sib-pairs (i.e. sib-pairs where both members occupy the same phenotypic extreme), only those at the extreme with an excess of the rarer allele are informative. Since prior information on allele frequencies is seldom available, the safest strategy is to select concordant pairs at both extremes, as well as discordant pairs, for genotyping. The proportion of linkage information in a sample that can be retained by selecting the most informative 10% or 20% of the sample depends on the underlying genetic model, but in some cases can approach 80% or 90% (Eaves and Meyer, 1994). Even so, the detection of a QTL by linkage analysis is probably only feasible if the proportion of total phenotypic variance explained by the QTL is at least about 10%.

The analysis of selected samples is straightforward if a likelihood approach is used, provided that a fairly accurate estimate of the overall phenotypic covariance matrix is available or can be obtained from the complete phenotypic data prior to selection. Since selection is through phenotypic data only, it is sufficient to constrain the variance component parameters to be consistent with the estimated variances and covariances in the population.

5.9   Conclusions

Continuous and quasi-continuous traits present a greater degree of difficulty than simple Mendelian characters for genetic analysis. This is especially true for humans because experimental crosses are unethical. Nevertheless, by studying twins and other familial material, it is possible to discriminate genetic from environmental sources of variation. The methodology has evolved from analysis of variance, to linear regression and structural equation models, enabling more complex causal models involving multiple variables to be tested. Complex segregation analysis attempts to identify a major locus within the genetic component, by an amalgamation of quanitative genetic and classical Mendelian methods, but is handicapped by the problems of ascertainment, sensitivity to violation of model assumptions, and limited statistical power. With the availability of marker genotype information, however, the identifi- cation of the loci that contribute to the genetic component of quantitative traits is becoming increasingly feasible.

References

Aitken A C (1934): Note on selection from a multivariate normal population. *Proceedings of the Edinburgh Mathematical Society B*, **4**, 106–10.

Amos C I (1994): Robust variance-components approach for assessing genetic linkage in pedigrees. *American Journal of Human Genetics*, **54**, 535–43.

Amos C I and Williamson J A (1993): Robustness of the maximum-likelihood (LOD) method for detecting linkage. *American Journal of Human Genetics*, **52**, 213–14.

Amos C I, Elston R C, Wilson A F and Bailey-Wilson J E (1989): A more powerful robust sib-pair test of linkage for quantitative traits. *Genetic Epidemiology*, **6**, 435–49.

Bailey N T J (1951a): The estimation of the frequencies of recessives with incomplete multiple selection. *Annals of Eugenics*, **16**, 215–22.

Bailey N T J (1951b): A classification of methods of ascertainment and analysis in estimating the frequencies of recessives in man. *Annals of Eugenics*, **16**, 223–25.

Bateson W (1901): Introductory note to experiments in plant hybridization by Gregor Mendel. *Journal of the Royal Horticultural Society*, **26**, 1–32.

Bentler P (1986): Structural equation modelling and Psychometrika: an historical perspective on growth and achievements. *Psychometrika*, **51**, 35–51.

Bernstein F (1925): Zusammenfassende Betrachtungen uber die erblichen Blutstrukturen des Menschen, **37**, 237–69.

Blackwelder W C and Elston R C (1985): A comparison of sib-pair linkage tests for disease susceptibility loci. *Genetic Epidemiology*, **2**, 85–97.

Bodmer W F (1986): Human genetics: the molecular challenge. *Cold Spring Harbour Symposium of Quantitative Biology*, **51**, 1–13.

Bollen K A (1989): *Structural Equations with Latent Variables*. New York: Wiley.

Bonney G E (1984): On the statistical determination of major gene mechanisms in continuous human traits: regressive models. *American Journal of Medical Genetics*, **18**, 731–49.

Bonney G E (1986): Regressive logistic models for familial disease and other binary traits. *Biometrics*, **42**, 611–25.

Bonney G E (1992): Compound regressive models for family data. *Human Heredity*, **42**, 28–41.

Bonney G E, Dunston, C-M and Wilson J (1989): Regressive logistic models for ordered and unordered polychotomous traits: application to affective disorders. *Genetic Epidemiology*, **6**, 211–15.

Botstein D, White R L, Skolnick M H and Davies R W (1980): Construction of a genetic linkage map in man using restriction fragment length polymorphisms. *American Journal of Human Genetics*, **32**, 314–31.

Cannings C and Thompson E A (1977): Ascertainment in the sequential sampling of pedigree. *Clinical Genetics*, **12**, 108–211.

Cannings C, Thompson E A and Skolnick M H (1978): Probability functions on complex pedigrees. *Advances in Applied Probability*, **10**, 26–61.

Carter C O (1969): Genetics of common disorders. *British Medical Bulletin*, **25**, 52–57.

Chiano M N and Yates J R W (1995): Linkage detection under heterogeneity and the mixture problem. *Annals of Human Genetics*, **59**, 83–95.

Chotai J (1984): On the lod score method in linkage analysis. *Annals of Human Genetics*, **48**, 359–78.

Clerget-Darpoux F, Bonaiti-Pellie C and Hochez J (1986): Effects of misspecifying genetic parameters in lod score analysis. *Biometrics*, **42**, 393–99.

Cloninger C R, Rice J and Reich T (1979): Multifactorial inheritance with cultural transmission and assortative mating. II. A general model of combined polygenic and cultural inheritance. *American Journal of Human Genetics*, **31**, 176–98.

Collins A and Morton N E (1991): Significance of maximum lods. *Annals of Human Genetics*, **55**, 39–41.

Cottingham Jr R W, Idury R M and Schaffer A A (1993): Faster sequential genetic linkage computations. *American Journal of Human Genetics*, **53**, 252–63.

Crittenden L B (1961): An interpretation of familial aggregation based on multiple genetic and environmental factors. *Annals of the New York Academy of Sciences*, **91**, 739–80.

Crow J F and Kimura M (1971): *An Introduction to Population Genetics Theory*. New York: Harper & Row.

Curnow R N and Smith C (1975): Multifactorial models for familial diseases in man. *Journal of the Royal Statistical Society*, **137**, 131–69.

Curtis D (1994): Another procedure for the preliminary ordering of loci on two-point lod scores. *Annals of Human Genetics*, **58**, 65–75.

Curtis D and Gurling H (1993): A procedure for combining two-point scores into a summary multipoint map. *Human Heredity*, **43**, 173–85.

Curtis D and Sham P C (1994): Using risk calculation to implement an extended relative pair analysis. *Annals of Human Genetics*, **58**, 151–62.

Curtis D and Sham P C (1995): Model-free linkage analysis using likelihoods. *American Journal of Human Genetics*, **57**, 703–16.

Davie A M (1979): The singles method for segregation analysis under incomplete ascertainment. *Annals of Human Genetics*, **41**, 507–12.

Davies S, Schroeder M, Goldin L R and Weeks D E (1996): Nonparametric simulation-based statistics for detecting linkage in general pedigrees. *American Journal of Human Genetics*, **58**, 867–80.

De la Chapelle A (1993): Disease gene mapping in isolated human populations: the example of Finland. *Journal of Medical Genetics*, **30**, 857–65.

DeFries J C and Fulker D W (1985): Multiple regression analysis of twin data. *Behavior Genetics*, **15**, 467–73.

Devlin B, Risch N and Roeder S (1996): Disequilibrium mapping: composite likelihood for pairwise disequilibrium. *Genomics*, **36**, 1–16.

Donner A (1986): A review of inference procedures for the intraclass correlation coefficient in the one-way random effects model. *International Statistical Review*, **54**, 67–82.

Eaves L J (1977): Inferring the causes of human variation. *Journal of the Royal Statistical Society, Series A*, **140**, 324–55.

Eaves L and Meyer J (1994): Locating human quantitative trait loci: guidelines for the selection of sibling pairs for genotyping. *Behavior Genetics*, **24**, 443–55.

Editorial (1901): *Biometrika*, **1**, 1–6.

Edwards A W F (1984): *Likelihood*. Cambridge: Cambridge University Press.

Edwards J H (1960): The simulation of Mendelism. *Acta Geneticae Medicae et Gemellogiae (Roma)*, **10**, 63–70.

Edwards J H (1969): Familial predisposition in man. *British Medical Bulletin*, **25**, 58–64.

Edwards J H (1976): The interpretation of lod scores in linkage analysis. *Human Gene Mapping*, **3**, 289–93.

Elston R C and Sobel E (1979): Sampling considerations in the gathering and analysis of pedigree data. *American Journal of Human Genetics*, **31**, 62–69.

Elston R C and Stewart J (1971): A general model for the analysis of pedigree data. *Human Heredity*, **21**, 523–42.

Everitt B S (1995): *The Cambridge Dictionary of Statistics in the Medical Sciences*. Cambridge: Cambridge University Press.

Ewens W J and Shute N C E (1986): A resolution of the ascertainment sampling problem. *Theoretical Population Biology*, **30**, 388–412.

Eysenck H J and Eysenck S B G (1975): *Manual of Eysenck Personality Questionnaire*. San Diego: Digits.

Falconer D S (1965): The inheritance of liability to certain diseases estimated from the incidence among relatives. *Annals of Human Genetics*, **29**, 51–76.

Falconer D S and Mackay T F C (1996): *Introduction to Quantitative Genetics*, fourth edition. Harlow: Longman.

Falk C T and Rubinstein P (1987): Haplotype relative risk: an easy reliable way to construct a proper control sample for risk calculations. *Annals of Human Genetics*, **51**, 227–33.

Faraway J (1993): Distribution of the admixture test for the detection of linkage under heterogeneity. *Genetic Epidemiology*, **10**, 75–83.

Farmer A E, McGuffin P and Gottesman I I (1987): Twin concordance for DSM-III schizophrenia: scrutinising the validity of the definition. *Archives of General Psychiatry*, **44**, 634–41.

Feingold E, O'Brown P and Siegmund D (1993): Gaussian models for genetic linkage analysis using complete high-resolution maps of identity by descent. *American Journal Human Genetics*, **53**, 234–51.

Fisher R A (1918): The correlation between relatives on the supposition of Mendelian inheritance. *Transactions of the Royal Society of Edinburgh*, **52**, 399–433.

Fisher R A (1934): The effect of methods of ascertainment upon the estimation of frequencies. *Annals of Eugenics*, **6**, 13–25.

Fisher R A (1952): Statistical methods in genetics. *Heredity*, **6**, 1–12.

Froemel E C (1971): A comparison of computer subroutines for the calculation of the tetrachoric correlation coefficient. *Psychometrika*, **36**, 165–74.

Fulker D W (1988): Genetic and cultural transmission in human behaviour. In B S Weir, E J Ewen, M M Goodman and Namkoong (Eds), *Proceedings of the Second International Conference on Quantitative Genetics* (pp. 318–40). Sunderland, MA: Sinauer.

Fulker D W and Cherny S S (1997): An improved multipoint sib-pair analysis of quantitative traits. *Behavior Genetics*, **26**, 527–32.

Galton F (1875): The history of twin, as a criterion of the relative powers of nature and nurture. *Fraser's*, Nov 566–76.

Galton F (1877): Typical laws of heredity. *Nature*, **15**, 492–95, 512–14, 532–33.

Galton F (1889): *Natural Inheritance*. London: Macmillan.

Galton F (1890): Kinship and correlation. *North American Review*, **150**, 419–31. Reprinted in *Statistical Science*, **4**, 81–86.

Galton F (1897): The average contribution of each several ancestor to the total heritage of the offspring. *Proceedings of the Royal Society, London*, **LXI**, 401–13.

Galton F (1908): *Memoirs of My Life*. London: Methuen.

Goldgar D E (1990): Multipoint analysis of quantitative genetic variation. *American Journal of Human Genetics*, **47**, 957–67.

Goldin L R (1992): Detection of linkage and under heterogeneity: comparison of the two-locus vs. admixture models. *Genetic Epidemiology*, **9**, 61–66.

Goldin L R and Weeks D E (1993): Two-locus models of disease: comparison of likelihood and nonparametric linkage methods. *American Journal of Human Genetics*, **53**, 908–15.

Greenberg D A (1990): Linkage analysis assuming a single-locus mode of inheritance for traits determined by two loci: inferring mode of inheritance and estimating penetrance. *Genetic Epidemiology*, **7**, 467–79.

Greenberg D A and Hodge S E (1989): Linkage analysis under 'random' and 'genetic' reduced penetrance. *Genetic Epidemiology*, **6**, 259–64.

Grimmett G R and Stirzaker D R (1992): *Probability and Random Processes*. Oxford: Clarendon Press.

Gruneberg H (1952): Genetical studies on the skeleton of the mouse. IV. Quasi-continuous variations. *Journal of Genetics*, **51**, 95–114.

Guo S W and Thompson E A (1992): Performing the exact test of Hardy-Weinberg proportion for multiple alleles. *Bimoetrics*, **48**, 361–72.

Hamdan M A (1970): The equivalence of tetrachoric and maximum likelihood estimates of ρ in 2×2 tables. *Biometrika*, **57**, 212–15.

Hardy G H (1908): Mendelian proportions in a mixed population. *Science*, **28**, 49–50.

Haseman J K and Elston R C (1972): The investigation of linkage between a quantitative trait and a marker locus. *Behavior Genetics*, **2**, 3–19.

Hasstedt S J (1982): A mixed model likelihood approximation on large pedigrees. *Computing in Biomedical Research*, **15**, 295–307.

Hasstedt S J (1991): A variance components/major locus likelihood approximation on quantitative data. *Genetic Epidemiology*, **8**, 113–25.

Hasstedt S J (1993): Variance components/major locus likelihood approximation for quantitative, polychotomous, and multivariate data. *Genetic Epidemiology*, **10**, 145–58.

Hastbacka J, de la Chapelle A, Kaitila I, Sistonen P, Weaver A and Lander E (1992): Linkage disequilibrium mapping in isolated founder populations: diastrophic dysplasia in Finland. *Nature Genetics*, **2**, 204–11.

Hastbacka J, de la Chapelle A, Mahtani M M, Clines G, Reeve-Daly M P, Daly M, Hamilton B A, Jusumi K, Trivedi B, Weaver A, Coloma A, Lovett M, Buckler A, Kaitila I and Lander E S (1994): The diastrophic dysplasia gene encodes a novel sulphate transporter: positional cloning by fine-structure disequilibrium mapping. *Cell*, **78**, 1073–87.

Heath A C, Kessler R C, Neal M C, Hewitt J K, Eaves L J and Kendler K S (1993): Testing hypotheses about direction of causation using cross-sectional family data. *Behavior Genetics*, **23**, 29–50.

Hill W G and Weir B S (1994): Maximum-likelihood estimation of gene location by linkage disequilibrium. *American Journal of Human Genetics*, **54**, 705–14.

Hippocrates (1849): *The Genuine Works of Hippocrates* (translated by Francis Adams). London: The Syndenham Society.

Hodge S E (1984): The information contained in multiple siblings pairs. *Genetic Epidemiology*, **1**, 109–22.

Hodge S E (1993): Linkage analysis versus association analysis distinguish between two models that explain disease marker associations. *American Journal of Human Genetics*, **52**, 135–143.

Hodge S E (1994): Reply to Suarez and Hampe and Spielman *et al*: cosegregation, association, and linkage. *American Journal of Human Genetics*, **54**, 560–63.

Hodge S E and Elston R C (1994): Lods, wrods, and mods: the interpretation of lod scores calculated under different models. *Genetic Epidemiology*, **11**, 329–42.

Holmans P (1993): Asymptotic properties of affected-sib-pair linkage analysis. *American Journal of Human Genetics*, **52**, 362–74.

Holzinger K J (1929): The relative effect of nature and nurture influences on twin differences. *Journal of Educational Psychology*, **20**, 241–48.

Jacquard A (1978): *Genetics of Human Populations*. San Francisco: Freeman, Cooper & Co.

James J (1971): Frequency in relatives for an all-or-none trait. *Annals of Human Genetics*, **35**, 47–49.

Jinks J L and Fulker D W (1970): Comparison of the biometrical genetical, MAVA, and classical approaches to the analysis of human behaviour. *Psychological Bulletin*, **73**, 311–49.

Joreskog K G (1969): A general approach to comfirmatory maximum likelihood factor analysis. *Psychometrika*, **34**, 183–202.

Joreskog K G (1970): A general method for analysis of covariance structures. *Biometrika*, **57**, 239–51.

Joreskog K G (1971): Simultaneous factor analysis in several populations. *Psychometrika*, **36**, 409–26.

Joreskog K G and Sorbom D (1986): *LISREL: analysis of linear structural relationships by the method of maximum likelihood.* Chicago: National Educational Resources.

Joreskog K G and Sorbom D (1988): *PRELIS – A program for multivariate data screening and data summarization. A Preprocessor for LISREL*, second edition. Mooresville, Indiana: Scientific Software, Inc.

Kaplan N L and Weir B S (1995): Are moment bounds on the recombination fraction between a marker and a disease locus too good to be true? Allelic association mapping revisited for simple genetic diseases in the Finnish population. *American Journal of Human Genetics*, **57**, 1486–98.

Kaplan N J, Hill W G and Weir B S (1995): Likelihood methods for locating disease genes in nonequilibrium populations. *American Journal of Human Genetics*, **56**, 18–32.

Karlin S and Liberman U (1978): Classifications and comparisons of multilocus recombination distributions. *Proceedings of the National Academy of Science, USA*, **75**, 6332–36.

Kempthorne O (1957): *An Introduction to Genetic Statistics.* New York: Wiley.

Kirk D B (1973): On the numerical approximation of the bivariate normal (tetrachoric) correlation coefficient. *Psychometrika*, **38**, 259–68.

Knapp M, Seuchter S A and Baur M P (1995a): Linkage analysis in nuclear families, I. Optimality criteria for affected sib-pair tests. *Human Heredity*, **44**, 37–43.

Knapp M, Wassmer G and Baur M P (1995b): The relative efficiency of the Hardy–Weinberg equilibrium-likelihood and the conditional on parental genotype-likelihood methods for candidate-gene association studies. *American Journal of Human Genetics*, **57**, 1476–85.

Kosambi D D (1944): The estimation of map distances from recombination values. *Annals of Eugenics*, **12**, 172–75.

Kruglyak L and Lander E S (1995a): A non-parametric approach for mapping quantitative trait loci. *Genetics*, **139**, 1421–28.

Kruglyak L and Lander E S (1995b): Complete multipoint sib pair analysis of qualitative and quantitative traits. *American Journal of Human Genetics*, **57**, 439–54.

Kruglyak L and Lander E S (1995c): High-resolution genetic mapping of complex traits. *American Journal of Human Genetics*, **56**, 1212–23.

Kruglyak L, Daly M J and Lander S (1995): Rapid multipoint linkage analysis of recessive traits in nuclear families, including homozygosity mapping. *American Journal of Human Genetics*, **56**, 519–27.

Kruglyak L, Daly M J, Reeve-Daly M P and Lander L S (1996): Parametric and nonparametric linkage analysis: a unified multipoint approach. *American Journal of Human Genetics*, **58**, 1347–63.

Lalouel J M (1977): Linkage mapping from pair-wise recombination data. *Heredity*, **38**, 61–77.

Lalouel J M and Morton N E (1981): Complex segregation analysis with pointers. *Human Heredity*, **31**, 312–21.

Lalouel J M, Rao D C, Morton N E and Elston R C (1983): A unified model for complex segregation analysis. *American Journal of Human Genetics*, **35**, 816–26.

Lander E and Kruglyak L (1995): Genetic dissection of complex traits: guidelines for interpreting and reporting linkage results. *Nature Genetics*, **11**, November.

Lander E S and Green P (1987): Construction of multilocus genetic maps in humans. *Proceedings of the National Academy of Science USA*, **84**, 2363–67.

Lander E S, Green P, Abrahamson J, Barlow A, Daly M J, Lincoln S E and Newburg L (1987): MAPMAKER: an interactive computer package for constructing primary genetic linkage maps of experimental and natural populations. *Genomics*, **1**, 174–81.

Lange K and Elston R C (1975): Extensions to pedigree analysis. I. Likelihood calculations for simple and complex pedigrees. *Human Heredity*, **25**, 95–105.

Lange K, Weeks D and Boehnke M (1988): Programs for pedigree analysis: MENDEL, FISHER, and dGENE. *Genetic Epidemiology*, **5**, 471–72.

Lathrop G M, Lalouel J M, Julier C and Ott J (1984): Strategies for multilocus linkage analysis in humans. *Proceedings of the National Academy of Science, USA*, **81**, 3443–46.

Lathrop G M, Lalouel J M, Julier C and Ott J (1985): Multilocus linkage analysis in humans: detection of linkage and estimation of recombination. *American Journal of Human Genetics*, **37**, 482–98.

Levene H (1949): On a matching problem arising in genetics. *Annals of Mathematical Statistics*, **20**, 91–94.

Li C C and Mantel N (1968): A simple method of estimating the segregation ratio under complete ascertainment. *American Journal of Human Genetics*, **20**, 61–81.

Liang K Y (1993): Hypothesis testing under mixture models: application to genetic linkage analysis. Technical Report No. 759. Department of Biostatistics, Johns Hopkins University.

Liberman U and Karlin S (1984): Theoretical models of genetic map functions. *Theoretical Population Biology*, **25**, 331–46.

Macdonald A M (1996): An epidemiological and quantitative genetic study of obsessionality. PhD Thesis, Institute of Psychiatry, University of London.

MacLean C J, Morton N E and Lew R (1975): Analysis of family resemblance. IV. Operational characteristics of segregational analysis. *American Journal of Human Genetics*, **27**, 365–84.

MacLean C J, Morton N E and Elston R C (1976): Skewness in commingled distributions. *Biometrics*, **32**, 695–99.

MacLean C J, Ploughman L M, Diehl S R and Kendler K S (1992): A new test for linkage in the presence of locus heterogeneity. *American Journal of Human Genetics*, **50**, 1259–66.

MacLean C J, Bishop D T, Sherman S L and Diehl S R (1993a): Distribution of lod scores under certain mode of inheritance. *American Journal of Human Genetics*, **52**, 354–61.

MacLean C J, Sham P C and Kendler K S (1993b): Joint linkage of multiple loci for a complex disorder. *American Journal of Human Genetics*, **53**, 353–66.

Martin N G and Eaves L J (1977):. The genetical analysis of covariance structure. *Heredity*, **38**, 79–95.

Mather K (1938): Crossing-over. *Biological Reviews of the Cambridge Philosophical Society*, **13**, 252–92.

Mather K and Jinks J L (1977): *Introduction to Biometrical Genetics*. Ithaca, New York: Cornell University Press.

McDermott A (1973): The frequency and distribution of chiasmata in man. *Annals of Human Genetics*, **37**, 13–20.

McKusick V A (1994): *Mendelian Inheritance in Man*, 11th edn. Baltimore: Johns Hopkins University Press.

Mendel G, De Vries H, Correns C and Tschermak E V (1950): The birth of genetics. *Genetics*, **35** (supplement), 1–47.

Morton N E (1955): Sequential tests for the detection of linkage. *American Journal of Human Genetics*, **7**, 277–318.

Morton N E (1956): The detection and estimation of linkage between the genes for elliptocytosis and the Rh blood type. *American Journal of Human Genetics*, **8**, 80–96.

Morton N E (1958): Segregation analysis in human genetics. *Science*, **127**, 79–80.

Morton N E (1959): Genetic tests under incomplete ascertainment. *American Journal of Human Genetics*, **11**, 1–16.

Morton N E and MacLean C J (1974): Analysis of family resemblance. III. Complex segregation analysis of quantitative traits. *American Journal of Human Genetics*, **26**, 489–503.

Mourant A R (1954): *The Distribution of the Human Blood Groups*. Oxford: Blackwell.

Neale M C (1993): *Mx: statistical modelling*. Box 710 MCV. Richmond, VA 23298-0710, USA (neale@sruby.vcu.edu).

Neale M C and Cardon L R (1992): *Methodology for Genetic Studies of Twins and Families*. Dordrecht: Kluwer Academic.

Neale M C, Heath A C, Hewitt J K, Eaves L J and Fulker D W (1989): Fitting genetic models with LISREL: hypothesis testing. *Behavior Genetics*, **19**, 37–49.

Neel J V and Schull W J (1954): *Human Heredity*, Chicago: University of Chicago Press.

O'Connell J R and Weeks D E (1995): The VITESSE algorithm for rapid exact multilocus linkage analysis via genotype set-recording and fuzzy inheritance. *Nature Genetics*, **11**, 402–408.

Ohta T and Kimura M (1969): Linkage disequilibrium at steady state determined by random genetic drift and recurrent mutation. *Genetics*, **63**, 229–38.

Ott J (1974): Estimation of the recombination fraction in human pedigrees: efficient computation of the likelihood for human linkage studies. *American Journal of Human Genetics*, **26**, 588–97.

Ott J (1976): A computer program for linkage analysis of general human pedigrees. *American Journal of Human Genetics*, **28**, 528–29.

Ott J (1992): Strategies for characterising highly polymorphic markets in human gene mapping. *American Journal of Human Genetics*, **51**, 283–90.

Pearson K (1900): *The Grammar of Science*, second edition. London: A&C Black.

Pearson K (1901): On the correlations of characters not quantitatively measurable. *Philosophical Transactions of the Royal Society of London, A*, **195**, 1–47.

Pearson K (1903a): The law of ancestral heredity. *Biometrika*, **2**, 211–36.

Pearson K (1903b): On the influence of natural selection on the variability and correlation of organs. *Philosophical Transaction of the Royal Society of London, A*, **200**, 1–66.

Pearson K and Heron D (1913): On theories of association. *Biometrika*, **9**, 159–315.

Pearson K and Lee A (1901): On the inheritance of characters not capable of exact quantitative measurement. *Philosophical Transactions of the Royal Society of London, A*, **195**, 79–150.

Penrose L S (1935): The detection of autosomal linkage in data which consist of pairs of brothers and sisters of unspecified parentage. *Annals of Eugenics*, **6**, 133–38.

Penrose L S (1959): *Outline of Human Genetics*. London: Heinemann.

Ploughman L M and Boehnke M (1989): Estimating the power of a proposed linkage study for a complex genetic trait. *American Journal of Human Genetics*, **44**, 543–51.

Price B (1950): Primary biases in twin studies: a review of prenatal and natal difference-producing factors in monozygotic twins. *American Journal of Human Genetics*, **2**, 293–52.

Raine D N, Cooke J R, Andrews W A and Mahon D F (1972): Screening for inherited metabolic disease by plasma chromatography (Scriver) in a large city. *British Medical Journal*, **3**, 7–13.

Rao D C, Morton N E and Yee S (1974): Analysis of family resemblance. II. A linear model for familial correlation. *American Journal of Human Genetics*, **26**, 331–59.

Rao D C, Morton N E and Yee S (1976): Resolution of cultural and biological inheritance by path analysis. *American Journal of Human Genetics*, **28**, 228–42.

Rao D C, Keats B J D, Morton N E, Yee S and Lew R (1979): Variability of human linkage data. *American Journal of Human Genetics*, **30**, 516–29.

Reich T, James J W and Morris C A (1972): The use of multiple thresholds in determining the mode of inheritance of semi-continuous traits. *Annals of Human Genetics*, **36**, 163–84.

Rice J, Cloninger C R and Reich T (1978): Multifactorial inheritance with cultural transmission and assortative mating. I. Description and basic properties of the unitary models. *American Journal of Human Genetics*, **30**, 618–43.

Risch N (1983): A general model for disease-marker association. *Annals of Human Genetics*, **47**, 245–52.

Risch N (1989): Linkage detection tests under heterogeneity. *Genetic Epidemiology*, **6**, 473–80.

Risch N (1990a): Linkage strategies for genetically complex traits II. The power of affected relative pairs. *American Journal of Human Genetics*, **46**, 229–41.

Risch N (1990b): Linkage strategies for genetically complex traits III. The effect of marker polymorphism on analysis of affected relative pairs. *American Journal of Human Genetics*, **46**, 242–53.

Risch N and Lange K (1979): An alternative model of recombination and interference. *Annals of Human Genetics*, **43**, 61–70.

Risch N and Giuffra L (1992): Model misspecification and multipoint linkage analysis. *Human Heredity*, **42**, 77–92.

Risch N and Zhang H (1995): Extreme discordant sib pairs for mapping quantitative trait loci in humans. *Science*, **268**, 1584–89.

Risch N and Zhang H (1996): Mapping quantitative trait loci with extreme discordant sib pairs: sampling considerations. *American Journal of Human Genetics*, **58**, 836–43.

Rubinstein P, Walker M, Carpenter C, Carrier C, Krassner J, Falk C and Ginsberg F (1981): Genetics of HLA disease associations: the use of the haplotype relative risk (HRR) and the 'haplo-delta' (Dh) estimates in juvenile diabetes from three racial groups. *Human Immunology*, **3**, 384.

Sandkuijl L A (1989): Analysis of affected sib-pairs using information from extended families. *Multipoint mapping and linkage based upon affected pedigree members: genetic analysis workshop 6*. New York: Alan R Liss.

Schaid D J and Sommer S S (1993): Genotype relative risks: methods for design and analysis of candidate-gene association studies. *American Journal of Human Genetics*, **53**, 1114–26.

Schervish M J (1984): Multivariate normal probabilities with error bound. *Applied Statistics*, **33**, 81 (correction, **34**, 103).

Schork N J (1993): Extended multipoint identity-by-descent analysis of human quantitative traits: efficiency, power, and modelling considerations. *American Journal of Human Genetics*, **53**, 1306–19.

Schork N J, Boehnke M, Terwilliger J D and Ott J (1993): Two-trait-locus linkage analysis: a powerful strategy for mapping complex genetic traits. *American Journal of Human Genetics*, **53**, 1127–36.

Searle S R, Casella G and McCulloch C E (1992): *Variance Components*. New York: Wiley.

Self S G and Liang K Y (1987): Asymptotic properties of maximum likelihood estimators and likelihood ratio tests under nonstandard conditions. *Journal of the American Statistical Association*, **82**, 605–10.

Shaikh S, Collier D A, Sham P C, Ball D, Aitchison K, Vallada H, Smith I, Gill M and Kerwin R W (1996): Allelic association between a Ser-9-Gly polymorphism in the dopamine D3 receptor gene and schizophrenia. *Human Genetics*, **97**, 714–19.

Sham P C and Curtis D (1995): An extended transmission/disequilibrium test (TDT) for multiallele marker loci. *Annals of Human Genetics*, **59**, 323–36.

Sham P C, MacLean C J and Kendler K S (1994): Two-locus versus one-locus lods for complex traits. *American Journal of Human Genetics*, **55**, 855–56.

Sham P C, Curtis D and MacLean C J (1996): Likelihood ratio tests for linkage and linkage disequilibrium: asymptotic distribution and power. *American Journal of Human Genetics*, **58**, 1093–95.

Sham P C, Zhao J H and Curtis D (1997): Optimal weighting scheme for affected sib-pair analysis of sibship data. *Annals of Human Genetics*, **61**, 61–69.

Smith C A B (1959): Some comments on the statistical methods used in linkage investigations. *American Journal of Human Genetics*, **11**, 289–304.

Spencer N, Hopkinson D A and Harris H (1964): Quantitative differences and gene dosage in the human red cell acid phosphatase polymorphism. *Nature*, **201**, 299–300.

Spielman R S, McGinnis R E and Ewens W J (1993): Transmission test for linkage disequilibrium: the insulin gene region and insulin-dependent diabetes mellitus (IDDM): *American Journal of Human Genetics*, **52**, 506–16.

Spielman R S, McGinnis R E and Ewens W J (1994): The transmission/disequilibrium test detects cosegregation and linkage. *American Journal of Human Genetics*, **54**, 559–60.

Stigler S M (1989): Francis Galton's account of the invention of correlation. *Statistical Science*, **4**, 73–79.

Strachan T and Read A P (1996): *Human Molecular Genetics*. Oxford: BIOS Scientific Publishers.

Sturt E (1976): A mapping function for human chromosomes. *Annals of Human Genetics*, **40**, 147–63.

Suarez B K and Hampe C L (1994): Linkage and association. *American Journal of Human Genetics*, **54**, 554–59.

Suarez B K and Hodge S E (1979): A simple method to detect linkage for rare recessive diseases: an application to juvenile diabetes. *Clinical Genetics*, **15**, 126–36.

Suarez B K and Van Eerdewegh P (1984): A comparison of three affected-sib-pair scoring methods to detect HLA-linked disease susceptibility genes. *American Journal of Medical Genetics*, **18**, 135–46.

Suarez B K, Rice J P and Reich T (1978): The generalised sib-pair IBD distribution: its use in the detection of linkage. *Annals of Human Genetics*, **42**, 87–94.

Terwilliger J D (1995): A powerful likelihood method for the analysis of linkage disequilibrium between trait loci and one or more polymorphic marker loci. *American Journal of Human Genetics*, **56**, 777–87.

Terwilliger J and Ott J (1992): A haplotype-based 'haplotype relative risk' approach to detecting allelic associations. *Human Heredity*, **42**, 337–46.

Terwilliger J D and Ott J (1994): *Handbook of Human Linkage Analysis*. Baltimore: Johns Hopkins University Press.

Vieland V J and Hodge S E (1995): Inherent intractability of the ascertainment problem for pedigree data: a general likelihood framework. *American Journal of Human Genetics*, **56**, 33–43.

Vogel F and Motulsky A G (1986): *Human Genetics, Problems and Approaches*, second edition. Berlin: Springer-Verlag.

Wald A (1947): *Sequential Analysis*. New York: John Wiley.

Watson J D, Hopkins N H, Roberts J W, Steitz J A and Weiner A M (1987):

Molecular Biology of the Gene, Fourth edition. Menlo Park: Benjamin/ Comings.

Weeks D E and Lange K (1988): The affected-pedigree-member method of linkage analysis. *American Journal of Human Genetics*, **42**, 315–26.

Weeks D E, Lathrop G M and Ott J (1993): Multipoint mapping under genetic interference. *Human Heredity*, **43**, 86–97.

Weeks D E, Lehner T, Squires-Wheeler E, Kaufmann C and Ott J (1990): Measuring the inflation of the lod score due to its maximisation over model parameter values in human linkage analysis. *Genetics Epidemiology*, **7**, 237–43.

Weinberg W (1908): Uber den Nachweis der Vererbung beim Menschen. *Jahreshefte des Vereins fur vaterlandische Naturkunde in Wuttemberg*, **64**, 368–82.

Weiner A S (1943): *Blood Groups and Transfusion*. Thomas, Springfield. Reprinted in 1962 by Hafner, New York.

Whittemore A S and Halpern J (1994a): Probability of gene identity by descent: computation and application. *Biometrics*, **50**, 109–17.

Whittemore A S and Halpern J (1994b): A class of tests for linkage using affected pedigree members. *Biometrics*, **50**, 118–27.

Williamson J A and Amos C I (1995): Guess LOD approach: sufficient conditions for robustness. *Genetic Epidemiology*, **12**, 163–76.

Woolf B (1955): On estimating the relation between blood group and disease. *Annals of Human Genetics*, **19**, 251–53.

Wright S (1921): Correlation and causation. *Journal of Agricultural Research*, **20**, 557–85.

Wright S (1968): *Evolution and the Genetics of Populations. Vol. 1. Genetics and Biometric Foundations*. Chicago: University of Chicago Press.

Yule G U (1902): Mendel's laws and their probable relations to intra-racial heredity. *The New Phytologist*, **1**, 193–207.

Yule G U (1912): On the methods of measuring association between two attributes. *Journal of the Royal Statistical Society*, **75**, 579–642.

Zhao L P, Thompson E and Prentice R (1990): Joint estimation of recombination fractions and interference coefficients in multilocus linkage analysis. *American Journal of Human Genetics*, **47**, 255–65.

Author Index

Subject Index